国家卫生和计划生育委员会"十三五"英文版规划教材
全国高等学校教材

供临床医学专业及来华留学生(MBBS)双语教学用

# Physical Medicine and Rehabilitation Pocket Companion

# 康复医学 改编教学版
Annotated Edition

**Marlís González-Fernández, Jarrod David Friedman**

**主　编** 虞乐华
**Chief Editor** Lehua Yu

**副主编** 吴　毅　　藏　磊　　许　涛
**Vice Chief Editor** Yi Wu　　Lei Zang　　Tao Xu

人民卫生出版社
·北　京·

The original English language work: *Physical Medicine and Rehabilitation Pocket Companion*, By Marlís González-Fernández, MD, PhD, Jarrod David Friedman, MD, ISBN: 978-1-933864-53-2, has been published by: Demos Medical Publishing, an imprint of Springer Publishing Company, LLC

Princeton, NJ, USA

Copyright © 2011 All rights reserved.

This bilingual Chinese/English edition is published by People's Medical Publishing House Co., Ltd through arrangement with Springer Publishing Company, LLC., and is for distribution in the People's Republic of China only.

## 图书在版编目（CIP）数据

康复医学 / 虞乐华主编. -- 北京：人民卫生出版社，2025. 1. --（临床医学专业英文版教材）. -- ISBN 978-7-117-37451-4

Ⅰ. R49

中国国家版本馆 CIP 数据核字第 2025Q5B518 号

| | | |
|---|---|---|
| 人卫智网 | www.ipmph.com | 医学教育、学术、考试、健康，购书智慧智能综合服务平台 |
| 人卫官网 | www.pmph.com | 人卫官方资讯发布平台 |

图字：01-2023-2545 号

**康 复 医 学**
Kangfu Yixue

主　　编：虞乐华
出版发行：人民卫生出版社（中继线 010-59780011）
地　　址：北京市朝阳区潘家园南里 19 号
邮　　编：100021
E - mail：pmph @ pmph.com
购书热线：010-59787592　010-59787584　010-65264830
印　　刷：三河市潮河印业有限公司
经　　销：新华书店
开　　本：850×1168　1/16　　印张：16
字　　数：496 千字
版　　次：2025 年 1 月第 1 版
印　　次：2025 年 2 月第 1 次印刷
标准书号：ISBN 978-7-117-37451-4
定　　价：78.00 元

打击盗版举报电话：010-59787491　E-mail：WQ @ pmph.com
质量问题联系电话：010-59787234　E-mail：zhiliang @ pmph.com
数字融合服务电话：4001118166　E-mail：zengzhi @ pmph.com

## 编者（按姓氏笔画排序）

马跃文　　中国医科大学附属第一医院
Yuewen Ma　The First Hospital of China Medical University

王于领　　中山大学附属第六医院
Yuling Wang　The Sixth Affiliated Hospital, Sun Yat-sen University

白定群　　重庆医科大学附属第一医院
Dingqun Bai　The First Affiliated Hospital of Chongqing Medical University

刘元标　　南京医科大学第二附属医院
Yuanbiao Liu　The Second Affiliated Hospital of Nanjing Medical University

刘四海　　中国康复研究中心（北京博爱医院）
Sihai Liu　China Rehabilitation Research Center (Beijing Boai Hospital)

许　涛　　华中科技大学同济医学院附属同济医院
Tao Xu　Tongji Hospital, Tongji Medical College, Huazhong University of Science and Technology

杜　青　　上海交通大学医学院附属新华医院
Qing Du　Xinhua Hospital Affiliated to Shanghai Jiao Tong University School of Medicine

吴　毅　　复旦大学附属华山医院
Yi Wu　Huashan Hospital, Fudan University

郑朝旭　　中国医学科学院肿瘤医院
Zhaoxu Zheng　Cancer Hospital Chinese Academy of Medical Sciences

单春雷　　上海交通大学医学院
Chunlei Shan　Shanghai Jiao Tong University School of Medicine

袁　华　　空军军医大学西京医院
Hua Yuan　Xijing Hospital, Air Force Medical University

倪国新　　厦门大学附属第一医院
Guoxin Ni　The First Affiliated Hospital of Xiamen University

殷　樱　　重庆医科大学附属第二医院
Ying Yin　The Second Affiliated Hospital of Chongqing Medical University

曾　岩　　北京大学人民医院
Yan Zeng　Peking University People's Hospital

谢　青　　上海交通大学医学院附属瑞金医院
Qing Xie　Ruijin Hospital, Shanghai Jiaotong University School Of Medicine

虞乐华　　重庆医科大学附属第二医院
Lehua Yu　The Second Affiliated Hospital of Chongqing Medical University

廖维靖　　武汉大学中南医院
Weijing Liao　Zhongnan Hospital of Wuhan University

缪　萍　　广州医科大学附属第二医院
Ping Miao　The Second Affiliated Hospital of Guangzhou Medical University

藏　磊　　首都医科大学附属北京朝阳医院
Lei Zang　Beijing Chaoyang Hospital, Capital Medical University

1995 年，我国首次招收全英文授课医学留学生，到 2015 年，接收临床医学专业 MBBS（Bachelor of Medicine & Bachelor of Surgery）留学生的院校达到了 40 余家，MBBS 院校数量、规模不断扩张；同时，医学院校在临床医学专业五年制、长学制教学中陆续开展不同规模和范围的双语或全英文授课，使得对一套符合我国教学实际、成体系、高质量英文教材的需求日益增长。

为了满足教学需求，进一步落实教育部《关于加强高等学校本科教学工作提高教学质量的若干意见（教高［2001］4 号）》和《来华留学生医学本科教育（英语授课）质量控制标准暂行规定（教外来［2007］39 号）》等相关文件的要求，规范和提高我国高等医学院校临床医学专业五年制、长学制和来华留学生（MBBS）双语教学及全英文教学的质量，推进医学双语教学和留学生教育的健康有序发展，完善和规范临床医学专业英文版教材的体系，人民卫生出版社在充分调研的基础上，于 2015 年召开了全国高等学校临床医学专业英文版规划教材的编写论证会，经过会上及会后的反复论证，最终确定组织编写一套全国规划的、适合我国高等医学院校教学实际的临床医学专业英文版教材，并计划作为 2017 年春季和秋季教材在全国出版发行。

本套英文版教材的编写结合国家卫生和计划生育委员会、教育部的总体要求，坚持"三基、五性、三特定"的原则，组织全国各大医学院校、教学医院的专家编写，主要特点如下：

1. 教材编写应教学之需启动，在全国范围进行了广泛、深入调研和论证，借鉴国内外医学人才培养模式和教材建设经验，对主要读者对象、编写模式、编写科目、编者遴选条件等进行了科学设计。

2. 坚持"三基、五性、三特定"和"多级论证"的教材编写原则，组织全国各大医学院校及教学医院有丰富英语教学经验的专家一起编写，以保证高质量出版。

3. 为保证英语表达的准确性和规范性，大部分教材以国外英文原版教科书为蓝本，根据我国教学大纲和人民卫生出版社临床医学专业第八轮规划教材主要内容进行改编，充分体现科学性、权威性、适用性和实用性。

4. 教材内部各环节合理设置，根据读者对象的特点，在英文原版教材的基础上结合需要，增加本章小结、关键术语（英中对照）、思考题、推荐阅读等模块，促进学生自主学习。

本套临床医学专业英文版规划教材共 38 种，均为国家卫生和计划生育委员会"十三五"规划教材，计划于 2017 年全部出版发行。

In 1995, China recruited overseas medical students of full English teaching for the first time. Up to 2015, more than 40 institutions enrolled overseas MBBS (Bachelor of Medicine & Bachelor of Surgery) students. The number of MBBS institutions and overseas students are continuously increasing. At the meantime, medical colleges' application for bilingual or full English teaching in different size and range in five-year and long-term professional clinical medicine teaching results to increasingly demand for a set of practical, systematic and high-qualified English teaching material.

In order to meet the teaching needs and to implement the regulations of relevant documents issued by Ministry of Education including "Some Suggestions to Strengthen the Undergraduate Teaching and to Improve the Teaching Quality" and "Interim Provisions on Quality Control Standards of International Medical Undergraduate Education (English teaching)", as well as to standardize and improve the quality of the bilingual teaching and English teaching of the five-year, long-term and international students (MBBS) of clinical medicine in China's higher medical colleges so as to promote the healthy and orderly development of medical bilingual teaching and international students education and to improve and standardize the system of English clinical medicine textbooks, after full investigation, People's Medical Publishing House (PMPH) held the writing discussion meeting of English textbook for clinical medicine department of national colleges and universities in 2015. After the repeated demonstration in and after the meeting, PMPH ultimately determined to organize the compilation of a set of national planning English textbooks which are suitable for China's actual clinical medicine teaching of medical colleges and universities. This set will be published as spring and autumn textbooks of 2017.

This set of English textbooks meets the overall requirements of the Ministry of Education and National Health and Family Planning Commission, the editorial committee includes the experts from major medical colleges and universities as well as teaching hospitals, the main features are as follows:

1. Textbooks compilation is started to meet the teaching needs, extensive and deep research and demonstration are conducted across the country, the main target readers, the model and subject of compilation and selection conditions of authors are scientifically designed in accordance with the reference of domestic and foreign medical personnel training model and experience in teaching materials.

2. Adhere to the teaching materials compiling principles of "three foundations, five characteristics, and three specialties" and "multi-level demonstration", the organization of English teaching experts with rich experience from major medical schools and teaching hospitals ensures the high quality of publication.

3. In order to ensure the accuracy and standardization of English expression, most of the textbooks are modeled on original English textbooks, and adapted based on national syllabus and main content of the eighth round of clinical medicine textbooks which were published by PMPH, fully reflecting the scientificity, authority, applicability and practicality.

4. All aspects of teaching materials are arranged reasonably, based on original textbooks,the chapter summary, key terms (English and Chinese), review questions, and recommended readings are added to promote students' independent learning in accordance with teaching needs and the characteristics of the target readers.

This set of English textbooks for clinical medicine includes 38 species which are among "13th Five-Year" planning  textbooks of National Health and Family Planning Commission, and will be all published in 2017.

## 全国高等学校临床医学专业第一轮英文版规划教材·教材目录

| 教材名称 | |
|---|---|
| 1 人体解剖学 | Human Anatomy |
| 2 生理学 | Physiology |
| 3 医学免疫学 | Medical Immunology |
| 4 生物化学 | Biochemistry |
| 5 组织学与胚胎学 | Histology and Embryology |
| 6 医学微生物学 | Medical Microbiology |
| 7 病理学 | Pathology |
| 8 医学分子生物学 | Medical Molecular Biology |
| 9 医学遗传学 | Medical Genetics |
| 10 医学细胞生物学 | Medical Cell Biology |
| 11 病理生理学 | Pathophysiology |
| 12 药理学 | Pharmacology |
| 13 临床药理学 | Clinical Pharmacology |
| 14 人体寄生虫学 | Human Parasitology |
| 15 流行病学 | Epidemiology |
| 16 医学统计学 | Medical Statistics |
| 17 核医学 | Nuclear Medicine |
| 18 医学影像学 | Medical Imaging |
| 19 临床诊断学 | Clinical Diagnostics |
| 20 实验诊断学 | Laboratory Diagnostics |
| 21 内科学 | Internal Medicine |
| 22 外科学 | Surgery |
| 23 妇产科学 | Obstetrics and Gynaecology |
| 24 儿科学 | Pediatrics |
| 25 神经病学 | Neurology |
| 26 精神病学 | Psychiatry |
| 27 传染病学 | Infectious Diseases |

## 全国高等学校临床医学专业第一轮英文版规划教材 · 教材目录

| | 教材名称 | |
|---|---|---|
| 28 | 皮肤性病学 | Dermatovenereology |
| 29 | 肿瘤学 | Oncology |
| 30 | 眼科学 | Ophthalmology |
| 31 | 康复医学 | Rehabilitation Medicine |
| 32 | 医学心理学 | Medical Psychology |
| 33 | 耳鼻咽喉头颈外科学 | Otorhinolaryngology-Head and Neck Surgery |
| 34 | 急诊医学 | Emergency Medicine |
| 35 | 法医学 | Forensic Medicine |
| 36 | 全球健康学 | Global Health |
| 37 | 中医学 | Chinese Medicine |
| 38 | 医学汉语 | Medical Chinese |

# Contributors

**Lisa S. Barrett, MD**
Medical Director
Inpatient Rehabilitation Medicine
Marietta Memorial Hospital
Marietta, Ohio

**Katherine E. Binder**
Staff Prosthetist
Dankmeyer, Inc.
Linthicum, Maryland

**Erik Stanton Brand, MD, MSc**
Chief Resident
Department of Physical Medicine
    and Rehabilitation
The Johns Hopkins University
    School of Medicine
Baltimore, Maryland

**Martin B. Brodsky, PhD**
Assistant Professor
Department of Physical Medicine
    and Rehabilitation
The Johns Hopkins University
    School of Medicine
Baltimore, Maryland

**Melanie Brown, MD**
Medical Director for Brain Injury
    Rehabilitation
Department of Physical Medicine
    and Rehabilitation
Sinai Hospital of Baltimore
Baltimore, Maryland

**Maggi A. Budd, PhD, MPh**
Clinical Rehabilitation
    Neuropsychologist
Department of Spinal Cord Injury
VA Boston Health Care System
Boston, Massachusetts
Clinical Rehabilitation
    Neuropsychologist
Department of Psychiatry
Harvard Medical School
Cambridge, Massachusetts

**Michael Lang Bushby**
Lifebridge Health
Courtland Gardens Nursing &
    Rehabilitation Center
Baltimore, Maryland

**SriKrishna Chandran, MD**
Chief Resident
Department of Physical Medicine
    and Rehabilitation
The Johns Hopkins University
    School of Medicine
Baltimore, Maryland

**Maria Eppig, DO**
Resident Physician
Department of Physical Medicine
    and Rehabilitation
Sinai Hospital of Baltimore
Baltimore, Maryland

**Dorianne Rachelle
    Feldman, MD**
Assistant Professor
Department of Physical Medicine
    and Rehabilitation
The Johns Hopkins University
    School of Medicine
Baltimore, Maryland

**Heidi A. Frere, DPT**
Senior Physical Therapist
    Rehabilitation
Children's Memorial Hospital
Chicago, Illinois

**Jarrod David Friedman, MD**
Pain Management Physician
Boca Raton, Florida

**Melissa Gong, DO**
Chief Resident
Department of Physical Medicine
    and Rehabilitation
Sinai Hospital of Baltimore
Baltimore, Maryland

**Marlís González-
    Fernández, MD, PhD**
Department of Physical Medicine
    and Rehabilitation
The Johns Hopkins University
    School of Medicine
Baltimore, Maryland

**Mark S. Hopkins, PT, CPO,
    MBA, BS**
Clinical Director
Dankmeyer, Inc.
Adjunct Faculty
Department of Physical Medicine
    and Rehabilitation
The Johns Hopkins University
    Medical School
Baltimore, Maryland

**Maribeth Gorman Jankowski, BS**
Senior Occupational Therapist
Department of Occupational
    Therapy
Children's Memorial Hospital
Chicago, Illinois

**John M. Jones, DO, MEd**
Chair, Osteopathic Principles and
    Practice
William Carey University College
    of Osteopathic Medicine
Hattiesburg, Mississippi

**Phong Kieu, MD**
Senior Resident
Department of Physical Medicine
    and Rehabilitation
The Johns Hopkins University
    School of Medicine
Baltimore, Maryland

**Barbara J. de Lateur**
Distinguished Service Professor
Department of Physical Medicine
    and Rehabilitation
The Johns Hopkins University
    School of Medicine
Baltimore, Maryland

**Scott J. Lepre, MD**
Clinical Associate
Department of Physical Medicine
  and Rehabilitation
The Johns Hopkins University
  School of Medicine
Baltimore, Maryland

**Zachary Martin, MD**
Plastic and Reconstructive
  Surgery
Good Samaritan Hospital
Baltimore, Maryland

**Rosemary Martino, MH, MSc, PhD**
Associate Professor
Department of Speech Language
  Pathology
University of Toronto
Affiliated Scientist
Health Care and Outcomes
  Research
Toronto Western Research
  Institution
Toronto, Ontario, Canada

**Robert Samuel Mayer, MD**
Vice Chair, Education
Department of Physical Medicine
  and Rehabilitation
The Johns Hopkins University
  School of Medicine
Baltimore, Maryland

**Nathan J. Neufeld, DO**
Resident Physician
Department of Physical Medicine
  and Rehabilitation
The Johns Hopkins University
  School of Medicine
Baltimore, Maryland

**Bryan O'Young, MD**
Clinical Associate Professor
Department of Rehabilitation
  Medicine
New York University School of
  Medicine
Attending Physician
Rusk Institute of Rehabilitation
  Medicine
New York University Langone
  Medical Center
New York, New York

**Andrew Sears, PhD**
Professor and Chair
Department of Information
  Systems
University of Maryland
Baltimore, Maryland

**Lauren T. Shapiro, MD**
Instructor
Department of Physical Medicine
  and Rehabilitation
The Johns Hopkins University
  School of Medicine
Baltimore, Maryland

**Kenneth H. Silver, MD**
Vice Chair, Clinical Affairs
Department of Physical Medicine
  and Rehabilitation
The Johns Hopkins University
  School of Medicine
Baltimore, Maryland

**Kerry J. Stewart, EdD**
Professor of Medicine
Division of Cardiology
Director
Clinical and Research Exercise
  Physiology
Director
Hopkins Institute for Clinical and
  Translational Research Exercise
  and Body Composition Core
The Johns Hopkins University
  School of Medicine
Baltimore, Maryland

**Katherine Dawn Travnicek, MD**
Resident
Department of Physical Medicine
  and Rehabilitation
Johns Hopkins School of
  Medicine
Baltimore, Maryland

**Sue Carol Verrillo, BSN, MSN, RN**
Nurse Manager
Department of Physical Medicine
  and Rehabilitation
The Johns Hopkins Hospital
Baltimore, Maryland

**Christine L. Yantz, PhD**
Psychologist
Department of Psychology
Gaylord Specialty Healthcare
Wallingford, Connecticut

**Mark A. Young, MD**
Department of Physical Medicine
  and Rehabilitation
The Johns Hopkins University
  School of Medicine
Chair, Physical Medicine and
  Rehabilitation
The Workforce and Technology
  Center
Maryland Division of
  Rehabilitation Service
State of Maryland Department
  of Education
Baltimore, Maryland

**Michael J. Young**
University of Maryland
Baltimore, Maryland

**Richard D. Zorowitz, MD**
Associate Professor
Department of Physical Medicine
  and Rehabilitation
The Johns Hopkins University
  School of Medicine
Chairman
Physical Medicine and
  Rehabilitation
Johns Hopkins Bayview Medical
  Center
Baltimore, Maryland

# 改编版前言

  我们很高兴为来华留学生呈现这本改编版的英文教材《康复医学》。本教材各章的编者来自全国各大知名医学院和医院的康复医学领域专家，他们渊博的学识和丰富的临床经验能够帮助来华学习康复医学的留学生全面、深入地了解康复医学。该教材的内容经过精心策划，保留了英文原版教材"原汁原味"的核心内容，涵盖了康复医学领域的各大主题，研究者特别感兴趣的主题和其他参考学习资源。除此之外，改编版还增加了更丰富的内容，每章增加了概要、重要术语、思考题，既能促进课堂学习又能培养学生课外自学能力，为学生提供了坚实的康复医学理论知识学习和实践经验，使学习者学习体验更加全面，以此增强学习者对康复医学的理解，从而培养学生思辨能力、激发学生进一步探索康复医学学科的兴趣。

  我们要衷心感谢编委会的全体成员，他们为编写这本教材贡献了他们的专业知识、宝贵时间和精力。他们的集体智慧和经验为确保本教材的内容质量和真实性起到了重要作用。我们还要感谢所有为本教材慷慨分享见解和知识的贡献者，他们的无私分享使本教材成为康复医学学生宝贵的学习资源。我们希望这本《康复医学》改编版教材能成为来华留学生学习临床医学的宝贵工具，也成为康复医学双语教学的参考。我们真诚地希望这本教材能为康复医学领域的知识、技能传承和优秀医疗人才培养作出贡献。

  全书经过编者互审、提出意见、多次修改，尽管全体编写人员努力进行了整合和审定，但由于水平、时间有限，不足之处在所难免。我们诚挚地恳请广大读者和同道们不吝赐教，以便再版时进一步完善。

主编 虞乐华

# Adaptation Preface

We are pleased to present the adapted version of the English textbook *Physical Medicine and Rehabilitation Pocket Companion* for international students studying clinical medicine in China. Editors of this adapted version are experts from various prestigious medical schools and hospitals in the field of rehabilitation medicine across the country. With their profound knowledge and rich experience in rehabilitation medicine, the adapted version aims to provide international students a comprehensive and in-depth understanding of rehabilitation medicine. With a complicated plan, the adapted version preserves the authentic learning experience for learners by covering major topics in rehabilitation medicine, discussing topics that are of particular interest in the field of rehabilitation medicine, and listing learning resources for further study and reference. In addition, to enrich students' learning experience, the adapted version provides students with knowledge-based learning and practical experience by adding more informative resources, including summary,important terminology and review questions at the end of each chapter to both facilitate classroom learning and cultivate students' independent learning ability. As a result, students are motivated to think critically and explore the field of rehabilitation medicine as their learning experience is enriched, and their understanding about rehabilitation is enhanced.

We would like to express our gratitude to the esteemed members of the editorial board, who have contributed their expertise, time, and effort to the creation of this textbook. Their wisdom and experience have been instrumental in ensuring the quality and authenticity of the content. We would also like to thank all the contributors who have generously shared their insights and knowledge to make this textbook a valuable resource for students studying rehabilitation medicine. We hope that the adapted version of *Physical Medicine and Rehabilitation Pocket Companion* will serve as a valuable tool for international students studying clinical medicine, as well as a reference for bilingual teaching in the field of rehabilitation medicine. It is our sincere belief that this textbook will contribute to the transmission of knowledge and skills as well as the cultivation of competent healthcare professionals in the field of rehabilitation medicine.

The entire book has undergone thorough peer review and multiple revisions. Although all authors have made efforts to integrate and review the content, limitations are inevitable due to varying levels of expertise and time constraints. We sincerely invite readers and colleagues to kindly offer your valuable insights and suggestions so that we can further improve the textbook in subsequent editions.

Professor Lehua Yu
**Chief Editor**

# *Preface*

Finding small (but crucial) information is important in clinical practice particularly for residents who are required to learn, incorporate, and utilize vast amounts of information on a daily basis. Physical medicine and rehabilitation residents also have the unique challenge of mastering a field that covers multiple medical and nonmedical disciplines that are not normally taught in great detail during medical school. There are many excellent and comprehensive books on physical medicine and rehabilitation (PM&R); even books devoted to single rehabilitation topics, but finding the right information at the right time can be elusive for trainees and practitioners alike.

For those at an early stage in their career (students or residents), this book will provide an introduction to the PM&R patient care approach and a bird's eye view of critical topics. For those at later stages of their career, it should provide easy access to facts and core information on areas of rehabilitation medicine that have not been visited recently. To that end, we chose to divide the book into three sections. The first section introduces the reader to the spectrum of rehabilitation practice. The second section provides an overview on the scope of practice of allied health professionals who are part of the rehabilitation team. Rehabilitation topics and practice areas are discussed in section three.

We are optimistic that this book will be a useful tool for medical students, residents, and the seasoned practitioner.

Marlís González-Fernádez, MD, PhD
Jarrod David Friedman, MD

# CONTENTS

# *REHABILITATIVE STRATEGIES*

The goal of rehabilitation, the guiding principle, and the rehabilitative strategies to accomplish the goal collectively provide a theoretical construct that will allow the practitioner to systematize the approach to the rehabilitation of individual patients, regardless of diagnosis. With this construct in mind, rehabilitative tactics can be applied.

## ■ GOAL

The goal of rehabilitation is to optimize the health, function, and ability to participate in desired activities in the family, work, recreation, and community.

## ■ GUIDING PRINCIPLE

Woven throughout rehabilitation is the guiding principle of anticipatory management. Although no 2 patients with any given disease or injury are exactly alike, there are enough similarities that certain patterns can be discerned in the natural history of the condition. Patients and providers can thus be spared the distress of enduring typical complications, which may cause a deterioration of health and prevent or delay return to function and participation.

## ■ STRATEGIES

I would suggest that the first and the best rehabilitative strategy, whenever possible to apply, is primary prevention. This is not ordinarily considered a part of rehabilitation and is certainly not the province solely of rehabilitative medicine, but surely prevention is preferable to "picking up the pieces" after a stroke, spinal injury, traumatic brain injury, heart attack, malaria, burn, or other condition has occurred.

The second strategy is reduction of the pathologic process to a minimum. Here, early care is of great importance to the ultimate functional outcome.

The third strategy, and the first one commonly considered a rehabilitative strategy, is prevention of secondary complications (sometimes expressed as secondary disability). This strategy often challenges time-worn concepts of bed rest as a treatment and, instead, promotes early mobilization to prevent pressure ulcers, deconditioning, contractures, loss of bone mass, and depression, to name a few.

The fourth strategy is enhancement of the function of the affected systems - basically attempting to repair the damage done. Attempting to strengthen weakened limbs in a patient with stroke would be an example of this strategy.

The fifth strategy is enhancement of the function of the unaffected systems. This overlaps with the sixth strategy, which is compensation or compensatory techniques. Examples of these strategies include strengthening the upper body of a person with paraplegia (fifth) and strengthening the less affected side of a person with stroke (sixth).

The seventh is cognitive and behavioral intervention. A person with spatial-perceptual impairment may learn to "talk himself through" a transfer or dressing or other task.

The eighth strategy is environmental adaptation. This may be temporary, employed before the first 7 strategies have had their full effect. More often, they change as rehabilitation progresses.

## ■ TACTICS

The tactics or techniques employed in rehabilitation are numerous. They are what are usually considered rehabilitation. The tactics and techniques are the means by which the goal is achieved and the strategies accomplished. In earlier times of multidisciplinary rehabilitation, certain tactics were considered the territory of certain disciplines. I would submit that in true interdisciplinary rehabilitation, practitioners of one discipline may have primary responsibility for one strategy and the associated tactics, but other team members will be actively involved. For example, the psychologist may have primary responsibility for helping the patient incorporate certain behaviors in his/her repertoire (such as frequent pressure-relief maneuvers in the patient with spinal cord injury), but other team members, including family and friends, will need to reinforce the behaviors by a smile or the word "Good" when a wheelchair pushup is observed. Wheelchair transfers may be taught in the physical or occupational therapy gym, but nursing will need to ensure that the patient does these transfers in her room. This interdisciplinary approach helps the patient transition from "can do" to "does."

## ■ SUMMARY

The theme of this paper is "Rehabilitative Strategies" for rehabilitation treatment. The author proposes that the goal of rehabilitation is to optimize the health, function, and ability to participate in desired activities in the family, work, recreation, and community. The author emphasizes that with this theoretical framework, rehabilitation treatments can be systematically applied to patients with different diagnoses. The paper points out that rehabilitative strategies can be achieved through prevention of secondary injury, reduction of pathology to a minimum, and cognitive and behavioral intervention. Additionally, the paper introduces the guiding principle of anticipatory management, which suggests that by judging the natural progression of the disease, typical complications that may cause deterioration of health and prevent or delay return to function and participation can be avoided. In summary, this paper emphasizes the importance of rehabilitation therapy and provides practical advice and strategies to achieve treatment goals.

## ■ IMPORTANT TERMINOLOGY

rehabilitative strategies　康复策略
multidisciplinary rehabilitation　多学科康复
interdisciplinary approach　跨学科方法
psychology　心理学
physical therapy　物理治疗
occupational therapy　作业治疗
nursing　护理

natural history   自然病史
typical complications   典型并发症
cognitive   认知
behavioral intervention   行为干预
primary prevention   一级预防
environmental adaptation   环境适应
trauma   创伤

## ■ REVIEW QUESTIONS

1. What are the different approaches to rehabilitative strategies mentioned in the article, and how can they be used to systematically approach rehabilitation for individual patients?
2. How important is the interdisciplinary approach to rehabilitative strategies, and what roles can multidisciplinary teams play in ensuring successful patient outcomes?
3. What are some of the typical complications that may arise during rehabilitation, and how can anticipatory management strategies be used to anticipate and avoid these complications?
4. What are some of the cognitive and behavioral interventions that can be used to assist patients with spatial-perceptual impairments during rehabilitation?
5. Can you provide examples of environmental adaptations that may be employed during the rehabilitation process, and how might these environmental adaptations change as rehabilitation progresses?

（王于领）

# REHABILITATION DOCUMENTATION

## ■ INTRODUCTION

Well-written, accurate, and comprehensive documentation is key to optimal patient assessment and management as well as serving as justification for a patient's admission to, and continued stay, on a comprehensive inpatient rehabilitation service. Recent changes in medicare oversight of inpatient rehabilitation facilities (IRF) have heightened the necessity for physicians and other rehabilitation care providers to improve documentation in order to avoid denial of payment by auditors [1]. With the implementation of the DRG/DIP payment or Per-Diem Payment system, there is an increased need for physicians and other rehabilitation care providers to improve their records to provide a reasonable basis for using National Healthcare Security fund. Documentation at the preadmission, admission H&P, daily progress note, team conference, and discharge summary levels should support that services are reasonable, appropriate (in terms of efficacy, duration, frequency, and amount) for treatment of the patient's condition, as well as necessary to furnish the care on an inpatient hospital basis, rather than in a less intensive facility such as a skilled nursing facility (SNF) or on an outpatient or home-based basis. Templates, both electronic and written, are useful to facilitate the completion of such documentation requirements.

## ■ HISTORY AND PHYSICAL ADMISSION NOTE

The history and physical admission note (H&P) should clearly communicate the assessment and treatment plan of the admitting physician. The reviewer must be able to ascertain the reason for admission, the prior level of function, the therapies required, the anticipated course of treatment, and the expected goals [2,3].

*More specifically, the H&P serves as the detailed review of a rehabilitation patient's*
- Actively treated conditions
- Newly recognized conditions
- Resolving/resolved conditions
- Rehabilitation diagnosis (primary functional limitation, primary impairment, and cause)
- Complications and coexisting conditions
- Symptoms that will require treatment
- Chronic medical conditions
- Potential conditions that require preventive measures, restrictions, and/ or precautions
- Other functional deficits

*In addition, the H&P should support the medical and rehabilitation necessity of the IRF admission by*
- Describing the reason for admission to an IRF
- Providing evidence of the complexity of the planned interdisciplinary program

- Listing the interventions to be provided by each discipline (ie, Physical, Occupational, Speech Therapies, Nursing, Rehabilitation Nursing, and Case Management)
- Providing evidence that the patient will be able to tolerate, benefit from, and participate in the intensity of approximately 3 hours of therapy per day
- Detailing the need and plan for cross-disciplinary reinforcement of the medical, nursing, and therapy programs
- Demonstrating the complexity of medical and rehabilitation conditions that require both nursing assessment 24 hours a day and frequent physician visits and oversight
- Identifying the anticipated impact of coexisting medical conditions on the rehabilitation plan and how those medical issues alter the approach to treatment

The following characteristics apply to all documentation in the inpatient rehabilitation service, including the H&P: legibility, completeness, timeliness (payor and institutions may require certain documents to be in the patient's record within 24 or 48 hours), and authentication (physicians' and other clinicians' signatures are required on all their own documentation). As well, attending physicians need to co-sign and often document more detailed information along with documentation for other clinicians whose work they are responsible for (ie, residents and physician extenders). Additionally, the appropriate method to make corrections and alterations of the document should be corrected in the following manner: put a line through the documentation made in error; write the word error above the line; initial and date just after the word error; and finally, erasures, whiteout, or other cover-up techniques should never be used in patient medical records—they call into question the credibility of the entire record.

The physiatric history and physical admission note utilize the standard medical H&P as a platform from which to additionally document

an assessment of the patient's impairments, disabilities, and handicaps, as well to formulate a management plan of coordinated, multidisciplinary rehabilitation care. Key to a comprehensive Rehabilitation H&P is a detailed account of the patient's medical history that focuses on past and present medical conditions as well as past and present functional limitations and the resources available to maximize independence and functionality postdischarge (see Table 2.1).

The physical examination component of the admission note should be the documentation of a thorough examination that emphasizes the patient's neurological, musculoskeletal, and psychological status, while also examining more specifically aspects of gait, balance, and upper and lower extremity function. The physical examination needs to be tailored to the condition for which the patient is being admitted. For instance, an orthopedic patient with a total joint replacement does not necessarily require a comprehensive neurological examination.

The summary portion of the H&P admission note should include an active medical and functional problem list, along with a management plan that details the coordinated, multidisciplinary approach required for patients admitted to an IRF. The management plan should speak to justifying the admission as it relates to medical necessity standards. The H&P summary should also highlight the patient's anticipated activity and participation limitations, focusing on:

- Estimated length of stay
- Anticipated discharge setting
- Discharge functional goals
- Precautions (falls, cardiac, seizure, sternal, orthopedic).

If a resident physician or a physician extender (PA or NP) is involved, there should be a separate section for the PM&R attending physician's history, physical examination, and assessment information.

**TABLE 2.1** ▪ The Admission Inpatient Rehabilitation document should contain the following categories of the patient's history

---

Date of Admission
Referring Physician/Institution/Service Information
Consulting Physicians from Referral Institution
PCP
Reason for Admission
Primary Medical Diagnosis
Rehabilitation/Functional Diagnoses
History of Present Illness
Past Medical History
Past and Recent Medications Including Allergies
Social History Including
   Occupation
   Where patient lives or plans to live
   Type of residence including stairs, floor levels, outside access
   Family resources
   Tobacco, alcohol, drug abuse
Family Medical History
Functional history (prior to and current) including levels of proficiencies in upper and lower extremity ADLs, mobility, toileting, cognition, comprehension, and expression
Bladder and Bowel Function (prior to admission and current)
Diet and swallowing history (prior to admission and current)
Comprehensive review of systems
Laboratory and imaging data

---

## Daily Progress Notes

Progress notes must demonstrate frequent, direct, and medically necessary physician involvement for the entire IRF stay. This documentation should include any revisions to the expectations of the anticipated course and predicted functional gains. In addition to serving as an accurate current assessment of the status of the patient's medical problems and functional/rehabilitation progress, the progress note identifies the continuing necessity for a coordinated and comprehensive inpatient rehabilitation approach. This is accomplished by documenting a daily management plan that links specific medical or rehabilitation issues to prescribed treatments and involvement of the multidisciplinary team. For instance, the development of orthostatic hypotension in a stroke patient would require in addition to a medical plan for further medical assessment and treatment, documentation of how the therapist should modify the therapeutic plan for gait therapy and monitor vital signs, and nursing should institute and monitor response to compression stocking/wrapping. In addition, the daily note should include information regarding the patient's progress toward the stated rehabilitation goals, and if he/she was unable to attend or participate in rehabilitation therapies, the reason should be indicated. As inpatient rehabilitation reimbursement becomes subject to strict reviews of medical necessity documentation, it is imperative that the daily progress note document the continuing justification for the patient to remain on the rehabilitation service. This includes evidence in the note that progress is being made toward goal attainment, the patient is able to tolerate the intensity of services prescribed, and that coordinated multidisciplinary care requiring 24-hour rehabilitation nursing and frequent physician presence is being given.

A Physiatric Daily Progress note may be written in a SOAP format (symptoms, objective, assessment, plan) with inclusion of the patient's functional/rehabilitation status and progress in addition to addressing the active medical problems and plan of care. Typically this includes

1. Chief complaints and status of present illness

2. Relevant review of systems

3. Physical examination findings including vital signs

4. Results of recent and pertinent laboratory tests and imaging

5. An impression that focuses on the status of active medical problems and rehabilitation issues including the degree of progress accomplished

6. A plan of management for those active medical and rehabilitation problems with sufficient specificity as to both the individualized and coordinated nature of plan. For example, daily documentation for a patient whose leg spasticity is worsening may include not only the medical assessment of the type and degree of spasticity and the medication to be prescribed but also that management of the spasticity will additionally focus on nursing carrying through a stretching program in bed with appropriate splint application, and physical therapy will use ice and electrical stimulation to reduce tone and increase ankle range of motion.

## Documentation of Discharge from the Rehabilitation Inpatient Service

Hospital discharge or transfer of service summaries serve as the primary documents communicating a patient's care plan to the receiving medical or surgical service, subacute rehabilitation unit or facility, or an outpatient primary care or specialist provider. At times, these documents are the only form of clinical information that accompanies the patient to the next setting of care. Therefore, these summaries need to be of high quality including sufficient enough detail to permit safe and effective care to resume after the handoff from one practitioner to the other. The Joint Commission has published standard that specify expected components of hospital discharge summaries that include:

1. Reason for hospitalization (chief complaint and history of present illness)

2. Significant findings during the stay (primary diagnoses)

3. Procedures and treatments provided (hospital course, procedures and consultations)

4. Patient's discharge condition (the patient's health status at discharge)

5. Patient and family instructions if appropriate (discharge medications, activity orders, therapy orders, dietary instructions, plans for medical/surgical follow-up)

6. Attending physician signature of the discharge summary

Although the above applies to all types of medical and surgical discharges or transfer notes, the physiatric version needs to additionally focus on conveying critical information pertaining to the rehabilitation needs of the patient. The discharge summary reviews both the medical and the rehabilitation aspects of the hospital stay including functional deficits, barriers to further progress, progress/attainment of rehabilitation goals, and the type of discharge setting.

For program summaries of patient's being discharged to the home setting, it is critical to specify equipment already provided or being delivered including assistive devices, dwelling modifications suggested, the degree of physical assistance needed, and specifications for the frequency and duration of nursing and therapy services prescribed, either in the home or in an outpatient facility, and documenting appropriate training and education of the patient and family.

For those patients being discharged to a skilled nursing facility/ subacute rehabilitation program, rehabilitation instructions should focus on a detailed plan of medical and rehabilitation care that the receiving team of nurses and therapists can easily understand and institute. Recommendations for equipment and rehabilitation services have to be consistent with resources likely to be available in noncomprehensive rehabilitation settings.

Patients being transferred off a comprehensive rehabilitation service due to a need for urgent or more complex medical and surgical management should be accompanied by a Transfer Summary, which follows the principles of the rehabilitation discharge summary mentioned above. However, transfer summaries need to include detailed documentation as to why the patient requires changing services with up-to-date summary of the recent hospital course, up-to-date lists of medications, procedures, and laboratory and imaging findings. This transfer information needs to be sufficiently clear and comprehensive that the physician and nursing team assuming care can do so expeditiously and safely. Moreover, the summary must also detail recommendations for continued rehabilitation management as best can be accomplished on an acute medical-surgical service. Particular emphasis needs to be placed on bladder and bowel management, and skin care, as well as the importance of early mobilization and preserving joint range of motion. Suggestions should be made to restart rehabilitation therapies as soon as is medically feasible.

# ■ ELECTRODIAGNOSTIC REPORTS

Electromyography (EMG) and nerve conduction studies (NCS) performed by appropriately trained and experienced individuals are used to evaluate patients with neuromuscular disease and to diagnose the presence, distribution, and severity of neurological system pathology. The report that the electrodiagnostician produces after completion of the test serves as a communication instrument to the referring physician documenting the results and conclusions of the electrodiagnostic evaluation. EMG and NCS need to be performed and reported with consideration of the clinical context, not merely as isolated tests—in essence, an electrodiagnostic consultation. Electrodiagnostic studies should always be considered as an extension of the physical exam. The final diagnoses and subsequent clinical decisions made should reflect that. Thus, the EMG report should strive not to portray generalizations (ie, "suggest clinical correlation"), but rather to make a determination as to whether or not the results explain the patient's signs and symptoms. This is only possible if the electromyographer has discussed the history with the patient and done at least a focused physical examination.

The question arises what information should be included in the report and what is the best way to present that information. It is paramount that the electromyographer's final report be a concise and clearly written summary of relevant findings and interpretation. It is desirable that the report not be a lengthy list of every subtest result, irrespective of the clinical significance of those findings. This type of report is often due to the electromyographer's lack of certainty as to the clinical relevance of a given result. The EMG report should be concise, to the point, and understandable to the less sophisticated reader.

A good-quality EMG report should always include the actual waveforms of sensory, motor, and F-wave tests. This is in addition to the numerical data that are usually included in tabular format. Another important indicator of a good-quality study and report is the inclusion of temperature data. Whether or not the ideal temperature can be obtained, an EMG report without a temperature recorded offers incomplete and possibly inaccurate information.

The model report should include a description of the clinical problem for which the patient was referred, the electrodiagnostic tests performed and their results, and the diagnostic interpretation of the data. If the report only contains a conclusion but without supportive data, it is difficult for the referring clinician to determine whether the test results support the conclusions made and whether the diagnosed condition is worsening, improving, or stable. Normal reference values included adjacent to the specific results are desirable to allow the reader to verify why certain findings were reported as abnormal.

List of recommended components of a complete electrodiagnostic report [4-6]:

1. Patient's demographic data (name, age/birth date, gender) Also consider: height, weight, handedness

2. Clinic-based information: Hospital/patient number, electromyographer's name, referring physician, name of assisting technician or resident physician, testing location, date

3. Limb temperatures

4. Medical history including presenting problem, relevant past medical history, relevant medications (especially anticoagulants)

5. Brief physical examination findings

6. Other: obstacles to performing the complete test (ie, contraindications to performing parts of the test such as nerve conduction in face of a cardiac pacemaker, or needle EMG of certain muscles because of anticoagulation, or inability to test certain muscles/nerves due to difficulty in positioning)

7. Use nonnarrative, tabular formats to present NCS and Needle-EMG data

8. Nerve conduction study results. List the nerves and the side (right or left) studied, and include results for the following test parameters:

- name of nerve studied
- sites of stimulation
- distance between the distal stimulation site and the recording site, and distances between the various stimulation sites
- sensory peak distal latencies and peak-to-peak (or baseline-to-peak) amplitudes
- depending on preference, calculated sensory conduction velocity (determined from onset latencies)
- motor onset latencies and baseline-to-negative peak compound muscle action potential (CMAP) amplitudes
- calculated motor conduction velocities for specified nerve segment (ie, ulnar across elbow segment)

**Example of Motor Nerve Conduction Table of Results**

| Nerve | Side | Site (stim- record) | Distance (cm) | Latency (ms) | Amplitude (mV) | Segment | Conduction Velocity (m/s) |
|-------|------|---------------------|---------------|--------------|----------------|---------|---------------------------|
| Ulnar | Right | Wrist (W)-ADM | 8 | 3.8 | 8 | — | — |
|       |      | Below elbow (BE) | 28 |  | 7 | BE-W | 56 |
|       |      | Above elbow (AE) | 12 |  | 6.5 | AE-BE | 62 |

9. Other Nerve Conduction

- F-wave studies
  - Name of nerve studied (ie, ulnar)
  - Side of test
  - Stimulation and recording sites
  - Report minimum F-wave latency
- H-reflex studies
  - Name of the nerve studied (ie, tibial)
  - Side of test
  - Stimulation and recording sites
  - Report minimum H-reflex latency
  - (recorded H-wave amplitude is optional)
- Repetitive nerve stimulation
  - Sites of nerve stimulation and muscle recorded from
  - Indicate if stimulation was performed at rest or after exercise, and if after exercise, the duration of the exercise and the time since the exercise

- Indicate the rate of stimulation (ie, 3/s) and the number of stimuli in the pulse train
- Report the initial CMAP (M) amplitude, and the increment or decrement is calculated (% change of amplitude or area of the fourth or fifth M-wave to the first).

10. Needle electromyography

- Describe insertional, spontaneous, and voluntary activity for each muscle studied
- It is helpful, but optional, to associate each muscle tested with a corresponding peripheral nerve or root level of innervation.
- State whether the test utilized a monopolar or concentric needle. Divide the needle EMG findings per muscle according to spontaneous activity and voluntary activity
  - Spontaneous activity should include insertional activity (increased, decreased, or normal); fibrillations (0-4+); positive sharp waves (0-4+); fasciculations, complex repetitive discharges, other abnormal spontaneous activity noted (ie, myokymia, myotonia, cramps)
  - Voluntary activity should be divided into motor unit action potential (MUAP) amplitude and duration (increased, normal, or decreased), polyphasicity (normal or increased), and recruitment or firing pattern (normal, early, decreased). Indication of the fullness of the interference pattern with maximal effort should be described (full, incomplete, discrete, or single unit pattern)

Indication of factors limiting the needle examination of that muscle (ie, unable to relax; did not tolerate secondary to pain)

**Example of Needle EMG Table of Results**

☐ At rest          ☐ With activation

| Muscle | Innervation | Insertional | Fib | PSP | Fasic | CRD | Other |
|--------|-------------|-------------|-----|-----|-------|-----|-------|
| APB | Med/C8 | increased | 2+ | 2+ | none | OCC | none |

| Ampl | Duration | Polys | Recruitment | Interference | Comments |
|------|----------|-------|-------------|--------------|----------|
| increased | increased | increased | decreased | incomplete | pain limited |

11. The summary of results section of the report should not be a regurgitation of detailed individual data elements (already included in the table format presentation) but instead be a summarization of the findings with an attempt at recognized patterns of the results [7].

- For instance, "NCS show generalized borderline motor nerve conduction velocities with low amplitude sensory and motor responses. There is disproportionate focal slowing of conduction across the left elbow without amplitude loss comparing above and below elbow stimulation sites. Concentric needle examination demonstrated low-grade spontaneous activity in distal leg and arm muscles, with mildly increased MUAP amplitudes in several distal foot muscles."

12. The interpretation section of the report should tie the summary of results into a probable electrophysiological diagnosis, noting whether the findings are normal or abnormal (ie, This is an abnormal electrodiagnostic examination. The EMG findings suggest mild to moderate predominantly axonal, sensorimotor peripheral neuropathy with superimposed focal compression ulnar neuropathy at the right cubital tunnel).

# ■ SUMMARY

The theme of this article is "Rehabilitation Literature". The author suggests that well written, accurate, and comprehensive documents are the key to optimizing patient assessment and management, as well as the reason for patients to stay and continue to stay in comprehensive inpatient rehabilitation services. The author emphasizes the importance of rehabilitation documents for patient evaluation, management, and providing legitimacy for inpatient rehabilitation services, as they must be able to determine the reason for admission, previous functional levels, required treatment, expected treatment process, and expected goals. This article lists the content, format, and details that need to be noted in rehabilitation documents with a focus on the importance of medical history and physical admission records, daily progress records, and discharge documents. In addition, electromyography (EMG) and nerve conduction study (NCS) are used to evaluate patients with neuromuscular diseases and diagnose the existence, distribution and severity of nervous system pathology. The article also introduces the writing standards and key points of electrical diagnosis report. In summary, this article emphasizes the importance of rehabilitation literature and provides a detailed discussion of its important details.

## ■ IMPORTANT TERMINOLOGY

rehabilitation documentation　康复文书
the history and physical admission note　病史和住院体检记录
inpatient rehabilitation facilities　住院康复机构
skilled nursing facility　专业护理机构
physical examination　体格检查
daily progress notes　每日病程记录
documentation of discharge　出院记录
electrodiagnostic reports　电诊断报告
electromyography　肌电图
nerve conduction studies　神经传导检测

## ■ REVIEW QUESTIONS

1. Why is high-quality rehabilitation documentation important for patient assessment and management?
2. What is the purpose of reviewing the history and physical admission note in the rehabilitation work?
3. What should be included in the history and physical admission note?
4. What should be the focus of the daily progress notes?
5. What should be included in documentation of discharge from the rehabilitation inpatient service to ensure comprehensive rehabilitation management?
6. What are the key components of a good-quality EMG report?

## ■ REFERENCES

1. US Department of Health and Human Services, Centers for Medicare & Medicaid Services. Proposed Rule: Medicare: inpatient rehabilitation facility prospective payment system (2008 FY); update, [07-2241]. Fed Regist. 26230-26279.
2. Ganer B, Erickson R, et al. Clinical evaluation. In: Joel AD, Gans BM, Walsh NE, Bockenek WL, eds. Physical Medicine and Rehabilitation: Principles and Practice. 4th ed. Lippincott Williams & Wilkins; 2004.
3. Odell M, Lin C, Panagos A, Fung N. The physiatric history and physical examination. In: Braddom, ed. Physical Medicine and Rehabilitation, 3rd ed. Elsevier.
4. Jablecki C, et al. Reporting the results of needle EMG and nerve conduction studies: an educational report. Muscle Nerve. 2005.

5.  American Association of Neuromuscular and Electrodiagnostic medicine. Recommended policy for electrodiagnostic medicine. Muscle Nerve. 1999; 22:S101-S104.

6.  Dumitru D, Zwarts MJ. The electrodiagnostic medicine consultation: approach and report generation. In:Dumitru D,AmatoAA,Zwarts MJ,eds.Electrodiagnostic Medicine. 2nd ed. Philadelphia, PA: Hanley & Belfus; 2002:515-540.

7.  Smith B. What good is EMG to the patient and practitioner? Semin Neurol. 2003;23(3):335-342.

（马跃文）

# OUTPATIENT REHABILITATION: CLINICS AND PRACTICE

## ■ INTRODUCTION

Outpatient medicine is a key component of a physiatric practice. Clinics can be both a primary and secondary site in the care of our patients. An outpatient physician does not have to practice within a hospital setting or a university setting. Unlike an inpatient practice, the majority of outpatient clinics are not part of a university or hospital setting. This short chapter will give you some basic important information regarding outpatient clinics and outpatient medicine.

## ■ STATISTICS

Outpatient visits outnumber inpatient visit at a ratio of 3 : 1. According to the CDC US Health Report in 2009, US hospitals saw 102.2 million outpatients compared with 34.9 million discharges from the US hospital inpatient care facilities in 2006 [1]. The same report notes that in 2007, Medicare-reported physicians saw 994 million patient visits to their outpatient physician offices, whereas US hospital outpatient facilities saw only 89 million visits [1]. In general, physicians who plan to practice in an outpatient setting see and handle larger volumes of patients than inpatient attending physicians and must be capable of handling a higher patient load and be efficient doing so while ensuring that the health care they deliver is of the highest quality.

Despite the significantly higher volume of patients seen in the outpatient setting, the cost of care is lower. According to the CDC, 2007 national healthcare expenditures in the US totaled $2.2 trillion. Hospital costs accounted for 31% of these expenditures, while outpatient clinic costs accounted for 21%. This does not speak for the complexity of outpatient care, very much to the contrary.

## ■ OUTPATIENT PRACTICES

Physiatrists have a wide array of subspecialties to choose from. From neurologic disorders to musculoskeletal disease or even cardiopulmonary disease and the choice between pediatric and adult populations, physiatry can accommodate a wide variety of interests (Table 3.1). Specialization within physiatry is not necessary if a physician is interested in seeing a wide variety of patients with a host impairments and disability.

**TABLE 3.1** ▪ Types of clinics

| Common Clinics | Subtypes |
|---|---|
| Amputee | |
| Balance disorders | |
| Brain Injury | |
| Cancer | |
| Cardiopulmonary | • Cardiac<br>• Pulmonary |
| EMG/NCV | |
| Independent medical evaluation/<br>disability evaluations | |
| Gait | |
| General outpatient physiatry | |
| Musculoskeletal | • Arthritis and joint osteoporosis, etc. |
| Occupational/work | |
| Orthotics and prosthetics | |
| Pain management | • Interventional<br>• Noninterventional |
| Palliative care | |
| Pediatrics | • Numerous subclinics exist:<br>Cerebral palsy, gait, JRA,<br>neuromuscular clinic, etc. |
| Scoliosis | |
| Spasticity | • May be part of a spine, stroke, or<br>brain injury clinic or independent |
| Spine | • Spinal cord injury<br>• Scoliosis<br>• Conservative pain focus:<br>Radiculopathy, degenerative<br>or herniated disc disease |
| Sports medicine | |
| Stroke | |
| Wheel chair clinic | |

Only through experience can an individual choose which focus or subspecialty best suites his or her personality and intellectual interest. Anyone thinking of pursuing a career in outpatient physiatry is encouraged to obtain exposure to as many different fields as possible.

## ■ THE OUTPATIENT TEAM

A hallmark of acute inpatient rehabilitation is the provision of multidisciplinary care with a team approach. The outpatient setting is no different. Understanding and learning the different components is very important to best serve patients in an outpatient setting. The role of the physiatrist as coordinator of care becomes crucial in the outpatient setting when the care provided by different disciplines is in multiple locations.

In order to understand outpatient practice, it is useful to understand how a patient moves in and out of a given clinic. This is referred to as clinic flow dynamics. Although each clinic is different, the basic design is usually similar (Figure 3.1).

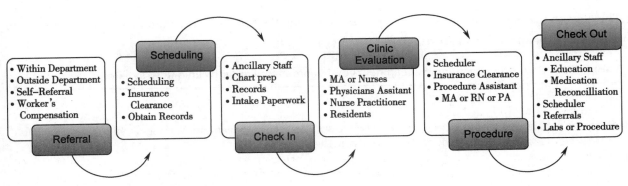

**Figure 3.1**   Basic outpatient clinic flow.

Clinic flow and the other logistical issues that will be mentioned might be considered obvious to some, while others find it difficult or think it is irrelevant. However, because many of these issues affect outpatient practice and are seldom taught during residency or medical school, we will provide a brief introduction.

## ■ CLINIC FLOW AND CLINICAL PRACTICE

Clinic flow and efficiency can have a significant impact on clinical practice for multiple reasons:

### 1. Clinic flow affects patient satisfaction and referrals

Understanding clinic flow can help to minimize or even prevent patient and physician frustration and dissatisfaction. For example, if a colleague needs a patient scheduled quickly into your clinic and you are not fully aware of the clinic's registration process or availability of appointments, you may tell him to just call the clinic without realizing that the process can take 15 minutes to 1 hour on the phone talking to 3 different people. Potentially, the next open appointment is 4 weeks away or worse than that, the clinic doesn't accept the patient's insurance. These issues lead to frustration on the referring physicians' part and can inevitably lead to less referrals. By understanding who schedules your patients and the registration process, you can better direct a colleague or a patient to the right person to facilitate flow. Knowing clinic flow is necessary to correct issues related to your patients' needs and treatment as they arise, thus minimizing or preventing patient and referring physician frustration and dissatisfaction.

### 2. Clinic flow affects availability of clinical services

If no clear procedures are in place for "walk-in's," urgent appointments, late-cancellations, and so on. clinical productivity is affected. Processes should be in place to fill all available appointment times and to reduce the time between the initial call and the scheduled appointment.

### 3. Clinic flow affects overall work satisfaction

Delays can be very frustrating to clinic staff and physicians alike. For example, a patient is scheduled for a follow-up appointment specifically to discuss laboratory or radiological results. On the day the patient comes for the appointment, the results are not available. The staff has to make last-minute phone calls or computer entries, which takes time and prevents them from performing other duties, slowing down the clinic flow, prolonging the clinic day, and delaying care of other patients. Clinic-flow analysis studies show that delays in an outpatient clinic are a key issue in patient and physician dissatisfaction (2). Constant delays unnecessarily reduce patient volumes, affecting overall productivity and staff satisfaction. By understanding clinic processes, problems can be minimized and processes optimized.

It is important to learn from experience and develop a practice style based on the specific practice's needs. The goal should always be efficiency while maintaining the highest quality of service and patient care.

There are also some basic questions that should be asked when working in a new outpatient clinic (Table 3.2).

These questions can guide the evaluation process. Investing the time to understand these issues as related to clinic flow dynamics is key in the delivery of patient care.

**TABLE 3.2** ▪ Common questions that can help you become familiar with clinic-flow dynamics

| Questions to Ask |
| --- |
| 1. How does the flow of your clinic work? |
| 2. What is each person's responsibility? That is, who checks in, who brings patients to clinic rooms, who takes vital signs? |
| 3. How long does your check-in process take? What is involved? |
| 4. What is the average wait time until a patient is actually ready for you to see them? |
| 5. What is the average wait time for new and return patients? Is the process the same or different? Can you add patients easily on to your schedule? That is, urgent visits or important referrals. |
| 6. What procedures require insurance clearance? What do not? |
| 7. What labs or X-rays can be done within your clinic? If any, what is the wait time? |
| 8. How many clinic rooms do you have to use? Do patients wait in the rooms or another area for procedures, labs etc? |
| 9. Given the requirements in some areas for medication reconciliation forms to be given to patient prior to leaving the clinic, how is this handled and how are medication prescriptions tracked and followed? |
| 10. Who is in charge of the ancillary staff? If you have a problem, who is in charge of resolving it? |

# ■ REFERRAL SOURCES

No physician can practice without patients. Physiatrist patient volumes are highly dependent on referrals. Understanding and maintaining referral sources is very important within the practice of physiatry. Referral sources can be both direct and indirect (Table 3.3).

Direct referrals are when a patient schedules a visit without another health care providers' intervention (self-referred). They might have been given your name by a friend, seen an advertisement, or read an informational brochure or an article. Indirect referrals are when another physician or health care provider refers a patient for evaluation.

**TABLE 3.3** ▪ Common referral sources

| Main Type of Referral | Sources Subtype |
| --- | --- |
| **DIRECT** | |
| 1. Self-referral | |
| | • Another patient |
| | • Internet search |
| | • Yellow pages |
| | • Newspaper, radio or TV information, or article |
| | • TV or radio ad |
| **INDIRECT** | |
| 2. Consults from another physician or practitioner | |
| | • Cardiology |
| | • Geriatrics |
| | • Neurology |
| | • Neurosurgery |
| | • Oncology |
| | • Orthopedics |
| | • Primary care |
| | • Pulmonary |
| | • Rheumatology |
| 3. Follow-up from an inpatient admission | |
| | • Your own patient |
| | • From MD within your group |
| | • From MD outside your group |

Continued

| Main Type of Referral | Sources Subtype |
| --- | --- |
| 4. Referral for specific test or procedures | Such as<br>• Driving evaluation<br>• Gait analysis<br>• Intramuscular injection<br>• NCV/EMG<br>• Neurocognitive testing<br>• Peripheral joint injection<br>• Swallowing evaluation<br>• Spinal injection<br>• Urodynamics |
| 5. Workers' compensation | • Direct from a company<br>• Insurance career<br>• Law firm<br>• Self-referred |

Reasons for referrals from other physicians or health care practitioners vary. Most commonly, a specialized evaluation or procedure is requested. Factors that may affect referrals include rapport with referral sources and availability of services (wait times). To establish relationships for continued referrals, it is important to understand the needs of the health care providers in the local community. Educating referral sources on how a particular practice can meet their needs will lead in turn to more referrals.

Once a patient has been seen, several steps will ensure continued referrals (Table 3.4):

1. All the questions in the referral and any specific requests should be answered.

2. Notes should be legible, easy to read, and organized.

3. Plan of care should be clear and simple. Respect the referring physician's time.

4. Make sure clinical reasoning is clearly stated for each recommendation. Notes are frequently reviewed by payers to determine if procedures or medications are medically necessary.

5. Communicate to the referring physician or support staff the results of your evaluation or testing/procedure promptly and without delay. This is extremely helpful and allows building a better relationship with referral sources.

**TABLE 3.4 ▪ Referrals appreciate prompt accurate communication of your evaluation and/or test results**

| Notes |
| --- |
| 1. Answer referral questions clearly |
| 2. Legible notes |
| 3. Organized concise notes & plan |
| 4. Recommendations clearly stated |
| 5. Goals clearly stated |
| **COMMUNICATION** |
| 1. Send notes promptly |
| 2. Ensure accuracy of notes |
| 3. Make phone calls when necessary |

## ■ GOALS OF AN OUTPATIENT PROGRAM

Understanding the clinic's philosophy and goals and the specific practitioner's goals is very important. Table 3.5 describes some common goals of an outpatient program. Understanding and clearly defining the goals of a clinic and practice are paramount to servicing patients and ensuring the highest quality of care and quality of life for the patient.

**TABLE 3.5** ▪ General principles of outpatient practice

1. Always note and determine the patients' goals.
   - Document goals
   - Determine if these goals are reasonable
   - If the goals are not reasonable, educate and establish reasonable goals with your patient.
   - Review and update goals during each visit.
   - Document when goals have been accomplished or reached.
2. Determine current pathologies.
3. Determine biomechanical dysfunction and neurologic impairments both direct and indirect.
   - Current
   - Future (when possible)
     - Example
       - Spinal Fusion: Commonly have pain in the future above and below the levels of fusion. This is likely secondary to biomechanical strain at these areas. Goal is to minimize through preventative education and biomechanical retraining to not overrotate or strain the areas above and below the fusion during activity and utilization of adaptive equipment to accomplish everyday tasks.
4. Determine methods and needs to optimize function.
   - Diagnostic testing
     - Balance testing
     - Functional evaluation
     - Neurocognitive evaluation
     - Functional radiological testing
     - Urodynamics testing
       EMG/nerve conduction
       Swallowing study
   - Equipment needs
     - Adaptive equipment
     - Bracing
     - Car adaptations
     - Ergonomics at home and work
     - Home equipment
     - Orthotics
     - Prosthetics
     - Work adaptation
   - Exercise
   - Interventional procedures: Injections, surgeries
   - Life style adaptation
   - Nutrition
   - Weight loss plan: Should include percentage of body fat
   - Smoking and drug cessation plan when relevant
5. Educate patient and family
6. Improve or at a minimum attempt to maintain current function and quality of life
7. Optimize and record medical history and current and past medications
   - Determine how they may contribute to
     - Functional impairment or improvement
     - Quality of life impairment improvement

## Basic Steps in an Outpatient Clinic

We discussed briefly clinic flow dynamics, but patient and physician flow dynamics are different (Figure 3.2).

The goal of this diagram is to help understand the steps involved in outpatient care because, regardless of the type of practice, an outpatient practice thrives on the delivery of high-quality care efficiently. This is very important in today's health care system, where we are to provide excellent care while being cognizant of reducing cost.

These steps are also important and a necessity for patient satisfaction. A smooth and efficient outpatient program is less frustrating for patients and health care practitioners.

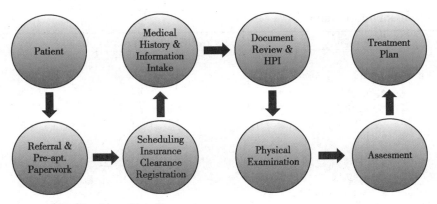

**Figure 3.2**   Basic patient flow.

Special considerations:

1. **Patient referral sheet obtained and reviewed. (Ideally prior to appointment)**

A patient referral sheet is the most common source of information when we see a patient. It is the basic form of communication from one department to another. In some settings, this is computerized; for others and many in nonhospital affiliated systems, the process still involves a piece of paper. It is usually faxed or emailed before the appointment, but on occasion it is brought in by the patients on the day of service. This referral sheet serves as confirmation to third-party payers of the referring practitioner's intent and may be the only means to legally show that you were asked to see the patient and may be reviewed by insurance companies or third parties for determination of payment for the services provided. It is important to review this sheet (personally or by an experienced staff member) to ensure that the questions to be answered are within the scope of the practice. Health care and patient advocates have noted inappropriate evaluations and referrals as a source of medical waste. Thus, this step will avoid unnecessary evaluations and improve utilization of health care resources.

2. **Clinic registration and insurance clearance**

This step is straightforward, but it can take a significant amount of time because of the paperwork and data entry required. This time is useful to ensure that patients brought and have filled out clinical information forms and have other supporting documents available. This step provides another checkpoint in clinic flow to help ensure that the face-to-face time spent in patient care is optimal.

3. **Patient intake**

Patient intake is the step that involves the initial data gathering performed before seeing the primary provider. In most outpatient clinics, this step is performed by physician extender (Table 3.6). Physician extenders improve clinic efficiency and can obtain basic information as described in Table 3.7. This information is then confirmed by the primary physician to ensure accuracy as well as interpret its relationship for inclusion in the evaluation. The physician should also obtain further details if needed.

**TABLE 3.6** ▪ Physician extenders

| Physician Extenders |
| --- |
| • Medical assistant |
| • Registered nurse |
| • Nurse practitioner |
| • Physician assistant |
| • Medical students |
| • Resident |
| • Fellow |

**TABLE 3.7** ▪ Basic patient information

| Item | Extender | Physician Inquiry |
|---|---|---|
| Basic Vitals | | |
| | • Age | |
| | • Height | |
| | • Weight | |
| | • Temp | |
| | • HR | |
| | • BP | |
| | • RR | |
| | • Pulse Ox | |
| | • Pain (VAS 0-10) | |
| Current Medication | • Prescription meds | Inquiry about allergy details |
| | • Supplements | Previous meds: opioids, anesthetics, neurologics |
| | • Allergies | |
| ROS | • Standard systems | Physician should review this and ask more focused questions related to patient problem |
| History | • Family | |
| | • Medical | |
| | • Surgical | |
| | • Obstetrical | |
| | • Home equipment | |
| | • Orthotics/prosthetics | |
| | • Mental health | Mood, impulsivity, sleep, buying habits, concentration, |
| |   • Hospitalization | suicidal thoughts, etc., especially in pts with risk factors |
| |   • Drug use | or central neurologic |
| |   • ETOH | |
| |   • Nicotine | |
| |   • drug abuse | |
| | • Social history | Housing, education, religion, work environment, driving/ transport, children/support |
| | • Legal history | • Active or settled case |
| | | • Situation: MVA, work, or personal injury |
| | | • Record all details and time frame |

#### 4. Main evaluation

The role of the physician in the outpatient setting is very similar to the role as an inpatient practitioner. A significant difference is that in the inpatient setting the primary diagnosis is usually known and we concentrate on treating the physiologic and biomechanical dysfunction associated with the patient's individual pathologies and known or unknown diagnoses. A significant portion of an outpatient practice setting is the evaluation of patients for the purpose of providing a diagnosis or to determine if a procedure is indicated.

A patient referred from an inpatient program usually has a clear diagnosis, and the effort is to focus on continued rehabilitative efforts building upon what was already started on an inpatient basis or to take rehabilitation to the next step. The primary focus is on function and quality of life while continuing to manage the patient's pathologies and disease processes and working to prevent or minimize progression.

Outpatient intake information (ie, HPI, medical history, and functional history) is similar to other care settings. The main difference is likely to be that the diagnosis, biomechanical dysfunction, and impairments are not known. Subsequently, the assessment and plan will differ. The assessment will need to restate the complaint and biomechanical or neurologic dysfunction along with the patient's stated goals (ie, I want to be pain-free, I want to eat regular food, or talk normal etc.) (Table 3.8). The assessment should be logical and orderly. If the pathologic diagnosis is not known, your assessment will need to justify your suspected diagnosis, the rationale for the differential diagnosis, subsequent evaluation, and treatment.

**TABLE 3.8** ▪ Physician's evaluation

| HPI | Summary of symptoms and historical data |
|---|---|
| | • Seek information from as many sources as possible<br>　• Patient<br>　• Family members<br>　• Medical records |
| Documentation | (Review all supportive documentation)<br>May or may not be part of HPI<br>• Hospital history and physical<br>• Hospital discharge summary<br>• Referring notes<br>• Diagnostic studies |
| Physical Examination | (Clinical findings)<br>• Initial: Complete but pertinent examination<br>• Follow-up: May be more focused |
| Assessment | (Thought process)<br>1. State the reason for the visit<br>　a. No need to restate the entire history<br>　b. Review key issues and facts concisely<br>2. Ensure you state the patient-stated goals<br>　Report your opinion and why goals are<br>　a. Reasonable<br>　b. Unreasonable<br>3. List outpatient current impairments<br>　a. Biomechanical<br>　b. Neurologic<br>　c. Musculoskeletal |
| Diagnoses | • List in order of significance |
| Treatment Plan | • Diagnostic testing<br>• Medications<br>• Equipment<br>• Therapies<br>　• Physical<br>　• Occupational<br>　• Psychology<br>　• Speech<br>　• Complementary<br>• Interventions<br>• Other consults/referrals<br>• Prognosis: Short/long term<br>• Work status<br>• Follow-up recommendations |

The differential diagnosis should be ordered starting with the most likely diagnosis. In patients who have multiple issues causing or related to the patient compliant, list the potential pathologies associated to each complaint. It is prudent to include in this section active comorbidities and relevant important lifestyles or behaviors (ie, obesity, smoking, sedentary lifestyle, drug abuse, among others).

In order to confirm the diagnostic impression, additional diagnostic testing is usually necessary. In cases where the diagnosis is already known, diagnostic testing may or may not be necessary. A justification statement for diagnostic tests is highly recommended (both for patient care and payment justification or even approval). Other plans should be listed out in an organized fashion with justification.

Proper communication and patient education is the final step and the most important. After reviewing with the patient the diagnosis and plan, the checkout process occurs.

The process and flow in outpatient physiatry is simple and yet covers a wide array of pathologies and disabilities. Currently, there is high demand for qualified board-certified physiatrists. As diagnostic and therapeutic technology continues to improve, the need for outpatient physiatrists will only continue to increase. Our field has the unique ability to combine the best of both diagnostic and therapeutic interventions on both inpatient and outpatient environments. The strengths of physiatric practice lies in our ability to integrate information, manage patients, and optimize biomechanical and physiological function while improving and/or maintaining quality of life.

## ■ SUMMARY

Outpatient rehabilitation is an important part of the practice of medicine. Unlike inpatient clinics, most outpatient clinics are not part of a university or a hospital. A hallmark of acute inpatient rehabilitation is the provision of multidisciplinary care in a team approach. Many factors affect the quality and the level of outpatient rehabilitation, while outpatient flow can affect patients' satisfaction and referrals, availability of clinical services, and clinical staffs' overall job satisfaction. The source of patients also has a great impact on outpatient rehabilitation. Patients may be referred directly from other hospitals, or may obtain information from friends, advertisements, media, etc. and seek treatment. All rehabilitation training requires professional evaluation. Outpatient rehabilitation also needs to follow certain goals and processes. In particular, it is necessary to pay attention to the patient's clinical information, insurance-related matters, patient intake, and pay attention to the role of outpatient doctors in rehabilitation, which is different from the responsibilities of resident doctors.

## ■ IMPORTANT TERMINOLOGY

outpatient rehabilitation 门诊康复
physiatrist 康复医师
clinic flow 门诊流程
patient satisfaction 患者满意度
patient referral 患者转诊
assessment 评估
differential diagnosis 鉴别诊断
quality of life 生活质量
patient education 患者教育
biomechanics 生物力学
musculoskeletal 肌肉骨骼
pain management 疼痛管理
urodynamics 尿动力学
swallowing evaluation 吞咽评估
neurocognitive evaluation 神经认知评估
gait analysis 步态分析
adaptive equipment 自适应设备

## ■ REVIEW QUESTIONS

1. Which subspecialties can physiatrists choose?

2. What is indirect referral?

3. What should we do to get continued referral?

4. What are the general principles of outpatient practice?

5. How to make assessment for outpatients?

## ■ REFERENCES

1. National Center for Health Statistics. Health, United States, 2009: With Special Feature on Medical Technology. Hyattsville, MD; 2010.

（白定群）

# NURSING HOME CARE AND SUBACUTE REHABILITATION

Frequently, patients unable to return home following acute hospitalization are discharged for subacute rehabilitation in skilled nursing facilities (SNFs) rather than being admitted for more intensive and coordinated treatment in an inpatient rehabilitation facility or unit (IRF/U). Subacute rehabilitation is well suited for individuals ready for discharge from an acute hospital service who may not yet be physically able to participate in full-day intensive therapy, such as elderly patients following hip fracture who are restricted from weight-bearing for 6 weeks, or stroke patients lacking the physical stamina or cognitive capabilities to benefit from 3 hours of rehabilitation therapy services daily. SNF-based rehabilitation programs may also be recommended for those who have made some progress in an IRF/U but require a longer period of lower intensity. rehabilitation to master additional tasks consistent with a safe return to the home setting. Subacute rehabilitation may also be appropriate for those recovering from unilateral hip or knee surgery, fractures, and other orthopedic conditions that do not require multidisciplinary, coordinated care and frequent treatment by a physician. Generally, individuals not ready for home-discharge, not requiring frequent physician management, not in need of, or unable to benefit from or tolerate more intensive, inter-disciplinary therapies, who are medically stable, motivated to participate and who show reasonable potential to achieve their rehabilitation goals within a relatively short time are candidates for subacute programs. Patients are typically admitted directly from an acute-care hospital once their condition has stabilized. Presently in subacute facilities, patients are grouped according to the amount of rehabilitation they required. These resource utilization groups (RUGs) are based on data from resident assessments and fall into 5 categories ranging from "Ultra High" with a minimum of 720 minutes of two therapy disciplines weekly to "Low" with a minimum of 45 minutes weekly of one therapy discipline provided over at least 3 days.

It has been reported that one third of all Medicare patients discharged from acute-care hospitals require postacute care. Thirteen percent of these patients are sent to SNFs, 11% to home care services, and 5% to IRF or LTAC. Despite the availability of different settings along an apparent continuum of service intensity, only 4% of the beneficiaries discharged used more than one postacute setting [1]. The need to clearly differentiate among the various levels and sites of rehabilitation care is an ongoing challenge in ongoing challenge in field of Physical Medicine and Rehabilitation, made more difficult by evolving regulatory oversight from the Centers of Medicare and Medicaid Services (CMS) [2]. The rapidly changing health care system has resulted in the modification of the traditional pathways through the continuum of rehabilitation medicine. As of this writing, most states in the country use a compliance rate of 60% for determining a hospital's eligibility for payment as a rehabilitation hospital or unit as a result of CMS's "75% rule"—enacted in 2004 as a gradual phase-in requiring that 75% of patients on a comprehensive IRU carry 1 of 13 core diagnoses as the reason prompting admission [3]. In addition, comprehensive rehabilitation programs are now being asked to return payments for hospital stays retroactively audited by CMS and found not to meet new "medical necessity" guidelines. Both the "60% rule" and "medical necessity" denials have forced IRF/Us to reduce or curtail admissions for patients with unilateral knee or hip replacements among other diagnoses, raising concern that such policies effectively limit access to appropriate rehabilitative care for some patients. Given the push by payers to discharge acutely hospitalized patients with rehabilitation needs to less-intensive settings (usually an SNF), it is critical that professionals in the rehabilitation field differentiate among the sites of care to ensure medically sensible placement of patients and appropriate reimbursement. Triage should result in selecting the right patient for the right treatment setting at the right time. A primary goal at completion of rehabilitation is the patient's return to living in the community, which could mean living at home independently, living with family, receiving home health care, or living in an assisted living residence (Table 4.1). It is also important to consider that when patients are discharged to a subacute or long-term nursing facility, the option exists for transfer back to an inpatient comprehensive rehabilitation facility or unit. This would be relevant only if improvement in their physical/cognitive status is consistent with participation in more intensive and complex rehabilitation training. For example, a transfer back to an IRF from a SNF program may be indicated for a stroke patient who initially could not tolerate intensive rehabilitation because of severe concurrent debility and lethargy, but has now after 3 weeks of subacute care has gained sufficient strength, endurance, and alertness to undertake 3 hours of an interdisciplinary therapy program.

**TABLE 4.1** ▪ Across-discipline comparison of IRF and skilled care

| Medical Discipline | Inpatient Rehabilitation | Subacute Rehabilitation |
|---|---|---|
| Physician | • Some active medical conditions not fully resolved<br>• Needs physician to oversee medical/rehab needs 5-7 d/wk | • Sufficiently resolved medical issues to be able to be managed by physician infrequently or off-site |
| Nursing | • Rehab nursing that deals with medical issues and promotes goals attainment<br>• Higher compliment of RN/LPN staff<br>• Documented patient/ family education<br>• Minimum 6 h/d | • Predominantly medical focus for staff<br>• Little or no family/ patient education<br>• Predominantly staffed with LPN overseeing aides<br>• 4 h/d |
| Therapy | • Two or more therapists (at least PT and OT)<br>• At least 3 h/d, 5 d/wk = 15 h/wk<br>• Groups <20% of therapy sessions | • May or may not receive therapies<br>• Only one therapy type permitted<br>• No minimum amount, maximum 6 h/wk |

As a general overview, the most intensive rehabilitation services today are provided at comprehensive IRUs within acute-care hospitals or at freestanding rehabilitation hospitals. Less-intense rehabilitative services are also administered in SNFs, at outpatient rehabilitation facilities, or at home through home health care. In addition, some patients who cannot tolerate 3 hours of daily rehabilitation therapy but still have long-term (>25 d length of stay) complicated medical and rehabilitative needs are discharged to chronic care in a long-term acute-care hospital (LTACH), for example, respiratory disease with ventilator-dependency, complicated wound care, and multisystem organ failure [4,5]. Also, patients who have lower-level rehabilitation needs, require only maintenance range of motion exercises and mobilization out of bed, and who have projected long-term institutional care needs may be discharged from the acute hospital directly to long term care in the nursing home setting.

The choice of the appropriate pathway for obtaining postacute rehabilitation care is typically made by the acute hospital's case manager or social worker, as a result of consultation with the treating physical or occupational therapist (PT/OT), the attending physician, the patient, and the patient's family. In some hospitals, rehabilitation medicine consultants, typically physiatrists, are available to make these recommendations (Figure 4.1).

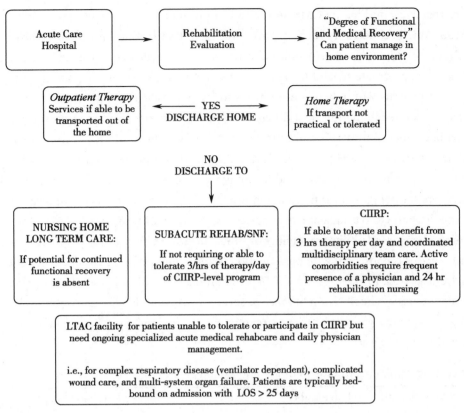

**Figure 4.1**    Determination of rehabilitation destinations.

Complicating this basic decision tree for rehabilitation program placement are the newer realities of admission justification along the "75% rule" and "medical necessity" guidelines. This requires the receiving IRF provide preadmission scrutiny of the referred patient ensuring IRF/U appropriateness. Consequently, admission staffs at IRFs have recently had to develop more sophisticated and detailed screening tools and documentation forms to help clarify the medical and rehabilitation justification for comprehensive integrated inpatient rehabilitation program (CIIRP) admission (see chapter on Hospital Forms).

A number of criteria typically guide which patients are admitted to SNF subacute rehabilitation versus CIIRP. The following factors help distinguish the 2 postacute-care settings:

## IRF/U entry criteria

1. Require at least 3 hours of any combination of physical, occupational, and speech therapy per day (the 3 h rule).

2. Require frequent care by a physician with rehabilitation training or experience related to the need to manage active medical comorbidities.

3. Require 24-hour care by a registered nurse with rehabilitation training or experience.

4. Require a coordinated care plan provided by a multidisciplinary team.

5. Be expected to achieve significant improvement over a reasonable period of time.

6. Have realistic rehabilitation goals that focus on achieving the maximum level of independent function.

7. Have a reasonable length of stay.

8. Generally (per 60% rule), patients' admitting diagnosis should predominantly be one of the following 13 categories:

■ Stroke

- Hip fracture
- Amputation
- Major multiple trauma
- Brain injury
- Spinal cord injury
- Congenital deformity
- Neurological disorders
- Burns
- Polyarticular rheumatoid arthritis
- Systemic vaculitides with joint inflammation
- Severe osteoarthritis of ≥3 weight-bearing major joints
- Complex total joint replacement (bilateral hip or knee, morbid obesity, or ≥85 years old)

## SNF Rehabilitation (subacute rehabilitation) entry criteria

1. No regulations for rehabilitation intensity or diagnoses.
2. Daily skilled nursing and/or rehab nursing.
3. 24-hour nursing service.
4. Prior minimum 3-day inpatient hospital stay for related illness or injury.
5. Practically, the required services can only be provided on an inpatient basis.
6. MD supervises care, with a required visit, other than for admission, only every 30 days or as required if a patient is experiencing a change in medical status. It is important to note that some subacute units in SNFs retain physiatrists who either provide PM&R consultation services or serve as the attending physician or even medical directors of these programs, often seeing the patient more frequently, between 1 and 3 times weekly.

*More specific differences between IRF and SAR/SNF levels of care include the following:*

1. An SNF is less likely than an IRF to have doctors and registered nurses on site at all times.
2. An SNF is more likely to have therapy aides or assistants provide rehabilitation treatments instead of licensed therapists.
3. Patients in an SNF are less likely to be discharged home and more likely to transition during their stay to long-term residents in that facility.
4. An IRF is more likely to have hospital-level resources on site such as laboratories, a pharmacy, or radiology rather than pharmacy and laboratory contracts, and portable x-ray machinery typical of most SNFs.
5. SNFs typically have a limited amount of space and equipment dedicated to rehabilitation therapies in contrast to more spacious and well equipped gyms seen in IRF.
6. SNFs are not as able to respond quickly to changes in a patient's medical status as are IRFs where highly skilled licensed professionals are always available.
7. IRFs have greater degrees of standardization of their rehabilitation programs and activities than SNFs due to licensing requirements.
8. Outcome measurements differ between the 2 care settings, with IRFs using IRF-PAI (patient assessment instrument) along with access to aggregated local, regional, and national data to manage their programs. SAR in SNF collect similar data but usually lack the sophisticated program evaluation tools.

Cost-effectiveness of care in subacute rehabilitation programs is still controversial. Comparative analyses between the 2 settings are difficult and must take into account both the direct costs as well as indirect subsequent costs such as hospital readmissions due to suboptimal medical stability. Some feel that much of the care provided in IRFs can be equally provided in SNFs; however, no accurate data exist to support such a policy.

In fact, a number of studies have suggested that for certain diagnoses, subacute care increases relative costs, lessens likelihood of discharge home, and increases risk of poor outcome and rehospitalization. Even though costs are considerably low on a daily basis in SNFs, the evidence comparing health outcomes is mixed [1,6-9]. Comprehensive stroke rehabilitation in IRFs has been shown to improve functional outcomes with a higher rate of return to community patients compared with patients treated at an SNF. Similarly, stroke patients discharged to SNFs had a higher mortality rate than that of patients referred to home health or IRF [10]. Outcomes for patients following orthopedic procedures are less clear, with no difference found in recovery of activities of daily living or return to community for patients with hip fracture treated in subacute SNFs compared with IRFs. However, others found that hip fracture patients experienced the most functional improvement when discharged to an IRF compared with SNF or home care and had significantly shorter lengths of stay [11]. The broad field of physical medicine and rehabilitation could benefit by more health services and outcomes research initiatives in this area.

It is important to consider that when patients are discharged either from acute medical or surgical services or from IRF/U to subacute or longer term nursing facilities, admission or readmission to hospital level rehabilitation may be indicated when or if clinical circumstances improve. For example, a transfer back to an IRF from an SNF program may be relevant for patients who need to gain strength and endurance before undertaking more complex and intensive rehabilitation (3 h/d).

A. Positive answers would support a comprehensive integrated inpatient rehabilitation program

1. Is the functional loss significant?

2. Does the patient have the ability or willingness to participate in multiple therapies per day?

3. Would the amount of achievable improvement likely alter postdischarge independence, improve safety, or decrease secondary complications?

4. Do support services exist to facilitate eventual community discharge or would functional improvement materially benefit the patient in a subsequent institutional setting (ie, SNF or NH)?

5. Are acute medical problems sufficiently controlled to allow primary focus on and involvement in the rehabilitation program?

B. Negative answers would support a subacute rehabilitation program (SNF)

1. Does the patient require rehabilitation nursing and/or more frequent or more accessible medical oversight than nonhospital level of rehab can provide?

2. Does the patient require multiple therapies coordinated within a common treatment plan, frequently reviewed and revised based on multidisciplinary input?

3. Is there need for cross-disciplinary reinforcement of therapies?

4. Does the rate of change of the patient's condition require frequent reevaluation/adjustment of the medical and rehabilitation care plan?

5. Would the time course for the achievement of goals be significantly affected by level of care chosen?

6. Is there a requirement for specialized equipment or assistive devices in the training or education program?

7. Will greater than 3 hours of therapy per day achieve goals more effectively than less than 3 hours daily?

8. Do behavioral health or psychological needs require regular assessment and treatment?

## ■ SUMMARY

The theme of this article is "Nursing Home Care and Subacute Rehabilitation". This article compares the differences between subacute rehabilitation patients sent to skilled nursing facilities (SNFs) between subacute rehabilitation patients sent to inpatient rehabilitation facilities or units (IRF/U) who are unable to return home after acute hospitalization. The author suggests that, compared to SNFs, IRF/U have a higher likelihood of providing better treatment outcomes for some subacute rehabilitation patients. However, due to evolving regulatory by insurance agencies, many patients are unable to be accurately placed in the appropriate level of rehabilitative care. Nevertheless, rehabilitation professionals (treating physical or occupational therapist, the attending physician) should make every effort to ensure that patients are placed in the appropriate treatment environment at the appropriate time to ensure medically justifiable placements and adequate reimbursement.

## ■ IMPORTANT TERMINOLOGY

nursing home care　养老院护理

subacute rehabilitation　亚急性康复

skilled nursing facility　专业护理机构

inpatient rehabilitation facility or unit　住院康复机构或部门

centers of medicare and medicaid services　医疗保险和医疗补助中心

long-term acute-care hospital　长期急性护理医院

## ■ REVIEW QUESTIONS

1.  What is subacute rehabilitation, and what type of patients is it best suited for?
2.  Why are patients sometimes sent to SNFs instead of IRF/U after an acute hospitalization?
3.  How do IRF and SAR/SNF levels of care differ from each other?
4.  Is cost-effectiveness of care in subacute rehabilitation programs still a controversy? If so, what are the direct and indirect subsequent costs?
5.  When is it appropriate to transfer a patient back to an IRF from an SNF program?

## ■ REFERENCES

1.  Walsh MB, Herbold J. Outcome after rehabilitation for total joint replacement at IRF and SNF: a case-controlled comparison. Am J of Phys Med Rehab. 2006;85(1):1-5.
2.  Gans B. There is a difference: distinguishing between IRH/U and SNF rehabilitation. Focus on Rehabilitation, Summer 2008;7(2):6.
3.  Centers for Medicare & Medicaid Services. Proposed Rule: Medicare: Inpatient rehabilitation facility prospective payment system (2008 FY); update [07-2241]. Fed Regist. 26230-26279.
4.  Zollar C. CMS publishes long-term care prospective payment system. AMRPA Magazine. 2002;5(7):37-42.
5.  Seneff MG, Wagner D, Thompson D, et al. The impact of long-term acutecare facilities on the outcome and cost of care for patients undergoing prolonged mechanical ventilation. Crit Care Med. February 2000;28(2):342-350.
6.  Prvu Bettger JA, Stineman MG. Effectiveness of multidisciplinary rehabilitation services in postacute care: State-of-the-science. A review. Arch Phys Med Rehabil. 2007;88:1526-1534.
7.  Deutsch A, et al. Outcomes and reimbursement of inpatient rehabilitation facilities and subacute rehabilitation programs for Medicare beneficiaries with hip fracture. Med Care. 2005;43:892-901.
8.  Deutsch A, et al. Poststroke rehabilitation: Outcomes and reimbursement of inpatient rehabilitation facilities and subacute rehabilitation programs. Stroke. 2006;37:1477-1482.
9.  Kane RL. Assessing the effectiveness of postacute care rehabilitation. Arch Phys Med Rehabil. 2007;88:1500-1504.

10. Kane R, Chen Q, Finch M, et al. Functional outcomes of posthospital care for stroke and hip fracture patients under Medicare. J Am Geriatr Soc. December 1998;46:1525-1533.
11. Munin M, Seligman K, Dew M, et al. Effect of rehabilitation site on functional recovery after hip fracture. Arch Phys Med Rehabil. 2005;86:367-372.

（王于领）

# PHYSICAL THERAPY

## ■ WHAT IS PHYSICAL THERAPY?

Physical therapy is a branch of rehabilitation medicine aiming at helping patients maintain, recover, or improve their physical abilities. including the treatment of any pain, disease, or injury by physical means. According to the Chartered Society of Physiotherapy (CSP), physical therapy is science-based, committed to extending, applying, evaluating, and reviewing the evidence that underpins and informs its practice and delivery. The exercise of clinical judgment and informed interpretation is at its core.

## ■ WHAT IS A PHYSICAL THERAPIST?

A physical therapist (PT) specializes in the evaluation and treatment of patients with functional limitations, impairments, and disabilities. Since 2002, all PT programs in the USA have been accredited at a master's degree level; moreover, the Commission on Accreditation in Physical Therapy Education (CAPTE) has mandated all these PT programs to offer the doctor of physical therapy (DPT) degree effective since December 31, 2015. The American Physical Therapy Association (APTA) reports that 96% of the professional PT programs already offer the DPT degree, as of February 2010. Moreover, the DPT is a clinical doctorate which augments the master of physical therapy (MPT) degree with continued training in differential diagnosis, pharmacology, radiology/imaging, and evidence-based practice. The DPT appeared to emerge concomitantly with the need for direct access to physical therapy without a physician referral. The rationale for direct access is for patients to receive more timely treatment while decreasing healthcare costs. The expectation is for the PT to refer to a physician when the patient's condition is outside the scope of PT practice.

In the USA, a physical therapist assistant (PTA) works under the direction and supervision of a licensed PT. The PTA provides select treatment interventions for the patient, collects data relevant to the treatment, and modifies select interventions to ensure patient safety or to progress the patient as directed by the PT. They must earn an associate degree from an accredited program. A passing score on a national examination is required for licensure for both PTs and PTAs in most states.

In April of 1983, the Chinese Rehabilitation on Medicine Research Society was formally established and then renamed the Chinese Association for Rehabilitation Medicine in 1988. At the beginning of the 1990s, some secondary specialized schools set up rehabilitation treatment education to alleviate the shortage of rehabilitation personnel; in 1989, Shanghai University of Sport began to recruit undergraduates in "sports health care and rehabilitation specialty" (then renamed "kinesiology"), authorized by the former State Education Commission. The students in this program were mainly allocated to the general hospital. In 2001, the Ministry of Education of the People's Republic of China formally added "rehabilitation treatment" into the formal academic education and classified it as a medical-related professional category. In the same year, Nanjing Medical

University began to recruit undergraduates in "rehabilitation treatment" first. Since then, an increasing number of colleges and universities have begun to set up this program. Students finishing 4 years of undergraduate courses will be awarded a bachelor of science; others finishing 3 years of systematic courses for rehabilitation treatment will get an Associate Degree. A physical therapist must pass the national certification examination administered by the National Health Commission of the People's Republic of China to get the PT qualifications.

In China, physical therapy was much more advanced compared with other subspecialties (such as occupational therapy, speech therapy, etc.). So far, in most Chinese universities, rehabilitation treatment education has been based on physical therapy. The physical therapy program in four universities (Kunming Medical University, West China Medical Center of Sichuan University, Fujian University of Traditional Chinese Medicine, and Shanghai University of Traditional Chinese Medicine) has been internationally certified by the World Confederation for Physical Therapy (WCPT). On the other hand, master's degrees related to rehabilitation medicine and therapy have been greatly improved in recent years, including the master of rehabilitation treatment, master of rehabilitation medicine, master of sport medicine, and master of kinesiology. Furthermore, PhDs co-supervised by West China Medical Center of Sichuan University and the Hong Kong Polytechnic University can be awarded doctoral degrees for physical therapy, occupational therapy, or orthopedic prosthetics.

## ■ WHERE DO PHYSICAL THERAPISTS PRACTICE?

Physical therapists practice in a variety of settings, working with patients that span age ranges from the neonate to the elderly. They may work in acute care hospitals; acute, sub-acute, or day rehabilitation centers; skilled nursing facilities; or outpatient facilities to name a few. The American Board of Physical Therapy Specialties (ABPTS) recognizes board-certified specialists in the following areas: cardiovascular and pulmonary, clinical electrophysiology, geriatrics, neurology, orthopedics, pediatrics, sports, and women's health physical therapy.

## ■ WHAT TYPES OF DISORDERS ARE APPROPRIATE FOR REFERRALS?

Physical therapists work with a wide variety of diagnoses which vary based upon the setting and area of specialty. Broadly speaking, physical therapists work with impairments involving the neuromuscular, musculoskeletal, integumentary, and cardiovascular/pulmonary systems. Examples of PT problems appropriate for referral are grouped by system and listed below. This list is adapted from the APTA's *Guide to Physical Therapist Practice*.

### Neuromuscular

    Impaired motor control
    Impaired neuro-motor development
    Impaired balance and coordination
    Compensatory movement strategies
    Gait deviations

### Musculoskeletal

    Postural alignment deviations

Impaired functional mobility (ie, bed mobility, transfers, ambulation, stair climbing, etc.)

Decreased joint mobility/range of motion(ROM)

Decreased strength

Decreased agility (ie, pivoting, running, jumping, climbing, etc.)

## Integumentary

Impaired integumentary integrity associated with superficial, partial thickness, and/or full-thickness skin involvement

## Cardiovascular/Pulmonary

Decreased endurance

Deconditioning

Impaired ventilation

Decreased ribcage or thoracic spine mobility

The interventional modalities used in physical therapy can be described as "3M", including physical modality therapy, manipulation therapy, and movement therapy [1]. Briefly speaking, physical therapists can use ultrasound, hot packs, cold compression, and electrical stimulation to reduce turgidity; and use traction and deep-tissue massage to relieve pain and improve flexibility and circulation. On the other hand, they may use prostheses crutches, wheelchairs, and other adaptive devices to improve mobility and dexterity, and they offer patients guidance in ways to use them.

## ■ PHYSICAL THERAPY ASSESSMENT AND TREATMENT

The *Guide to Physical Therapist Practice* describes the approach to patient management as follows: examination, evaluation, diagnosis, prognosis, and intervention PT examination begins by obtaining a detailed history from the patient followed by a systems review. It is important to assess the impact of the patient's medical history on his or her function [2]. The systems review may indicate a need for a referral to a physician or other health care provider. If the patient's medical condition is well managed and it is safe to continue the PT assessment, the PT will evaluate the patient, performing objective tests and measures to identify areas of functional limitations, and make clinical judgments based on the data gathered during the exam. The PT diagnoses the PT problems and prioritizes them based on the systems involved and the severity of limitation. A prognosis is made by determining the maximal level of function the patient may expect to attain and the time frame involved in completing this task [3]. PT intervention is then implemented accordingly.

In China, patients referring to physical therapy are often divided into outpatients (including referral) and inpatients (including consultation). For in- and out-patients, careful inquiry of history, the corresponding physical examination, laboratory examination, and imaging examination are necessary. Specialist doctors should make a clear and definite diagnosis, define the goals and requirements of the rehabilitation treatment or physiotherapy, and write the records of the determined rehabilitation programs. For patients who may be inappropriate for physiotherapy, promptly transferring to the relevant departments is necessary.

For a referral from other departments, clinical doctors should confirm that physiotherapy is necessary for the patient's recovery with the diagnosis and referral requirements written in the medical records. They also need to instruct the out-patient to register in the department of rehabilitation medicine. After physical examination and evaluation, determined treatment goals and plans should be defined by specialist doctors. Physical therapists then received a schedule for the physical intervention, which may consist of "3M". After necessary function assessments, the specific treatment will be implemented with corresponding records every time. Specialist physicians should check the progress of ongoing patients regularly; evaluate the treatment effects and define changes in the disease, modify the treatment plan, and review the specialist medical records. At the end of treatment, a brief summary is also needed.

## GOALS

PT treatment goals differ based upon the patient setting. It is important to discuss the patient's and/or family's goals for the patient's functional mobility so that they are incorporated into the PT goals appropriately.

### Inpatient

Inpatient PT goals focus on patient and family education as well as safe mobility to promote a safe discharge home. It is not necessarily to return to the prior level of function. The patient may require follow-up with inpatient rehabilitation or outpatient physical therapy to accomplish the goal of returning to the maximal level of function. Safe mobility may include bed mobility, transfers, ambulation, and stair climbing and involves education of the patient's caretakers if the patient requires assistance to complete a task. If the patient has stairs at home, it is important that the patient is able to perform stair climbing prior to his/her discharge home to promote safety in the home environment.

### Outpatient

The focus of outpatient PT is to habilitate the patient to achieve developmental skills previously unattained, or to rehabilitate the patient to return to his/her maximal level of function. This may include a return to sports in the athlete's case.

### Things to consider when writing an order for PT

- Prescriptions need to include diagnosis/reason for referral.
- Prescriptions need to include detailed descriptions, such as the type, frequency, time, and intensity for each chosen method.
- If indicated, identify ROM or weight-bearing restrictions—be as specific as possible.
- If weight bearing or ROM restrictions are to be placed, specifically state the length of time restrictions are to be maintained or the criteria for lifting or progressing the restrictions.
- If indicated, specify cardiac precautions or vital sign parameters.
- If indicated, note any positioning restrictions, including possible bracing needs.

Prescriptions are individualized. Please add or delete information as appropriate to meet the needs of each patient.

## ■ THE INDICATIONS AND CONTRAINDICATIONS OF DIFFERENT PHYSICAL THERAPY

Movement therapy is a rehabilitation treatment method that primarily uses functional training as a means of recovery, improvement, or reconstruction of bodily functions using both techniques and tools (apparatus). The indications and contraindications for movement therapy are as follows:

Indications: It can be used for muscle, connective tissue, and skin shortening, joint motion range reduction caused by soft tissue contraction, adhesion, or scar formation.

Contraindications: Inflammation of joint intra-articular or periarticular tissues, such as tuberculosis, infection, especially in the acute phase; recent fractures, muscle and ligament injuries; hematoma or other trauma within the tissue; severe osteoporosis; joint pain or muscle tension when stretched acutely after nerve injury or nerve anastomosis surgery within one month.

## Modality therapy

Modality therapy is the use of various physical methods such as electrotherapy, magnetic therapy, heat therapy, light therapy, and cryotherapy to treat patients. This therapy method can be used for many diseases, and the specific indications and contraindications are as follows:

Indications: Various acute and chronic pains, as well as diseases of the musculoskeletal system and nervous system.

Contraindications: Non-healing fractures, dislocations or tumors of joints, active infections; electrotherapy and magnetic therapy are contraindicated in patients with pacemaker implants; light therapy is contraindicated in photosensitive diseases.

## Manual therapy

Manual therapy refers to the use of hands-on therapy techniques such as massage, manipulation, traction, etc. by the physician. Manual therapy is mainly used for diseases of the musculoskeletal system, and the specific indications and contraindications are as follows:

Indications: Joint dysfunction caused by mechanical factors (non-neural), including joint pain, muscle tension, and spasms; joint motion reduction caused by immobilization; progressive joint movement limitation. Joint mobilization techniques play a major role in maintaining the existing range of motion, delaying disease progression, and preventing other adverse effects caused by inactivity.

Contraindications: Joint excessive motion, joint swelling (increased exudation), inflammation caused by trauma or disease, as well as malignant diseases and non-healing fractures

## ■ SUMMARY

A physical therapist (PT) specializes in the evaluation and treatment of patients with functional limitations, impairments, and disabilities. They work with patients from the neonate to the elderly in a variety of settings. A physical therapist works with impairments involving the neuromuscular, musculoskeletal, integumentary, and cardiovascular/pulmonary systems. The PT approaches to patient management including examination, evaluation, diagnosis, prognosis, and intervention, and PT treatment engagements differ based upon the patient setting.

## ■ IMPORTANT TERMINOLOGY

physical therapy  物理治疗
physical therapist  物理治疗师
doctor of physical therapy  物理治疗博士
master of physical therapy  物理治疗硕士
physical therapist assistant  助理物理治疗师
rehabilitation treatment  康复治疗
occupational therapy  作业治疗
speech therapy  言语治疗

orthopedic prosthetic   假肢矫形
movement therapy   运动治疗
manipulation therapy   手法治疗
physical modality therapy   物理因子治疗

## ■ REVIEW QUESTIONS

1. What is physical therapy?
2. What kind of settings does PT practice in?
3. What types of disorders are appropriate for referrals?
4. What does the "3M" mean in physical therapy?
5. What should be considered in an order for PT?

## ■ REFERENCES

1. Huang Xiaolin, Yan Tiebin. Rehabilitation Medicine. fifth edition. People's Medical Publishing House. 2013;35(35):98-99.
2. Massery, Mary. Advanced Pulmonary Course, 2010. Unpublished.
3. Guide to physical therapist practice. Phys Ther 1995;75(8): 713-716. 3.

（杜　青）

# OCCUPATIONAL THERAPY

## ■ WHAT IS OCCUPATIONAL THERAPY?

In 2012, the World Federation of Occupational Therapists (WFOT) defined "occupational therapy" as a client-centered health profession concerned with promoting health and well-being through occupation. The primary goal of occupational therapy is to enable people to participate in the activities of everyday life. Occupational therapists achieve this outcome by working with people and communities to enhance their ability to engage in the occupations they want to, need to, or are expected to do, or by modifying the occupation or the environment to better support their occupational goals.

According to the definition, occupational therapy is a specialty that (1) must be carried out with the guidance of certificated occupational therapists; (2) is based on the occupational activity; (3) aims to recover the ability to carry out the occupational activity; (4) emphasizes the patients' willingness in participating the treatments; (5) focuses on using the modified environment to ameliorate patients' disability or dysfunction[1].

## ■ WHAT IS AN OCCUPATIONAL THERAPIST?

Occupational therapists (OTs) are professionals who assess, treat, and educate individuals who have difficulties with the skills of everyday living including, but not limited to, self-care skills, fine motor skills, visual motor skills, social interactions, and sensory processing. In the USA, an OT must graduate from a program that is accredited by the US Accreditation Council for Occupational Therapy Education (ACOTE), complete a minimum of 24 weeks of clinical training, and sit for the national certification examination administered by the National Board for Certification in Occupational Therapy (NBCOT) of the US to use the OTR title. Most states also require state licensure, which may or may not include passing a test, and most states require ongoing professional continuing education. What's more, Occupational Therapy programs in America are Master's or Doctorate degree level programs; both may be entry-level or post-professional.

Furthermore, in the USA, an occupational therapy assistant (OTA) is a professional who works under the supervision of an OT to assist in the treatment of a patient. The OTA must graduate from a program that is accredited by ACOTE, complete a minimum of 16 weeks of clinical training, and sit for the national certification examination administered by NBCOT. Passing the certification exam allows the professional to use the COTA title. OTA programs consist of a 2-year associate's degree or a 1-year certificate from an accredited college or technical school. Most states also require state licensure which may or may not include passing a test, and most states require ongoing professional continuing education.

In October 1988, with the establishment of the Chinese Rehabilitation Research Center, occupational therapy was defined as a branch of rehabilitation treatment; and the occupational therapy education was performed as a sub-program of rehabilitation treatment education. So far, on the Chinese mainland, the occupational therapy program in two universities (West China Medical Center of Sichuan University and Shanghai University of Traditional Chinese Medicine) have been internationally certified by World Confederation for Occupational Therapy (WCOT).

## ■ WHERE DO OCCUPATIONAL THERAPISTS PRACTICE?

By the end of 2009, there were 107 000 OT jobs in the USA. The skills of an OT can be applied in a variety of areas including, but not limited to, acute care, inpatient rehabilitation, subacute rehabilitation, skilled nursing facility, day rehabilitation, mental health units and hospitals, schools, and a variety of outpatient settings. Each setting provides a distinct level of care, thus requiring a different intensity and purpose of therapy. As mentioned above, various settings may require a specialty level of training for the therapist. Occupational therapy consists of the following six sections: 1) functional OT which is defined as training for activities of daily living (ADL) including basic ADL and instrumental ADL; 2) vocational OT including pre-vocational evaluation, pre-vocational training, and vocational training; 3) entertainment activities including evaluation as well as treatment of play and recreation; 4) environmental intervention which means alleviating the dysfunction by improving the environment; 5) assistive technology; 6) OT consultation and education [1].

### The following are examples of the role an OT plays in various settings

**Neonatal Intensive Care Unit (NICU):** Work with parents, caregivers, and hospital staff to position the infant to promote typical movement patterns while limiting atypical patterns from developing, encouraging developmentally appropriate stimulus to foster typical development while promoting a sensory sensitive environment, and in some NICUs working on feeding skills. Please be aware that the roles of OT, physical therapy (PT), and speech-language pathology (SLP) in this environment may vary slightly. Specific skills such as feeding may be addressed by different disciplines in a particular unit. Inquiring about the discipline performing specific training in a particular unit might be necessary.

**Acute Care Hospital (for adults):** Work with patients and caregivers to promote the return to independence in everyday skills such as dressing, bathing, grooming, and eating. This includes working on strength and endurance tasks, muscle reeducation, and task modifications including the use of adaptive equipment as appropriate. The focus is to prepare the patient for return to home with possible referral to outpatient therapy or to prepare for a transfer to a rehabilitation unit or hospital for maximal recovery.

**Pediatrics:** Work with the children and their caregivers to promote age-appropriate skills in the areas of self-care (dressing, bathing, grooming, eating, etc.), play, and visual motor skills. As in the adult population, OT in acute care is to prepare for the next level of care whether it is return to home or to a more intensive therapy program.

It is not a standard practice to refer for rehabilitation services in an acute care setting to "continue" OT if the adult or child has been receiving outpatient services and is admitted for an acute medical issue (ie, a child with C.P. admitted for respiratory infection who receives outpatient OT does not need OT in the acute setting because she/he is missing their outpatient appointment or parent is requesting OT to continue). It would be appropriate if the acute care admission resulted in a change of functional status and the patient needed OT to teach/train the caregivers and/or patient strengthening exercises or adaptive techniques to return to the prior level of function.

**Rehabilitation Settings (unit in Acute Care Hospital or Rehab hospital):** This is an intensive, therapy-focused environment. Depending on state and federal regulations, there is a daily minimum of therapy hours a patient must participate in to be in this setting. The hours are typically divided amongst OT, PT, SLP, and possibly psychology services. The OT's role in this environment is functional independence. This means the goal is for the patient to return to an age-appropriate level of functioning. For adults, they will be able to complete their self-care skills (dressing, bathing, grooming, toileting, eating, and transfers), as well as participate in job-related activities and leisure activities safely and independently (with possible modifications and/or equipment use) as possible. With the ever-changing regulations, more rehabilitation programs are restricted on admission days based on diagnosis and progress with therapy. Patients who are unable to meet their goals of independence can transition to either subacute or outpatient settings.

**Subacute Care:** OTs work with patients whose progress is at a slower pace than allowable on a rehabilitation unit. In this environment, the OT's focus is consistent with that of a rehabilitation unit, but the goals are typically lower levels of functional outcome.

**Outpatient Settings:** There are a variety of outpatient settings including outpatient rehab clinics, schools, home health, hand clinics, and day rehab centers. The general role of the OT in these settings is to foster age-appropriate functional skills.

For adults, it is typically an exercise program to work on strength and endurance, muscle reeducation with possible use of modalities to assist the return of muscle strength, return to work programs (ergonomics, work simplification, joint protection), and higher level self-care skills (ie, cooking, laundry, balancing a checkbook, community reentry, and in some cases, driving). In some but not all clinics, it is the OT's role to do splinting as well.

For pediatrics, it can be an exercise program to work on strength and endurance, upper extremity muscle reeducation or muscle activation, promotion of typical patterns of movement, promotion of typical development and typical patterns of development, fine motor skill development (eg, handwriting skills, shoe tying, and other fasteners, manipulation skills), eye-hand coordination skills, visual motor skills, and self-care skills. In some clinics, the OT will work on feeding, while in other clinics the speech therapist will work on feeding, and there are even some clinics where there is a combined OT and speech domain to work on feeding skills. There are also therapists trained in the area of sensory processing dysfunction (also known as sensory integration or SI). There are some clinics devoted solely to this population.

# ■ WHEN IS IT APPROPRIATE TO REFER TO OCCUPATIONAL

It is appropriate to refer to occupational therapy when the patient demonstrates a decline in baseline function that impacts his or her level of independence with everyday skills. This decline in function or loss of skill may be a result of an injury (neurological or orthopedic), a progressive disease (eg, arthritis, multiple sclerosis, Alzheimer's disease), or an acute medical process such as cancer. It is also appropriate to refer to occupational therapy to focus on the acquisition of skills that were either not present or dysfunctional from birth. This is most common in the pediatric population for conditions such as developmental delays, cerebral palsy, spina bifida (multiple myeloma), sensory processing dysfunction, visual impairments, and birth injuries (eg, brachial plexus injuries, hypoxic-ischemic encephalopathy).

It is important to note that each state has its own requirements for a proper referral to occupational therapy. There are some states that have no specific requirements while others mandate a prescription from an authorized referral source such as a medical doctor, psychologist or psychiatrist, a dentist, an optometrist, or a podiatrist.

## Things to Consider When Writing an Order for OT

■ Occupational therapy and physical therapy are 2 separate disciplines that often work in tandem, however, require separate orders.

- Include diagnosis/reason for referral.
- If indicated, identify range of motion or weight-bearing restrictions.
- If indicated, specify cardiac precautions or vital sign parameters.
- If indicated, note any positioning restrictions, including possible bracing needs.

## WHEN IS A PATIENT DISCHARGED FROM OT?

There are several reasons for discharge. The most positive outcome is discharge because all goals are met. Other reasons for discharge include a plateau in recovery (no longer making progress), lack of compliance, lack of attendance in treatment, patient choosing to end services, and transition of services from one setting to another (eg, receiving outpatient services and qualifying to receive school-based services or transfer from acute to rehab). It is important to understand why a patient is being discharged from occupational therapy services, no matter what the setting.

### Examples of appropriate re-consult

- A patient was discharged from OT in an acute care setting but before hospital discharge and, while admitted, their functional status changes.
- If the patient is discharged from outpatient OT because all goals were met and it is determined during a follow-up appointment with a physician that there are more functional limitations or new functional limitations to be addressed.

### Examples of inappropriate re-consult:

- A patient was discharged from OT in an acute care setting after the patient and/or caregivers have been instructed on a home exercise program to help maintain his/her level of function during the patient's hospitalization, and the patient's level of function has not changed.
- If the patient is discharged from OT from an outpatient setting secondary to lack of progress or lack of participation (unless a significant change improves participation and likelihood of improvement. For example, weight-bearing restrictions are lifted).

## WHAT HAPPENS ONCE AN OT REFERRAL IS PLACED?

Inpatient: Once an order is received, the OT will do a chart review and call a member of the medical team to clarify any orders or precautions as needed. It is very helpful for precautions to be written on the prescription to forego any delays in the initiation of services. Once the chart review is complete, the OT will meet with the patient and begin the evaluation process. Once the evaluation is complete, the therapist will write a report and place it in the medical chart (pending the setting, it may be an electronic or paper chart). The therapist will include a plan of care, recommended frequency, possible consult recommendations, and possible discharge planning recommendations. The OT or OTA will then initiate the treatment plan as outlined in the evaluation report.

Outpatient: This prescription may be handed to the patient and/or caregiver to provide to the OT at the evaluation, or in some cases, may be entered into the electronic medical record for the OT to view at the evaluation if in the same facility. Whenever possible, the therapist will do a chart review prior to the evaluation. If no records are available to the therapist, the beginning of the evaluation will consist of an interview with the patient and/or caregiver to determine the history and progress. If there is insufficient information obtained during this interview process, the OT may stop the evaluation process and call a member of the patient's medical team to obtain any necessary medical information. Once the evaluation is complete, the therapist will then write up an evaluation report including evaluation findings, plan of care, and recommendations. Pending on the setting, the OT may send a summary of their findings, a full report, or a notification that a report is available to the referring physician.

## WHAT IS THE FREQUENCY OF OT?

Frequencies are determined by a variety of factors. There are some physicians who prefer to prescribe a certain number of visits, while other physicians allow the therapist to use their best discretion. The frequency is also, often times now, dictated by insurance. There may be protocols based on diagnosis or it may be from evidence-based practice recommendations. This is a good opportunity to talk with the OT to determine the best plan of care.

## METHODS OF OCCUPATIONAL THERAPY

Occupational therapy (OT) is a type of therapy that helps individuals with physical, mental, or cognitive disabilities to engage in daily activities and live more independently. There are several methods that occupational therapists use to help their patients:

**Activities of daily living (ADL) training:** This includes teaching patients the skills needed for basic tasks such as eating, grooming, bathing, and dressing.

**Instrumental activities of daily living (IADL) training:** This includes teaching patients how to perform more complex tasks such as cooking, cleaning, and managing finances.

**Assistive technology:** Occupational therapists may use specialized equipment such as wheelchairs, prosthetics, or communication devices to help patients carry out tasks they may not otherwise be able to do.

**Sensory integration therapy:** This approach is used to help patients with sensory processing difficulties by exposing them to different types of sensory stimuli in a controlled environment.

**Cognitive rehabilitation:** This involves exercises and activities designed to help patients improve their memory, attention, and problem-solving skills.

**Work-related therapy:** This involves helping patients return to work or find new employment after an injury or illness.

**Environmental modifications:** Occupational therapists can make recommendations for modifications to a patient's home or workplace to make it safer and more accessible.

The goal of occupational therapy is to help patients achieve greater independence and participate more fully in all aspects of their lives.

## SUMMARY

Occupational therapy provides support for people with health problems which set obstacles to their daily activities, such as dressing or getting to the shops and occupational therapists provide practical guidance for them. An OT should help people maintain, regain, or improve their independence by using different techniques and changing their environment with advanced types of equipment. He or she practices in a variety of settings, working with patients from the neonate to the elderly. It is appropriate to refer to occupational therapy when one shows a decline in baseline function which impacts his or her level of independence with everyday skills.

## ■ IMPORTANT TERMINOLOGY

occupational therapy    作业治疗

occupational therapist    作业治疗师

occupational therapist assistant    助理作业治疗师

rehabilitation treatment    康复治疗

functional OT    功能性作业治疗

Activities of Daily Living (ADL)    日常生活活动

basic ADL    基本日常生活活动

instrumental ADL    工具性日常生活活动

vocational OT    职业作业治疗

pre-vocational evaluation    就业前评定

pre-vocational training    就业前训练

vocational training    职业训练

evaluation of play and recreation    娱乐及游戏活动评定

treatment of play and recreation    娱乐及游戏活动治疗

environment intervention    环境干预

assistive technology    辅助技术

## ■ REVIEW QUESTIONS

1. What is the definition of occupational therapy and occupational therapist?
2. What kind of settings does OT practice in?
3. What does the occupational therapy contain?
4. What is needed to be considered in an order for OT?

## ■ REFERENCES

1. Huang Xiaolin, Yan Tiebin. Rehabilitation Medicine. fifth edition. People's Medical Publishing House. 2013; 35(35):123-124.

（杜　青）

# SPEECH-LANGUAGE PATHOLOGY

## ■ WHAT IS SPEECH-LANGUAGE PATHOLOGY

Speech-language pathology (SLP), also known as speech therapy (ST) in China, is one of the key professions under the umbrella of rehabilitation medicine. It is a profession involving assessment, treatment and research of various language/speech and communication disorders.

## ■ WHAT IS A SPEECH-LANGUAGE PATHOLOGIST?

Speech-language pathologists, or SLPs, are professionals who assess, diagnose, and treat individuals who have speech-language, voice, and swallowing disorders. At a minimum, SLPs have a Master's degree in communication disorders, a clinical fellowship following graduate school, and pass a national certification examination administered by the Educational Testing Service. Satisfactory completion of these 3 steps will earn an SLP the Certificate of Clinical Competence in Speech-Language Pathology (CCC-SLP) granted by the American Speech-Language Hearing Association (ASHA), the professional, scientific, and credentialing organization for audiologists, speech-language pathologists, and speech-language and hearing scientists. Earned credit through continuing education activities, combined with annual membership dues, will maintain this certification. Additionally, SLPs may be required to have state licensure, a requisite of which is ASHA certification.

Currently, people who want to work as speech-language pathologists in clinical settings, need to complete the national certification of rehabilitation therapists. Meanwhile, people who provide speech/language services in special education settings usually only hold a teacher certification.

## ■ IN WHAT SETTINGS DO SPEECH-LANGUAGE PATHOLOGISTS WORK?

By the end of 2009, there were over 120 700 ASHA-certified SLPs. With the capability of assessing, diagnosing, and treating patients from birth through senescence, SLPs may be found to work with any patient who is experiencing or is suspected to have communication and/or swallowing difficulties. Patients will range from children with developmental delays to adults who are intubated requiring mechanical ventilation, and to individuals who have stroke, progressive disease, and/or head and neck cancer. SLP professionals can be found in various settings, including public and private schools, private practice clinics, hospitals, rehabilitation facilities, extended care facilities/nursing homes, community clinics, and academic departments. You may also see SLPs conducting research in any of the above-named settings.

# ■ WHAT TYPES OF DISORDERS ARE APPROPRIATE FOR REFERRALS?

The types of disorders SLPs treat vary depending on the age of the patient and the nature of the disorder. SLPs habilitate, or treat patients to develop skills that were either not present or dysfunctional from birth. Likewise, SLPs also rehabilitate, or treat patients who have lost function in speech, language, voice, and swallowing as a result of a neurological injury (eg, stroke, traumatic brain injury), progressive disease (eg, Parkinson's disease, multiple sclerosis), orofacial and myofunctional disorders (eg, cleft lip/palate, tongue thrust), or head and neck cancer.

Within each of the broad classifications of communication and swallowing disorders are many types of dysfunction. It is important to characterize and distinguish the types of disorders within each of these classifications for a more complete understanding. Following are brief explanations for common disorders.

# ■ SPEECH DISORDERS

## Apraxia of Speech/Verbal Apraxia

This is a motor speech disorder affecting the planning for speech acts. A person with apraxia of speech fails to consistently execute speech correctly, due to problems unrelated to muscle weakness and changes in reflexes. This speech disorder is independent of movement, sensation, or language deficits. The primary characteristic is the inability to transition within and between segments of sounds resulting in extended durations of consonants and vowels. Distortions are perceived as sound substitutions and stress changes that may be changed within words, phrases, and sentences, with consistency of location within utterances and invariable in type.

## Articulation/Phonological Processes

These disorders are generally associated with young children; however, they are frequently seen in persons with aphasia and some degenerative diseases. They manifest themselves as difficulty in correctly producing specific sounds (eg, sound omissions, lisps), or sound patterns (eg, substituting "t" for "k," a process called "fronting" in which sounds made in the back of the mouth are made in the front of the mouth).

## Dysarthria

A muscular weakness and dyscoordination that results in reduced clarity of sounds, breaks in pitch, changes in nasality/voice resonance, alterations to the rhythm of speech, or disruption in the ability to produce air (ie, breathing) for voice. Often, dysarthria is described as slurred or slow speech that may be difficult to understand.

## Stuttering/Fluency

A disorder, in the absence of weakness, resulting in a disruption in the production of sounds. This problem can be characterized by repetition or prolongation of sounds, syllables, or words. Other disruptions may include an increase in word or sentence starters such as "umm. . ." or "uh. . .".

# ■ LANGUAGE DISORDERS

## Language-Based Learning Disabilities

These are disabilities specific to reading, writing, and spelling, having little to do with intelligence. Many language disorders are reflected in spoken and listening disorders as well as these literacy deficits. Dysfunctions in these areas may result in difficulties in reading or spoken comprehension (eg, following directions), expression of written thought, and writing letters/numbers (eg, naming).

## Aphasia

An acquired disorder from a neurological event that results in disordered uses of language in all of the following areas of language:(1) auditory comprehension, (2) reading comprehension, (3) spoken expression, and (4) written expression. Among the most common difficulties are reduced ability to follow conversation and directions (spoken or written), difficulty in identifying and/or naming objects, problems retrieving the correct words to express thought (spoken or written), and difficulty in coherent/cohesive writing.

## Right Hemisphere/Traumatic Brain Injury/Cognitive-Linguistic Impairments

This is an acquired communication disorder from stroke, brain injury, or progressive disease (eg, dementia) that may lead to any combination of impairments of memory, awareness/attention, visual-perceptual skills, problem solving/reasoning, thought organization, and use of language in social situations (ie, pragmatics).

## Voice And Voice Disorders

### Dysphonia

Simply stated, dysphonia involves an abnormality in the sound of the voice. Changes to the quality of voice (including resonance) may be the result of anatomical changes (eg, tracheotomy, laryngectomy, growths on the vocal folds such as nodules or polyps), neurological changes (eg, vocal fold paresis/paralysis), or other health issues affecting vocal fold tissue (eg, immunological issues). Sometimes, physical bases do not explain dysphonia, which is, instead, related to muscle use patterns. Examples of voice changes with dysphonia include hoarseness, "rough voice" and tremor or "shaky" voice.

### Resonance

This term addresses the quality of an individual's voice in terms of how the pharynx, nasal cavity, and oral cavity shape the sound vibrations produced by the vocal folds in the larynx. *Nasality* is a term used to describe, specifically, how the velum allows air to escape (or not) during speech. A hypernasal voice is one that sounds like someone is "talking through his/her nose" (ie, more air is escaping through the nose than normal). A hyponasal voice is one that sounds like someone is "all stopped up," a common quality of one's voice when someone has a cold.

### Intubation And Tracheostomy

Although a patient with a tracheostomy tube is not considered to have a voice disorder, a patient with a tracheostomy does require SLP services. These patients may be able to phonate (ie, produce voice) with the proper adjustments to these types of indwelling respiratory devices. In cases in which patients are not able to phonate, an SLP can assist with patient-to-caregiver communication by providing assistive devices.

### Laryngectomy

Patients with parts of the larynx or the entire larynx removed will need SLP services for potential voice and swallowing disorders. An SLP will provide pre- and post-operative assessment and counseling for voice and swallowing restoration, and the therapy required to improve the patient's functional outcomes in these domains. An SLP will assist in maximizing use of voice that may still remain or alternatively provide a different source for voice (ie, alaryngeal speech).

# ■ SWALLOWING DISORDERS

*Dysphagia* is the term used to refer to the symptom of difficulty related to swallowing (ie, "The patient complains of dysphagia.") and a patient's diagnosis of having a swallowing disorder. Many clinicians divide swallowing into 3 phases: (1) oral phase, (2) pharyngeal phase, and (3) esophageal phase. Although these phases serve the purpose of describing the location of the bolus of liquid or food, it is difficult to use "phases" to describe the precise location of the problem producing dysphagia. There is a large amount of overlap and interdependence between the different physiologic components of swallowing, thus, making it difficult to distinguish these phases. For purposes of explanation below, use of term "phases" refers to the location of the bolus.

## Feeding Disorders

This domain is an "adjunct" area for SLPs. Strictly speaking, feeding refers to how an individual functions to get food or drink "from the table to his/her mouth." Attention to the physical movements of this act are largely assessed and treated by an occupational therapist (OT). In concert with the OT, the SLP addresses cognitive-behavioral aspects of feeding. These aspects typically include reducing the amount of distractions during mealtimes (generally used with patients who have difficulties with focus/attention/concentration), the speed of feeding, the amount of food placed on the fork or spoon, the volume of drink ingested, and the manner of liquid transport (ie, spoon, cup, or straw).

## Oral Dysphagia

The oral phase can be subdivided into 2 functions: (1) oral preparatory phase and (2) oral propulsive phase. The manner in which the bolus is prepared for swallowing is highly dependent upon the type of food or liquid ingested. Liquids, for example, are not masticated.

During the oral preparatory phase, saliva is secreted, the bolus is manipulated (and masticated with solid food), and the food and/or drink mixed with saliva. This phase softens and lubricates solid boluses in preparation for transport from the oral cavity and through the pharynx and esophagus. Disorders in this phase may include difficulties with control and manipulation of the bolus, secretion of saliva, cleft lip/palate, and muscle strength for mastication.

During the oral propulsive phase, the now-prepared food and/or drink is placed on the blade of the tongue for transport posteriorly into the pharynx. Disorders in this phase may include difficulties with bolus control and with initiation of the propulsive sequence. The vocal folds close and breathing ceases during this phase in many individuals, this behavior often regarded as protective by clinicians and researchers. The cessation of breathing is in preparation for the movement of the bolus toward the pharynx, while the airway is still open and vulnerable to bolus entry.

## Pharyngeal Dysphagia

During the "pharyngeal phase" many physiologic events occur in rapid succession. The velum closes to prevent the bolus from entering the nasopharynx before the bolus is transported posteriorly from the oral cavity. The oral tongue and tongue base, in concert with the posterior pharyngeal wall, act as the primary forces behind the bolus, pushing it through the pharynx and into the esophagus. During tongue base retraction and pharyngeal contraction, the upper airway closes to prevent bolus entry into the larynx, the pharynx shortens for efficient bolus transport, and the pharyngoesophageal segment (an area in the pharynx that contains the upper esophageal sphincter) opens allowing the passage of the bolus into the esophagus. Once the bolus has been pushed through the pharynx and into the esophagus, the system returns to rest by closing the pharyngoesophageal segment, reopening the airway, relaxing the tongue, reopening the velum, and restoring normal breathing. Disorders of the pharyngeal phase include delayed initiation of the pharyngeal swallow, insufficient retraction of the velum, reduced tongue base retraction, reduced hyolaryngeal excursion, reduced pharyngeal contraction, and reduced pharyngoesophageal segment opening. These dysfunctions may result in pharyngeal residue, laryngeal penetration (entrance of the bolus into the airway while remaining superior to the vocal folds), and/or aspiration (movement of the bolus inferiorly through the vocal folds and into the lower airways).

## Esophageal Dysphagia

SLPs do not assess, diagnose, or treat esophageal disorders. However, with the assistance of a physician, SLPs are able to screen for difficulties with esophageal clearance, making appropriate recommendations for further testing related to esophageal motility and other esophageal dis orders, for which patients may be referred to gastroenterology, otolaryngology, and/or radiology services.

## ■ HOW ARE SPEECH-LANGUAGE, VOICE, AND SWALLOWING DISORDERS ASSESSED AND TREATED?

As with any type of therapy or treatment program, prognosis is highly dependent on the nature of the disorder, the severity of the disorder, an individual's cognitive functioning, cooperation and tenacity, support system, and ability to generalize SLP-trained behaviors to new contexts.

### Assessment and Treatment of Speech Disorders

Speech disorders are assessed through multiple approaches. In most cases, testing of the cranial nerves associated with speech (ie, V, VII, IX, X, and XII), along with an oral motor examination, are standard. Once cranial nerve testing is completed, an articulation and/or phonological inventory may be taken, depending on the case. Such assessments can range from the sound level (production of individual sounds) to elicited and narrative speech to determine the level of breakdown. For example, a patient might be able to produce a sound or group of sounds correctly in isolation or single syllable words, but have difficulty producing the same sounds in multiple syllable words or in conversational speech. When assessing individuals with dysarthria, a motor speech disorder, the SLP must take into account all subsystems of speech (ie, respiration, phonation, articulation, prosody, and resonance) and how they affect intelligibility and verbal expression. Treatment time may be short or long, depending on the severity of difficulties, and will target individual sounds, short phrases, sentences, and finally conversational speech. Each level of treatment will focus on transfer and maintenance from the earlier levels. Assistive devices such as communication boards may be able to assist the patient who is unintelligible, but still able to use language. Although "perfect" speech is the ideal goal, intelligible speech to express wants and needs efficiently may be an endpoint in therapy.

### Assessment and Treatment of Language Disorders

Language disorders span many different domains, among them morphology (meaningful word units, ie, root words, prefixes, suffixes), semantics (word meaning), and syntax (construction of phrases, clauses, sentences, paragraphs, stories). Additional areas of language include naming, comprehension (written or spoken), expression (written or spoken), calculations, and pragmatics (how language is used). Added into this broad area of language is executive function, or cognitive-linguistic impairments. Topics in this area include awareness, attention, and concentration; memory; initiation of appropriate actions (or inhibition of inappropriate actions); planning; problem solving; reasoning; and cognitive flexibility. Depending on the need, these evaluations might take a gestalt approach, reviewing many areas of language and/or cognitive-linguistic impairments within the same evaluation, or they may have a more directed approach to address specific needs. Treatment periods are often lengthy, but depend on the severity of the impairment. Focuses in therapy may be situational (eg, scripted for specific situations) or adaptive (ie, broad application to many different contexts). As with speech, assistive devices such as communication boards may assist in providing the opportunity for patients to express wants and needs. These devices are especially helpful when patients are mechanically ventilated or have unintelligible speech. Treatment decisions and goals will largely depend on each patient's comfort level, physical, and overall cognitive abilities.

## Assessment and Treatment of Voice

Voice is assessed in many different ways. Laryngoscopy, or viewing of the vocal folds will allow the professional to assess functional and/ or anatomical changes to the larynx that might be affecting voice. Stroboscopy, a type of laryngoscopy whereby a pulsed light allows for a sampled viewing of the vocal folds in motion, is one manner to assess vocal fold function. Other types of evaluations might include respiratory plethysmography, acoustic assessments (eg, pitch/frequency, volume/ loudness, and acoustic surrogates of voice quality), and inventories completed by the patient. Most voice therapy has a short duration and is designed to improve changes in vocal behaviors (ie, reduce abusive and maladaptive behaviors) and possibly lifestyle to improve the condition producing voice problems.

Voice assessment in patients with laryngeal cancer is similar to that described above. Treatment for these types of patients may be more involved and includes pre- and post-surgical assessments with counseling. In patients who have impaired voice or the vocal folds are removed, alaryngeal speech may be an option. Examples of alaryngeal speech include training for use of a prosthesis, an electrolarynx, and esophageal speech. Use of each of these techniques will depend on the surgery and remaining anatomy, use of additional medical and/ or oncological therapies (eg, radiation therapy, chemotherapy), and patient goals. Most SLP treatments for patients with laryngectomy have a short duration; however, there may be frequent clinical follow-up appointments. Extent of treatments (ie, surgery, radiation, chemotherapy), impairments in cognitive functioning, and patient compliance may increase the amount of therapy time.

## Assessment and Treatment of Dysphagia

There are 2 types of assessments typically completed by SLPs for dysphagia-clinical and instrumental. The clinical swallowing examination, often referred to as a "bedside swallowing evaluation" (BSE), is a noninstrumental evaluation. Often, it includes a detailed history of the patient's swallowing problems; a screening of the patient's cognitive functioning, including speech, language, and voice functions; a careful review of the motor and sensory functions of the patient's oral, pharyngeal, and laryngeal anatomy; and trial feedings when deemed appropriate. Two methods of instrumental examination are most common for the assessment of dysphagia-fiberoptic endoscopic evaluation of swallowing (FEES) and video fluoroscopic swallow study (VFSS). Whereas the BSE may not necessarily be conclusive, instrumental examinations are diagnostic and each provides greater detail of swallowing physiology and function than the BSE. However, there are considerations for each.

FEES uses a fiberoptic endoscope that is passed transnasally through the nasopharynx and into the upper pharynx past the velum to view swallowing function. This procedure may be used with or without a nasal decongestant and/or a topical anesthetic to ease passing of the endoscope. Once in place, the patient is asked to swallow various consistencies of liquids and food. The clinician is able to assess velum function, pharyngeal weakness, and pharyngeal sensory impairments during this assessment. Additionally, laryngeal penetration and aspiration may be viewed before the swallow is initiated and after the swallow is completed. Viewing pharyngeal and laryngeal function during the swallow is not possible because the light from the endoscope's light source bounces back into the lens of the endoscope during the pharyngeal swallow as the tongue base retracts, epiglottis inverts, and the pharynx contracts, effectively creating a "white-out period" when laryngeal structures cannot be seen and physiology cannot be assessed. Although this white-out period is a shortcoming of the procedure and FEES does not have a standardized scoring procedure, among the benefits of FEES are the ability to perform the procedure bedside without a time limit for completion of the examination and the use of real food.

The VFSS, sometimes called a modified barium swallow study (MBSS), allows for observation of the oral cavity, nasopharynx, oropharynx, larynx, pharynx, and esophagus to assess individual components of swallowing physiology. Patients arrive in the radiology department and are placed in the fluoroscope, typically, while seated or standing. Patients are then presented with varying volumes and consistencies of liquid barium and solid food coated with barium. Each swallow is observed and judgments of efficiency and physiology are made by the SLP. Most often, SLPs perform this evaluation collaboratively with a physician, most commonly a radiologist or physiatrist. Although much more physiologic function of the swallow can be observed using VFSS as compared to FEES, laryngeal penetration and aspiration during the swallow may be observed and compensatory strategies are directly viewed for their effectiveness, there are several clinical disadvantages of the procedure. Among the clinical disadvantages are radiation exposure leading to a limitation in observation time for swallowing physiology; consumption of foreign tastes, textures, substances (ie, barium); confined spaces for larger patients; and obstructed fluoroscopic views from positioning and hardware.

Treatment for dysphagia varies. Therapy may last from a few days to a few months, depending on severity. A home program is key to therapy in the outpatient setting. Impairments in cognitive functioning may increase the amount of therapy time.

## ■ METHODS OF SPEECH THERAPY

Speech therapy, is a type of therapy that helps individuals with communication or swallowing difficulties. There are various methods that speech therapists use to help their patients:

**Articulation therapy:** This involves exercises and activities designed to help patients improve their pronunciation of sounds and words.

**Language therapy:** This includes exercises and activities designed to help patients improve their understanding and use of language, including grammar, vocabulary, and social communication.

**Fluency therapy:** This involves helping patients who stutter or have other fluency disorders to speak more smoothly and confidently.

**Voice therapy:** This includes exercises and activities designed to help patients improve the quality of their voice, such as by addressing issues like hoarseness, breathiness, or pitch problems.

**Swallowing therapy:** This involves helping patients with swallowing difficulties, which can be caused by a variety of conditions such as stroke, brain injury, or neurological disorders.

**Cognitive-communication therapy:** This involves exercises and activities designed to help patients address cognitive-communication difficulties, such as memory, attention, and problem-solving skills related to communication.

**Alternative and augmentative communication (AAC):** This involves strategies and techniques for individuals who have difficulty with verbal communication, such as using pictures, gestures, or technology devices to communicate.

The goal of speech therapy is to help patients improve their communication skills and maximize their ability to express themselves and participate in all aspects of their lives. The specific methods used may vary depending on the individual's needs and condition.

## ■ SUMMARY

SLPs are professionals who are educated in the anatomy, neuroanatomy, physiology, and psychology of assessment and treatment for speech-language, voice, and swallowing disorders. Each of these areas provides important life functions, yet are often taken for granted. When disordered, these types of impairments may span the gamut from the mildest of difficulties to the most devastating of dysfunctions, possibly leading to medical and behavioral/mental disorders. A proper referral for SLP services for patients who experience these types of impairments may provide the improved function and improved quality of life your patient deserves.

## ■ IMPORTANT TERMINOLOGY

speech-language pathology   言语语言病理学
speech-language pathologists   言语病理学家
spraxia of speech   言语失用症
srticulation/phonological processes   发音 / 语音过程
disorders of articulation and phonology   发音和音韵障碍
dysarthria   构音障碍
stuttering   口吃
fluency   流畅
language-based learning disabilities   基于语言的学习障碍
aphasia   失语( 症 )
voice disorders   发声障碍
dysphonia   发音困难
hypernasal   鼻音过重
hyponasal   鼻音过轻
swallowing disorder   吞咽障碍
dysphagia   吞咽困难
oral dysphagia   口期吞咽障碍
pharyngeal dysphagia   咽期吞咽障碍
esophageal dysphagia   食管期吞咽障碍

## ■ REVIEW QUESTIONS

1. How do rehabilitation physicians cooperate with speech-language pathologists?

2. How many types of speech disorders are there? What are their features?
3. How many types of language disorders are there? What are their features?
4. How many types of voice disorders are there? What are their features?
5. How many phases are there in normal swallow process? What is the feature of each swallow disorder type?

（单春雷）

# *REHABILITATION PSYCHOLOGY*

Physiatrists' goal is to restore a person with injury, illness, or disability to maximum functioning by treating the whole person rather than the medical issue alone This is best accomplished through an interdisciplinary team that provides collaborative care[1]. Rehabilitation psychologists, as a part of this team, facilitate effective, integrated care with specialized knowledge of psychosocial and psychophysiological processes in tandem with other disciplines. Collaborative medical care that includes mental health services has been shown to reduce treatment time and overall costs[2] as well as improve patient outcomes and satisfaction[3,4]. Common psychological services in the rehabilitation setting include patient education and fostering self-management of chronic conditions, family and caregiver education and support, consultation with other care providers, program evaluation, and an array of psychotherapeutic interventions. This chapter outlines practical rehabilitation psychology applications to help rehabilitation teams better understand patients' experiences and best manage behavioral reactions and psychological processes during inpatient stays.

## ■ MODEL FOR REHABILITATION: INTERFACE BETWEEN PERSONAL, SOCIAL, AND ENVIRONMENTAL FACTORS

Rehabilitation psychology is founded on the premise that multiple causal pathways interact to produce physical and mental outcomes, and the whole person (eg, the various factors impacting outcomes) has to be treated [1,5]; even outcomes from the best surgical treatments will be affected by nonsurgical factors.

Kurt Lewin's classic psychological theory[6] that describes the cause of observable human behavior has been used in the context of rehabilitation[1]. The formula $B = f (P \times O \times E)$ translates into behavior (B) is a function of the person (P), the organic or biologic (O), and the environment (E). This formula encompasses the total situation that has to be taken into account for behavioral change to occur. For example, an individual's tendency to react (P) coupled with a family's adjustment and/or support or financial assets (E) within the context of physical problems (O) can have a tremendous positive or negative impact on the patient's behaviors and compliance with rehabilitation recommendations (B). Lewin's model supports the mission and essence of rehabilitation with convergence of multiple levels and expertise in the assessment, conceptualization, and treatment for each patient. This globalistic way of approaching a patient in rehabilitation is key to understanding all the potential factors that contribute to outcomes so that all patient needs can be addressed.

## ■ ASSESSMENT

Rehabilitation psychologists perform assessments to identify barriers to full participation in rehabilitation programs and possible obstacles for generalizing skills into the patient's home environment (Table 8.1). Psychological assessments are also helpful to determine what other services and supervision needs can be expected after discharge. Psychological assessments on an inpatient service are generally brief (ie, approximately 60 min) compared with outpatient services (ie, several hours). However, both can address issues such as poor adjustment, inadequate pain management, cognitive or emotional issues, or concurrent substance dependence[7].

Cognitive assessment (ie, neuropsychological assessment) is particularly important as cognitive impairments often substantially affect the rehabilitation adherence and functional outcomes[8]. This is achieved by a psychologist examining brain-behavior relationships through quantitative tests of cognitive abilities across several domains. Collectively, data are then interpreted in the context of each patient's unique history.

**TABLE 8.1** ▪ Components of brief psychological assessments for inpatient rehabilitation

- Clinical interview
  - Medical, psychiatric, social history
  - Substance use history
  - Estimate of premorbid functioning
- Behavioral observations, orientation, mental health screening
  - Depressive symptoms
  - Anxious symptoms
  - Hallucinations and/or delusions
  - Suicidality
- Current pain status (including expectations, fluctuations, and treatments)
- Cognitive screening
  - Attention
  - Learning and memory
  - Executive functioning (eg, planning, organizing, initiating, inhibiting)
  - Language
  - Visuospatial processing

# ■ INTERVENTIONS TO PROMOTE COLLABORATIVE CARE

## Rapport

Rehabilitation is most effective when it is patient centered and with a high degree of patient collaboration[1,9]. Studies of psychotherapy outcomes have shown that strong relationships between clinician and patient account for as much success as the specific therapeutic intervention[10]. Qualities of effective clinical relationships include a team mentality (ie, that the clinician is "on the patient's side"), clinician empathy (warmth, compassion, and understanding), and collaboration on goals[11].

Satisfactory communication between patient and doctor is essential for a collaborative relationship (Table 8.2). Patients expect to have their concerns attended to and investigated with interest and thoroughness. Any perception otherwise can leave a patient feeling unsafe and threatened, which can manifest into anger, distrust, or noncompliance. When confronted with a dissatisfied patient, it is important that the treatment providers keep their response in check (eg, feeling defensive, insulted, or disappointed) and be careful not to reciprocate with anger or withdrawal[12]. In these situations, an understanding, nonjudgmental response is most helpful. For example, "You seem angry, can you tell me more about it?" followed by listening to their response. Soliciting the patient's perspective on solving problems that arise is also often helpful. A typical exchange of this type may take an additional 50 seconds[12], which is likely a minor cost compared with major gains in trust and mutual satisfaction.

**TABLE 8.2** ▪ Components of respectful doctor-patient interactions

- Make eye contact at patient's level (eg, sit down)
- Adjust speaking pace, complexity, and volume based on individuals' needs
- Ask for patient's input, including questions or suggestions
- Expect some patients to require slower than typical interactions for accurate comprehension
- Check patient's understanding of discussed information by asking for a summary
- Encourage the patient's active role in recovery by praising observed milestones and/or activity

# ■ PATIENT REACTIONS AND TEAM RESPONSES TO POTENTIAL BARRIERS

Patient reactions to injury are not always predictable[13], so interventions must be tailored to each individual patient and within that individual's life context. Individuals entering rehabilitation can have a number of stressors that can affect outcome: fear of continual decline, anxiety and/or shame about new dependency, unfamiliar environment, difficulty understanding hospital procedures and health care policies, and loss of future plans or dreams. There is no universal response to crisis or disability[14] or identified discrete stages for adjustment[15]. However, there are shared elements and common rules for rehabilitation patients in which broad interventions can be applied (Table 8.3) [14]. Foremost, interventions are most effective when the collective team has similar understanding of the case, agrees with treatment recommendations, and applies techniques consistently.

**TABLE 8.3** ▪ Suggestions to manage problem behaviors

| Behaviors | Approaches to Better Manage | Example of Management |
|---|---|---|
| Frequent or excessive Pt(patient) demands *Recognize that coping skills may be limited and that these behaviors repel others at a time when the Pt is in most need of attention* | • Avoid judging or blaming the Pt and maintain an objective viewpoint<br>• Identify the need being expressed and how the environment may be reinforcing it<br>• Establish alternative contingencies<br>• Listen and offer reassurance; suggest other activities | • Pt rings call bell very often<br>• Nurse consistently comes when call bell used, but not at other times<br>• Nurse and Pt agree on scheduled times for nurse to check on Pt and reasons to use call bell otherwise<br>• After brief discussion, Pt expresses loneliness when nurse leaves; Pt and staff agree that Pt should call friends or family instead |
| Anger *Avoid becoming defensive* | • Listen to the complaint<br>• Elicit an explanation or experience that surrounds the anger<br>• Empathize<br>• If appropriate, apologize or problem solve | • Pt describes anger at being asked to participate in PT despite pain<br>• "How had you hoped that I could help you?"<br>• "Pain can make people want to rest and avoid movement, even when exercise is the way we know to lessen the pain."<br>• Discuss plan to schedule pain medications prior to PT |
| Agitation | • Use a calm, firm voice<br>• Reduce environmental stimulation (private room, low lights, limit visitors). Play soft music<br>• Avoid under- and overstimulation; use timeouts/distraction as necessary<br>• Contract with agreeable goals and consequences<br>• Schedule tasks when most rested<br>• Talk about their interests | • Pt is restless and irritable most of the time, particularly when in the gym<br>• Therapist plans to hold therapy in private, quiet space<br>• Team discuss goals and plan with patient upfront<br>• Calmly refer to and remind about agreed upon goals to encourage task completion<br>Refer to agreed upon goals, calmly, to encourage task completion |
| Apathy or silence | • Check for hearing or language barriers<br>• Assess mood<br>• Explain the need for collaboration for full benefits<br>• Collaborate on modest and reachable goals, create graph to chart progress | • Pt appears apathetic and does not agree or disagree with stated team goals<br>• Elicit Pt's input<br>• "Just like you, the team has the same goal of restoring a good amount of functioning."<br>• Chart, reinforce activity |

Continued

| Behaviors | Approaches to Better Manage | Example of Management |
|---|---|---|
| Suspiciousness | • Assess mental status and presence of delusions<br>• Ignore accusations<br>• Be factual and consistent across team members<br>• Write down factual information and place in Pt's view | • Pt believes the medical team wants to keep him sick because the team wants job security<br>• May be due to delirium or premorbid psychotic disorder; each needs to be assessed<br>• Refer to written information regarding rationale of treatment routinely and consistently |
| Decreased participation | • Check Pt's understanding<br>• Learn about personal reinforcers<br>• Highlight and chart progress to motivate | • Pt terminates each treatment session early with varying excuses (eg, fatigue, pain, expecting a visitor)<br>• Elicit input/ understanding<br>• Use reinforcers (praise, rest breaks, pep talks) |
| Impulsivity | Elicit Pt's feedback on the factors contributing to the behavior<br>• Focus on positive behaviors with praise<br>• Consistently (across team members and time) tell<br>Pt behaviors that are unacceptable | • Despite education about precautions, Pt gets out of bed on her own<br>• Use praise ("Thank you for using the call bell and waiting when you wanted to get up.")<br>• "Stay in bed until there is help, for safety." |
| Verbal outbursts | • Teach and rehearse a "pause factor": stop, think and organize thoughts before responding | • Pt becomes angry at an aide and reacts with name calling<br>• He later expresses regret and becomes apologetic<br>• Reinforce his interest in behavior change<br>• Practice taking pauses |

# ■ PSYCHOLOGICAL SYMPTOMS

The prevalence rate of emotional symptoms is not higher in rehabilitation populations than that in other medical populations[16], but medical populations overall have higher rates of emotional symptoms than the general population[17]. Rehabilitation psychologists can help identify psychological factors and apply appropriate interventions to accentuate assets and ameliorate negative effects on recovery. Table 8.4 lists some common psychological reactions to disability that could be barriers to rehabilitation, things to consider relating to these reactions, and suggested interventions.

**TABLE 8.4** ▪ Psychological issues and suggested intervention strategies

| Psychological Issues | Things to Consider | Intervention Suggestions |
|---|---|---|
| Noncompliance | Consider Pt readiness to change | Discern performance ability from inability |
| | Explore cultural expectations | Discuss reasons for discrepancy in goals and actions |
| | Assess for psychological issues (depression or anxiety) | Have Pt state potential negative consequences and the probability for these outcomes |
| | | Clarify the context of noncompliance (eg, how others respond and identify usual and potential consequences) |
| Depression / Low mood | Could reflect appropriate recognition of a problem The patient may feel isolated and alone or guilty<br>The patient may not fully understand medical status | Listen actively to lessen feelings of isolation/ loneliness and learn what contributes to the distress<br>Correct misinformation regarding fears or guilt<br>Highlight assets and progress<br>Focus on the positive aspects of the situation |

Continued

| Psychological Issues | Things to Consider | Intervention Suggestions |
|---|---|---|
| Anxiety (generalized) | Mild episodes are normal<br>Intense, frequent, or prolonged anxiety can be problematic<br>Can be due to lack of understanding of medical status or lack of control/ predictability | Teach smooth, deep breathing and educate about stress response<br>Add predictable routines to the schedule<br>Offer unhurried explanations of medical status and upcoming events<br>Plan activities incompatible with anxiety (play games/ watch movies) |
| Anxiety (specific) | Anxiety is a learned fear response that is experienced under conditions associated with unpleasantness | Brainstorm Pt-specific relaxation techniques (music; imagery of positive outcome with feared stimuli; deep breathing; mantras)<br>Educate that specific anxiety responses can be unlearned |
| Conversion reactions | Expression of psychological stress in a physical way | Treat with regular rehab with explicit expectations that Pt will be "healed" in X sessions with Y therapy<br>Consult with rehabilitation psychologist to ensure stressors can be addressed<br>Coordinate treatment team so that positive expectations and praise of progress are consistent |

## Cognitive Problems

At times, cognitive problems can be the main barrier to optimal patient-team collaboration and engagement in rehabilitation services. Table 8.5 lists some deficits that frequently present during rehabilitation and some strategies to improve functioning.

**TABLE 8.5** ▪ Cognitive issues and strategies to improve functioning

| Deficit | Strategies |
|---|---|
| Orientation or confusion or advanced dementia | Create familiarity and predictability in the environment, routines, and caretakers<br>Place calendar, clock, and familiar pictures in the environment<br>Have treatment goals written and placed for regular viewing<br>Talk in a slow, calm, soothing manner, and ensure you have Pt's attention<br>Do not expect information to be retained and understood<br>Reasoning will not be helpful |
| Attention | Reduce environmental distractions<br>Concentrate on one task at a time<br>Discourage conversation during therapy exercises<br>Organize therapy tasks hierarchically with repeated activation |
| Initiation | Check comprehension<br>Structure and routinize activities<br>Divide complex tasks into discrete steps<br>Create a chart of progress<br>Reinforce efforts and small successes |
| Memory | Use a calendar for future reminders, and log daily events for historical reminders<br>Provide written information and cues often<br>Use alarms or cues for designated tasks (eg, meds, cooking)<br>Involve and educate family early in the process |
| Communication | Use brief, direct sentences with few words<br>Response choices can be used to express answers if nonverbal |

Continued

| Deficit | Strategies |
| --- | --- |
| Speed of processing | Adjust expectations to reduce frustration |
| | Structure and fully prepare for tasks to improve efficiency |
| | Expect and schedule additional time |
| | Increase pauses between sentences to permit comprehension |
| Visuospatial | Position environment to ensure safety |
| | Ensure appropriate supervision for mobility tasks |
| Unawareness | Educate Pt about how impairments may affect daily functioning |
| | Ask Pt for expectation prior to task, then compare expectation to performance |
| | Remind of progress by listing specific improvements |
| | Chart improvements as tangible feedback |

## Physical Factors

Rehabilitation psychologists help teams not only with interventions relating to adjustment or cognitive problems but also with interventions that involve physical issues such as pain or sexuality. Rehabilitation psychologists often integrate both psychological and physical factors that may affect a patient's ability to fully engage in rehabilitation and offer suggestions when physical symptoms may affect a person's rehabilitation (Table 8.6). Pain can affect cognitive abilities, emotional coping, and/or social relationships, and pain contributes considerably to additional loss of function and related disability [18]; treatment will be compromised if either psychological or physical factors are neglected [19]. Psychosocial factors related to pain have been found to be better predictors of return to work than medical aspects of the patient and demands of the job [20]. Educating patients about factual medical benefits of activity and harm of inactivity is imperative for patients in acute rehabilitation. Otherwise, the impact of acute pain can go along a "psychological cascade," with progressively more (persistent) interference on one's physical and cognitive functioning and ultimately one's life satisfaction or identity (see Ref. [21] for elaboration).

**TABLE 8.6** ▪ Things to consider when physical factors affect rehabilitation

| Physical Factors | Things to Consider |
| --- | --- |
| Chronic pain | Schedule longer-acting medications to permit patients to focus on "other" things rather than prn (pro re nata: as needed) |
| | Educate about possible poor correlation between pain and pathology and benefits of activity and dangers of inactivity |
| | Educate about acute pain and chronic pain |
| | Acknowledge both physical (eg, it is uncomfortable) and psychological experiences (eg, frustration) |
| | Assess resting and procedural pain |
| | Rule out undermedication and consider aspects that may reduce effectiveness (eg, history of addiction) |
| | Encourage behavioral pain management (relaxation training, imagery, hypnosis, distraction, etc.) |
| Oversedation | Reduce or discontinue benzodiazepines, narcotics, or other sedative medications |
| Poor sleep | Open shades and discourage naps during the day |
| | Ask about sleep habits before hospitalization |
| | Encourage daytime activities; discourage daytime napping |
| | Use eye masks or ear plugs if applicable at night |
| | Limit late meals and caffeine intake |
| | Use soft music or relaxation strategies to reduce autonomic arousal |
| | Assess for depression or anxiety |
| | Be aware of the physical dependence possibility from frequent use of prescribed sleep aids and/or rebound insomnia |

Continued

| Physical Factors | Things to Consider |
| --- | --- |
| Inadequate food intake | Increase socialization during meal times to increase intake educate about nutrition's role in healing and recovery<br>Assess for depression and dental issues |
| Fatigue and related agitation | Space therapy times to reduce fatigue<br>When possible, schedule challenging therapies in half-h blocks<br>Limit visitations and environmental stimulation<br>Assess for sleep quality, depression, or anxiety problems |
| Substance use and abuse | Avoid blaming or punishing<br>Focus on education and dialog of options for behavior change<br>Fill the behavioral void by replacing bad habits (smoking while in the car) with new ones (singing songs on the radio; taking a "walk break" instead of smoke break) |
| Sexual problems | Use the PLISSIT model (Permission, Limited Information, Specific Suggestions, and Intensive Therapy) [22]<br>Address at least the first 2 during rehabilitation: raise the topic and offer a few basic facts<br>Provide referrals for further suggestions or counseling if the PT wishes |

# ■ CLINICAL APPLICATION OF COGNITIVE THERAPY

Cognitive therapy (CT) is a type of psychotherapy that focuses on changing negative thought patterns in order to reduce psychological distress. The theoretical basis of cognitive therapy lies in the premise that psychological disorders arise from erroneous cognition, which can lead to abnormal emotional responses such as depression and anxiety. By identifying and analyzing erroneous cognition, and replacing it with rational and realistic cognition, the suffering of patients can be alleviated, allowing them to better adapt to their environment. CT has been found to be effective for a range of mental health conditions, and can be used in a variety of clinical settings. Here are some examples of the clinical applications of cognitive therapy:

**Depression:** CT is often used to treat depression, as it can help individuals identify and change negative patterns of thinking that contribute to feelings of hopelessness and low self-esteem.

**Anxiety disorders:** CT can be effective for treating various anxiety disorders, such as generalized anxiety disorder, panic disorder, and social anxiety disorder. It helps individuals recognize and challenge irrational thoughts that contribute to anxiety.

**Post-traumatic stress disorder (PTSD):** CT can be used to treat PTSD by helping individuals process traumatic events and learn coping strategies to manage symptoms.

**Eating disorders:** CT has been found to be effective in treating eating disorders, such as anorexia nervosa and bulimia nervosa, by helping individuals challenge negative thoughts related to body image and food.

**Substance abuse:** CT can be used to treat substance abuse by helping individuals identify and challenge distorted thinking related to drug or alcohol use, and develop coping strategies to manage cravings and triggers.

**Obsessive-compulsive disorder (OCD):** CT can be effective in treating OCD by helping individuals identify and challenge obsessive thoughts and compulsive behaviors.

Cognitive therapy can be a versatile and effective treatment option for a wide range of mental health conditions. It can be adapted to meet the unique needs of each individual, and can be used in individual or group therapy settings.

# ■ SUMMARY

Given the complexity of each patient in the acute rehabilitation setting, rehabilitation psychologists can play a unique role in the treatment team. Physiatrists first should clarify their goal, which is to restore a person with illness or disability to maximum functioning by focusing on the whole person. And this could be achieved through an interdisciplinary team providing collaborative care. Assessment is the first step because it could help psychologists identify barriers to full participation in rehabilitation programs. The authors list some common issues in clinical work and the solutions to these issues. So, this chapter provides a brief framework for rehabilitation teams to better understand, assess, and treat patients to encourage collaborative care and optimize functional outcomes.

## ■ IMPORTANT TERMINOLOGY

rehabilitation psychology　康复心理学

Kurt Lewin's classic psychological theory　Kurt Lewin 经典心理学理论

psychological assessment　心理学评估

substance dependence　物质依赖

cognitive assessment　认知评估

cognitive impairments　认知功能障碍

orientation　定向力

dementia　痴呆

attention　注意力

memory　记忆力

communication　沟通

visuospatial deficit　视觉空间缺陷

chronic pain　慢性疼痛

oversedation　过度镇静

poor sleep　睡眠障碍

## ■ REVIEW QUESTIONS

1. Please briefly state the goal of physiatrists and their role in the rehabilitation team.
2. Please briefly describe the Kurt Lewin's classic psychological theory and give an example for its use in clinical practice.
3. Please list the common abnormal behaviors in patients, how to manage these issues and give some examples.
4. Please list the common psychological issues and give some suggested intervention strategies to them.
5. Please describe the common cognitive issues and strategies to improve these functions.

## ■ REFERENCES

1. Wright BA. Physical Disability: A Psychological Approach. New York, NY: Harper & Row; 1983.
2. van Orden MA, Hoffman T, Haffman J, et al. Collaborative mental health care versus care as usual in a primary care setting: a randomized controlled trial. Psychiatr Serv. 2009;60:74-79.
3. Blumenthal JA, Sherwood A, Babyak MA, et al. Effects of exercise and stress management training on markers of cardiovascular risk in patients with ischemic heart disease: a randomized controlled trial. JAMA. 2005; 293(13);1626-1634.
4. Bruns D, Disorbio JM. Assessment of biopsychosocial risk factors for medical treatment: a collaborative approach. J Clin Psy-

chol Med Settings. 2009;16;127-147.

5.   Havelka M, Lucanin JD, Lucanin D. Biopsychosocial model—The integrated approach to health and disease. Coll Antropol. 2009;33(1);303-310.

6.   Lewin K. Field theory and experiment in social psychology: concepts and methods. Am J Soc. 1939;44(6);868-896.

7.   Wegener ST, Kortte KB, Hill-Briggs F, et al. Psychologic assessment and intervention in rehabilitation. In: Braddom RL, ed. Physical Medicine and Rehabilitation. 3rd ed. Philadelphia, PA: Elsevier; 2006:63-91.

8.   Bosworth HB, Oddone EZ, Weinberger M. Patient Treatment Adherence: Concepts, Interventions, and Measurement. Mahwah, NJ: Taylor and Francis; 2005.

9.   Lopez MA, Mermelstein RJ. A cognitive-behavioral program to improve geriatric rehabilitation outcome. Geront. 1995;35(5);696-700.

10.   Wampold BE. The Great Psychotherapy Debate: Models, Methods, and Findings. Mahwah, NJ: Erlbaum; 2001.

11.   Norcross JC, Hill CE. Compendium of empirically supported therapy relationships. In: Koocher GP, Norcross JC, Hill SS, eds. Psychologists' Desk Reference. Oxford, UK: Oxford University Press, 2005.

12.   Beckman HB. Difficult patients. In: Feldman MD, Christensen JF, eds. Behavioral Medicine in Primary Care: A Practical Guide. 2nd ed. New York, NY: Lange Medical Books/McGraw-Hill; 2003.

13.   Wortman CB, Silver RC. The myths of coping with loss. J Consult Clin Psych. 1989;57(3):349-357.

14.   Greif E, Matarazzo RG. Behavioral Approaches to Rehabilitation. New York, NY: Springer; 1982.

15.   Rodin G, Voshart K. Depression in the medically ill: an overview. Am J Psychiatry. 1986;143(6):696-705.

16.   Weissman MM, Meyers JK. Affective disorders in a US urban community, the use of research diagnostic criteria in an epidemiological survey. Arch Gen Psychiatry. 1978;35(11):1304-1311.

17.   Rusin MJ, Johngsma AE. The Rehabilitation Psychology Treatment Planner. New York, NY: John Wiley & Sons; 2001.

18.   Stanos S, Tyburski M, Harden R. Management of chronic pain. In: Braddom RL, ed. Physical Medicine and Rehabilitation. 3rd ed. Philadelphia, PA: Elsevier, 2006:951-988.

19.   Turk DC, Monarch ES. Biopsychosocial perspective on chronic pain. In: Turk DC, Gatchel RJ, eds. Psychological Approaches to Pain Management: A Practitioner's Handbook. New York, NY: Guilford Press; 2002: 3-29.

20.   Blyth FM, March LM, Nicholas MK, Cousins, MJ. Chronic pain, work performance and litigation. Pain. 2003;103;41-47.

21.   Morley SJ, Eccleston C. The object of fear in pain. In: Asmundson JG, Vlaeyen J, Crombez G, eds. Understanding and Treating Fear of Pain. Oxford University Press; 2004:163-188.

22.   Annon J. The Behavioral Treatment of Sexual Problems. Vol. 1. Honolulu, HI: Enabling Systems, Inc; 1974.

（单春雷）

# REHABILITATION NURSING

## ■ INTRODUCTION

Acute inpatient rehabilitation nursing is a specialty, just like intensive care unit (ICU) nursing. Instead of juggling vasoactive drips and watching monitors and hemodynamic parameters like the ICU nursing, the rehabilitation nurse is concerned about how patients adapt to a permanent impairment, integrating coping mechanisms into their daily routines to achieve as full and productive a life as possible and maximizing their functionality. The rehabilitation team is just as specialized and skilled as the ICU team but in a different skill set. The unique role of the rehabilitation nurse is to act as team coordinator to keep all members focusing on the aforementioned goals, because outside of the 3 hours of therapy a day, the rest of the patients' day is under the supervision of the nursing staff. This chapter discusses some of the key individual components of the rehabilitation nurse's role in an acute inpatient rehabilitation program.

## ■ CORE MEASURES

Rehabilitation nursing is much more comprehensive than simply administering medications or doing bladder scans. Today's rehabilitation nurse needs to be cognizant of clinical benchmarks, best practices, core measures and so on. How will stakeholders be apprised of the quality of the program, and how will defects be addressed through quality improvement initiatives? What benchmarks will be maintained, and how will the hash marks be moved forward? These are all questions that need nursing/patient data collected and analyzed to identify and differentiate among system barriers, process issues, and communication/teamwork defects.

Typical core measures usually include Functional Independence Measure (FIM UDS) change, 90-day mortality, 90-day rehospitalization, "bounce-backs" to acute care hospital within 72 hours of admission to the rehabilitation unit, and number of falls per month.

The FIM takes specific training of the nursing staff in order to ensure the accuracy of the assessed measures and make sure the staffs can apply the algorithms uniformly from shift to shift. Nursing shift report needs to include falls, voided volume, episodes of incontinence and urination during the shift, how much the patient assisted in bathing and dressing the upper body and lower body, and how much help was needed in transferring (ie, minimal, moderate, maximum assist, contact guard, or supervision, and making sure everyone is using the same definition). These above are included in the comprehensive data reported for each patient, resulting in accurate FIM reports.

90-day mortality and rehospitalization monitor the appropriateness of the admission into the acute inpatient rehabilitation program. A rate higher than region or nation would indicate that the preadmission evaluation of the patient needs to be reviewed and perhaps admission criteria into the acute inpatient rehabilitation program need to be reviewed. A much stronger signal of a program is a monthly review of all "bounce-backs" to an acute care hospital within 72 hours of admission to the acute inpatient rehabilitation program. This review will immediately identify procedural deficiencies, facilitate discussion between nurses and leadership on how to correct deficiencies and correct them The investment on nursing staff administrative time to review charts and carving out time to discuss the findings with the medical leadership benefits the overall health of the program.

# ■ TEAMWORK AND COMMUNICATION

Nursing works closely with the attending physicians and the resident physicians in rehabilitation units. Both health care providers have a major impact on each other's efficiency, effectiveness, and workflow. An effective communication tool can be a written document (sign-out) available on a common source (usually electronic) and updated daily by each team member. This document could greatly improve patient's safety and communication between the disciplines could possibly decrease length of stay by informing colleagues of the patient's progress (or lack thereof), which otherwise might be missed. Essential test results, treatment plans, or outstanding "to do" lists are examples of things that could be passed on from shift to shift.

Communication skills can also be learned through teamwork and communication workshops. Some communication skill examples include using the SBAR (situation, background, assessment, recommendation) framework for taking/giving reports to other units, using the 2-attempt rule before going up the chain of command, or using the DESC script for interpersonal conflict cases.

# ■ CLINICAL ISSUES

## Pain Management

Pain management is a challenge in an inpatient rehabilitation setting for multiple reasons. Some patient's pain might never have been adequately controlled. Other patients could have had controlled pain but when their exercise/therapy time is tripled from 1 hour or less a day to 3 hours a day, their pain increases with the increased demand on their body. Another subset of patients could have an added psychogenic component to their pain that needs to be identified and addressed through the services of neuropsychology or pain management. The literature is starting to address the issues of persistent pain and how to screen for this specific and troublesome patient care issue in older adults [1].

Nursing should accomplish patients' pain assessments every 4 hours and reassessments within 2 hours of administering oral pain medication. Nursing staff have the best overall picture of how much short acting pain medicine the patient is using, whether or not a long-acting agent needs to be added or increased, the effectiveness of the pain-relieving agent, and any untoward effects. Effectively tracking pain and response to treatment is critical for optimizing pain management and is crucial information for the prescribing practitioner.

## Bowel and Bladder Training

Bowel and bladder training is essential in any rehabilitation effort. The more proactive nursing is to schedule time for bowel and bladder training, the better the results [2]. It is just as important to schedule this time as it is to schedule physical therapy or occupational therapy. The more consistent nurses are from shift to shift to toilet the patient on the same schedule, the better the outcome. Nurses can minimize or prevent urinary tract infections by toileting every 3 to 4 hours, watching intake/output and lab values and verifying that the patient is emptying their bladder completely through follow-up post void residual bladder scans [3]. The rehabilitation nurse has to assess if bowel incontinence is a newly acquired deficit in self-care or a chronic/permanent deficit. Does bowel training involve an ostomy or is there an underlying infection like Clostridium difficile (*C.diff*)? After thorough assessment, a plan needs to be made to help the patient adapt to this self-care need, in order to assist them in regaining some measure of control over their body. It takes a sensitive, listening, and empathetic nurse to help the patient work through these issues during their short stay. The nurse needs to be part teacher, part coach, and part salesperson to gain the patient's trust and cooperation to initially participate in a bowel regimen and eventually independently maintain it. Repeated communication from shift to shift and standardized care are the key to helping the patient regain as much of this functionality as possible. Nursing also needs to schedule this time on an equal basis with other therapy times.

Nursing needs to be vigilant about assessing for *C. diff*, watching lab results, documenting numbers of and characteristics of each stool, and reporting this information to the health care provider. Good hand hygiene and minimizing the sharing of equipment, like shower chairs, is essential in eradicating outbreaks of nosocomial infections.

Awareness of the effects of prescribed medications on bowel function is critical. Some medications cause constipation, and others can cause diarrhea; the nurse should be able to differentiate between an untoward medication effect and an allergic reaction. The patient and family will need to be educated when the best bowel program is achieved and how they will need to continue at home.

## Skin

A majority of patients come to acute inpatient rehabilitation after some sort of surgery or trauma. Various incision sites, drains, and catheters have to be managed and scheduled into the daily care regimen. In addition to these, pressure ulcers should be monitored, assessed, and a treatment plan need to be developed by physicians and wound care specialists. One study indicated that the most common parameters for predicting the occurrence of pressure ulcers are men with moist, edematous skin, with a previous episode of centralized circulation dysfunction that resulted in mottled or reddened skin [4].

The wound care team must work closely with the nursing staff, particularly on complicated or infected wounds. Wound measurements (length × width × depth) and the color of the wound base should be documented. The nursing staff usually communicates the degree of effectiveness of the wound care regimen to health care providers and makes recommendations for changes, if needed. Nursing also works in conjunction with therapy to verify that the patient has the correct wheelchair cushion for pressure relief, reinforces pressure relieving techniques, and schedules treatments like pulse lavage. Individual patients might also need a specialized pressure relieving mattress overlay or specialty beds to assist in the management of their wounds. Close to discharge, nursing has to assess what modalities the patient will need at home and arrange for the inclusion of this equipment at home. Nursing and wound care work are in conjunction with nutritionists, the patient, and their family to maximize their nutrition to facilitate healing. The final step is patient and family teaching of the continuing needed therapies at home.

Surgical incisions are also addressed by rehabilitation nurses. These can present within a wide spectrum of healing. Some incisions are simple, needing only minimal care. Other incisions can become problematic, necessitating rehospitalization for a washout and a full course of intravenous antibiotics. Rehabilitation nurses need to be vigilant in identifying any signs or symptoms of infection as early as possible. Early intervention can mean the difference between staying on the rehabilitation unit with oral antibiotics or having to terminate rehabilitation for acute care management. As previously mentioned, communication needs to be clear and specific regarding the progress or lack of progress in the patient's wound healing.

## Mobility

Physical therapists and nurses have to work closely to treat mobility difficulties in order to maximize the patient's progress without compromising their safety. Rehabilitation nurses should have hands-on training on adaptive equipment like beasy boards, patient lift devices, as well as transfer techniques and other specific plans for mobility [5]. The benefit of this training comes in the off hours, which nursing can reinforce the skills the patient learned in their therapy sessions.

Therefore, nursing not only needs to be instructed in proper techniques for any transfers but also needs the instructions for adapting to specific limitations in mobility that any particular patient might have or include the use of adaptive equipment, such as a splint used for shoulder subluxation, an ankle foot orthosis (AFO) for foot drop, or use of multipodus boots at night. Nursing and therapy must work collaboratively to determine when the patient shows signs of being ready to challenge their deficit or impairment. These patients are the ones that benefit from co-treat sessions. For example, nursing could even move a stroke patient with neglect to a room with a furniture orientation, which forces the patient attention to their neglected side.

One of the biggest challenges rehabilitation nurses face is encouraging the patient to practice newly acquired skills for balance, gait, and ambulation while being aware of and staying within their individual safety parameters. The literature has reported that the higher the patient's level of impulsivity and the lower their safety awareness or situational awareness then the higher their fall rate. It is a constant effort to maintain safety while practicing newly acquired skills [6].

## Falls, Sitters, and Restraints

Part of the complexity of decreasing fall rates can be addressed through technology, but state-of-the art technology can only be as effective as its consistent use by the staff. If the bed alarms are not turned on or sounding alarms investigated promptly, then technology doesn't matter. Part of the goals in rehabilitation is to increase the functionality and independence, but increasing independence might put the patient at a higher fall risk [7]. Hourly rounding is important to address the 3 most cited reasons for falls: toileting, pain, and positioning. The literature suggests that it is important to identify the fall risk factors present for each patient and reduce them as much as possible or eliminate them [8]. A risk assessment on each patient should identify extrinsic and intrinsic factors, as well as environmental factors [9]. The most commonly restrained patients are those who had had a stroke [10]. Increasing cognitive impairment and slower ambulation speed place patients at higher risk of falls regardless of any fall reduction initiatives [11].

## Other

The rehabilitation nurse has to consult closely with the dietician and ancillary support team to monitor nutrition status via laboratory values, trending intake/output, weights, and response to therapy. Nutritional management can be further complicated by swallowing disorder and the presence of a gastrostomy tube.

When a gastrostomy tube is present, nursing needs to report the volume of residual feeding in the stomach each shift and how well the patient is tolerating the tube feed and work to transition the patient from continuous feeds to cyclic feeds to bolus feeds, if possible. Nursing must keep a watchful eye on the hydration status of the patient, as this is often overlooked. The main means of monitoring hydration are by trending renal laboratory values, checking skin turgor daily, and following 24-hour intake/output trends and blood pressures.

# ■ SUMMARY

Rehabilitation nursing is complex, in that, the care a rehabilitation nurse gives is multidisciplinary. The rehabilitation nurse collaborate with the attending physicians and the resident physicians, consults doctors, communicates with patients and their families and advocates to maximize patient, clinical, and financial outcomes. Priorities have to be reassessed throughout any given shift and essential data shared with all appropriate members of the team.

# ■ IMPORTANT TERMINOLOGY

ankle foot orthosis (AFO)   踝足矫形器

bladder training   膀胱功能训练

bowel training   肠道功能训练

bowel incontinence   大便失禁

clinical benchmarks   临床基准

cognitive impairment   认知障碍

foot drop   足下垂

Functional Independence Measure (FIM)   功能独立性评测

gastrostomy tube   胃造口管

swallowing disorder   吞咽障碍

neuropsychology   神经心理学

nosocomial infections   院内感染

nutritional management   营养管理

pain management   疼痛管理

pressure ulcer   压疮

rehabilitation uursing   康复护理

risk of falls   跌倒风险

shoulder subluxation   肩关节半脱位

urinary tract infections   尿路感染

# ■ REVIEW QUESTIONS

1. What makes rehabilitation nursing different from general nursing?
2. What is the significance of taking core measures in rehabilitation nursing?
3. What complications can occur after long-term immobilization?
4. What programs does clinical rehabilitation nursing include and how to implement these programs respectively?
5. What are the common causes of leading to voiding dysfunction?
6. How to decide the classification and grading of pressure ulcer?

# ■ REFERENCES

1. McLennon SM. Evidence-based guideline: persistent pain management. J Gerontol Nurs. 2007;5-14.
2. Roe B, Milne J, Ostaszkiewicz J, Wallace S. Systematic reviews of bladder training and voiding programmes in adults: a syn-

opsis of findings on theory and methods using metastudy techniques. J Adv Nurs. 2006;57:3-14.

3.  Ostaszkiewicz J. Incomplete bladder emptying in frail older adults: a clinical conundrum. Int J Urol Nurs. 2007;1:87-91.

4.  Compton F, Hoffman F, Hortig T, et al. Pressure ulcer predictors in ICU patients: nursing skin assessment versus objective parameters. J Wound Care. 2008;17:417-424.

5.  Nelson A, Harwood KJ, Tracey CA, Dunn KL. Myths and facts about safe patient handling in rehabilitation. Rehabil Nurs. 2008;33:10-17.

6.  Kneafsey, R. A systematic review of nursing contributions to mobility rehabilitation: examining the quality and content of the evidence. JCI. 2007;16: 325-340.

7.  Gilewski MJ, Roberts P, Hirata J. Discriminating high fall risk on an inpatient rehabilitation unit. Rehabil Nurs. 2007;32:234-240.

8.  Nazarko L. Falls part 1: causes and consequences. BJHCA. 2008;2:381-384.

9.  Hignett S, Masud T. A review of environmental hazards associated with in-patient falls. Ergonomics. 2006;49:605-616.

10. Gallinagh R, Nevin R, McIlory D, et al. The use of physical restraints as a safety measure in the care of older people in four rehabilitation wards: findings from an exploratory study. Int J Nurs Stud. 2002;39:147-156.

11. Rabadi MH, Rabadi FM, Peterson M. An analysis of falls occurring in patients with stroke on an acute rehabilitation unit. Rehabil Nurs. 2008;33:104-109.

（谢　青）

# *ANTICOAGULATION/VENOUS THROMBOEMBOLISM*

## ◼ INTRODUCTION

Venous thromboembolism (VTE) refers to deep vein thrombosis (DVT) and pulmonary embolism (PE). In the United States, the annual incidence of VTE is estimated to exceed 600 000 with nearly 300 000 fatalities[1], making it the most common preventable cause of hospital-related death [2]. Indeed, in 2001, the US Agency for Healthcare Research and Quality found that appropriate use of VTE prophylaxis was the most highly rated safe practice among 79 safe practices evaluated for impact and effectiveness. Unfortunately, only 50% of VTE events found at autopsy were diagnosed clinically before death. Hence, prevention and early diagnosis and treatment are critical [3].

### Risk Factors

Risk factors for VTE are major trauma, immobility, paresis, malignancy, previous VTE, increasing age, pregnancy and postpartum period, acute infection, heart failure, respiratory failure, obesity, and smoking [4]. The vast majority of rehabilitation inpatients fit into at least one of these categories. Thus, it is incumbent upon physiatrists to be adept in the prevention, early diagnosis, and treatment of VTE.

### Prevention

Only 33% of inpatients in US hospitals receive appropriate VTE prophylaxis [5]. The American College of Chest Physicians (ACCP) has established the most widely used guidelines [6]. These guidelines have been developed on evidence-based medicine but are not without controversy. Below are some alternative diagnosis-specific guidelines. Most vary little from the ACCP guidelines.

### Orthopedic Surgery

The American Academy of Orthopedic Surgery (AAOS) has published alternative guidelines, which reflect the concern among some orthopedic surgeons over the risk of postoperative hematomas in joint replacement patients placed on low molecular weight heparins (LMWH) [7]. The main difference between the ACCP and AAOS guidelines is that the AAOS guidelines allow for the optional use of high-dose aspirin in total knee replacements, whereas the ACCP guidelines advise against this practice.

### Complex Medical

In a meta-analysis of hospitalized internal medicine patients, LMWH and unfractionated heparin (UFH) 5000 units subcutaneously 3 times daily were found to be equally efficacious in preventing DVT with similar risks of bleeding[8]. The effect on the incidence of PE in that study could not be determined due to inadequate sample size. In neurosurgical patients, a meta-analysis of 18 studies indicated that LMWH could prevent VTE in patients without a contraindication to its use, whereas intermittent compression devices (ICDs) could also prevent VTE when there was a contraindication. Furthermore, UFH had a higher risk of VTE complications [9].

## Traumatic Brain Injury

A survey of NIDRR Brain Injury Model Systems revealed no clear consensus about VTE prophylaxis; only 56% of centers routinely used anticoagulants prophylactically [10]. The same study reported an incidence of fatal PE of 0.42 per practice year, emphasizing the need for guidelines [10].

## Spinal Cord Injury

Guidelines have been released for the prevention of VTE in cervical spinal cord injury (SCI) [11]. The use of LMWH prophylaxis in SCI patients undergoing acute rehabilitation resulted in a drop in the incidence of VTE from 21% to 7.9% compared with the use of low-dose UFH [12].

## Cancer

The US National Comprehensive Cancer Center Network released guidelines in 2007 recommending anticoagulation for VTE prophylaxis in all hospitalized cancer patients under active therapy who do not have contraindications [13].

## Intermittent Compression Devices

ICDs have some effectiveness in preventing DVTs when used alone compared with no intervention and should be used when there are contraindications to anticoagulation. The use of ICDs was substantially less effective than pharmacologic prophylaxis but did add additional benefit when used in combination with anticoagulation[14]. In stroke patients, no benefit to the use of mechanical prophylaxis has been demonstrated [15].

## Inferior Vena Cava Filters

Inferior vena cava filters (IVCFs) can be used to prevent a DVT from propagating to a PE in patients with contraindications to anticoagulation. However, there is no demonstrated benefit to using them as a primary prophylaxis [16].

## Prevention Saves Lives

The rigorous implementation of ACCP guidelines can result in a dramatic decrease in the incidence of VTE. In one study, the application of the ACCP guidelines in an academic hospital rehabilitation unit resulted in a 6-fold decrease in VTE events [17].

# ■ DIAGNOSIS

Diagnosis of VTE is notoriously difficult. Up to 70% of fatal PE is first diagnosed at autopsy [18]. It is optimal to diagnose VTE at the stage of DVT, as PE frequently results in sudden death.

## Diagnosing DVT

The gold standard for the diagnosis of lower limb DVT is venography. However, it is seldom used clinically outside the research setting as noninvasive testing, especially venous Doppler ultrasound (US), has such high positive and negative predictive values (PPVs and NPVs). It has an even higher NPV (99.5%) when duplex color technology is used [19]. This has become the optimal test for diagnosing DVT in patients with symptoms, that is, unilateral lower limb swelling or sudden onset of calf pain.

## What About D-Dimer?

Some have advocated the use of D-dimer to screen symptomatic patients prior to ordering a US. This may have some utility in the outpatient setting in patients at low risk [20]. However, in postoperative patients, it is of little benefit because the PPV is so low, and false positives are so frequent [21].

## Surveillance Dopplers

On first glance, it might make sense to screen all high-risk patients for VTE with US upon admission to the rehabilitation unit. Indeed, in a survey of NIDRR Brain Injury Model Systems, 50% of facilities did so [10]. However, this practice has been shown to be costly and ineffective [22]. It is not recommended under the ACCP guidelines [6].

## Diagnosing PE

Physicians need to maintain a high level of suspicion for PE, particularly in rehabilitation inpatients, who typically carry a high risk [23]. One widely used system for stratifying diagnostic suspicion for PE is the Wells rule. It has been revised into a simplified form, which carries similar validity in identifying patients with a high probability of PE upon further testing [24].

Basically, the presence of more than one of the following signs and symptoms should trigger a physician to order diagnostic testing for PE: clinical signs of DVT, tachycardia, immobilization in the last month, previous VTE, hemoptysis, malignancy, and an alternative diagnosis are less likely than PE.

## Diagnostic Testing for PE

Pulmonary angiography is the gold standard for diagnosing PE, but similar to venography, it is seldom used in clinical settings as noninvasive testing has nearly matched its sensitivity and specificity [19]. Ventilation-perfusion scintographic studies (V/Q) can have diagnostically definitive results in most patients, but a subset of patients will have intermediate probability scans [25]. Therefore, increasingly clinicians rely on spiral computerized tomography in patients who do not have a contraindication to this test (the primary contraindications being renal insufficiency or dye allergy) [19].

## ■ TREATMENT

Physiatrists are often the first physicians to initiate treatment of VTE in hospitalized patients. The advent of LMWH in the last decade has allowed the treatment of VTE with less intensive monitoring than UFH given intravenously. Dosages are weight based and far higher than prophylactic dosing. While baseline laboratory tests (CBC, aPTT, PT/INR, BMP) are advisable, there is no need to monitor aPTT as with UFH intravenously. This substantially simplifies care and reduces total cost [26].

## American College of Physicians (Acp)/American Academy of Family Physician (AAFP) Guidelines

The joint guidelines from the ACP and the AAFP[27] recommend the preferential use of LMWH for DVT and find equal efficacy for the use of LMWH and UFH for PE. The exceptions are patients with renal insufficiency, who should be treated with UFH, and patients with contraindications to anticoagulation (eg, active bleeding, thrombocytopenia, hereditary bleeding disorder).

## Treatment of Patients with Contraindications TO ANTICOAGULATION

Patients who cannot be anticoagulated can be safely treated with IVCFs[16]. These now are removable in cases where long-term use is not needed. It should be remembered that IVCFs do not treat DVT and indeed may worsen edema and pain; they frequently lead to post-thrombotic syndrome. What they are intended to do is to prevent the propagation of DVT to PE. They are not recommended for prophylactic use [6]. The ACP/AAFP guidelines recommend that most cases of DVT, and perhaps some cases of PE, can be safely treated in the outpatient setting [27]. The implication for physiatrists is that most patients with acute DVT, and perhaps some with hemodynamically stable PE, can be managed on the rehabilitation unit without transfer to acute care.

## Bed Rest and Compression Hose

Traditionally, physicians have recommended bed rest and the removal of compression devices for several days after DVT, for fear of propagation to PE. This appears to be bad advice, at least according to a retrospective study in Italy [28]. DVT patients who were immobilized and did not receive compression devices actually had a higher risk of developing PE subsequently.

## Long-Term Management

A systematic review of management of VTE [29] recommends 3 months of treatment with a vitamin K antagonist (Warfarin) for VTE in patients with transient risk factors (eg, postoperatively) and 12-month patients with "unprovoked" VTE or those with ongoing risk (eg, tetraplegia). LMWH was found to be an equally efficacious alternative, especially in cancer patients. The use of below knee compression stockings after DVT reduces the incidence of post-thrombotic syndrome by 50% [30].

## ICD codes

- 2010: 453.40—Acute venous embolism and thrombosis of unspecified deep vessels of lower extremity.
- 2010: 453.41—Acute venous embolism and thrombosis of deep vessels of proximal lower extremity.
- 2010: 453.42—Acute venous embolism and thrombosis of deep vessels of distal lower extremity (ie, the calf, lower leg NOS, peroneal, and tibia).
- 2010: 453.8—Other venous embolism and thrombosis of other specified veins (eg, upper extremity vein).
  If DVT is documented as a postoperative complication or iatrogenic, first assign code 997.2, followed by
- 451.11: Iatrogenic pulmonary embolism and infarction.
- 451.12: Septic pulmonary embolism (first code the underlying infection).
- 451.19: Other pulmonary embolism and infarction.

## ■ SUMMARY

This chapter focuses on the prevention and early diagnosis and treatment of VTE. VTE is comprised of two entities, DVT and PE. VTE has significant morbidity and mortality for both the inpatient and outpatient population. Indeed, the appropriate implementation of VTE prophylaxis can result in a dramatic decrease in the incidence of VTE.

The vast majority of inpatients, accompanied with at least one of these risk factors for VTE, are necessary to receive appropriate VTE prophylaxis. Although there are some alternative diagnosis-specific guidelines, the ACCP guidelines is most widely used. The ACCP guidelines advise LMWH as routine pharmacologic prophylaxis. However, for patients with a contraindication to anticoagulation therapy, intermittent compression devices have some effectiveness in preventing DVTs, and IVCFs can be used to prevent a DVT from propagating to a PE. As for the diagnosis of VTE, venous Doppler ultrasound has become the optimal test about PE, V/Q and spiral computerized tomography can be ordered by a physician to diagnosis PE if necessary, pulmonary angiography is the gold standard. Ultimately, with respect to the treatment of VTE, ACCP guidelines recommend the preferential use of LMWH. Dosages are weight based and far higher than prophylactic dosing. However, patients with renal insufficiency should be treated with unfractionated heparin and patients with contraindications to anticoagulation can be safely treated with IVCFs. For the discharged patients, long-term management are necessary, including pharmacologic anticoagulation and mechanical therapy.

## ■ IMPORTANT TERMINOLOGY

venous thromboembolism, VTE    静脉血栓栓塞
deep vein thrombosis, DVT    深静脉血栓
pulmonary embolism, PE    肺栓塞
low molecular weight heparin, LMWH    低分子量肝素
unfractionated heparin, UFH    普通肝素
inferior vena cava filter, IVCF    下腔静脉滤器
anticoagulation    抗凝
prophylaxis    预防
trauma    创伤
malignancy    恶性肿瘤
autopsy    尸检
contraindication    禁忌证
venography    静脉造影术
thrombocytopenia    血小板减少症
ultrasound    超声
hematoma    血肿
edema    水肿
swelling    肿胀
calf pain    小腿疼痛

## ■ REVIEW QUESTIONS

1.  What is the differential diagnosis, and what are the possible risk factors for DVT and PE?
2.  What is the best way to diagnose or exclude DVT and PE?
3.  What is the appropriate initial therapy for DVT; when is hospitalization not required?
4.  What is the recommended long-term treatment for DVT and PE?
5.  When should one screen for the presence of a hypercoagulable state, not only in the patient, but also in family members?

# ■ REFERENCES

1. Anderson FA, Zayaruzny M, Heit JA, Fidan D, Cohen AT. Estimated annual numbers of US acute-care hospital patients at risk for venous thromboembolism. Am J Hematol. 2007;82(9):777-782.

2. Michota FA. Bridging the gap between evidence and practice in venous thromboembolism prophylaxis: the quality improvement process. J Gen Intern Med. 2007;22(12):1762-1770.

3. Laporte S, Mismetti P, Decousus H, et al; RIETE Investigators. Clinical predictors for fatal pulmonary embolism in 15,520 patients with venous thromboembolism: findings from the registro informatizado de la enfermedad TromboEmbolica venosa (RIETE) registry. Circulation. 2008;117(13): 1711-1716.

4. Alikhan R, Cohen AT, Combe S, et al; MEDENOX study. Risk factors for venous thromboembolism in hospitalized patients with acute medical illness: analysis of the MEDENOX study. Arch Intern Med. 2004;164(9): 963-968.

5. Amin AN, Stemkowski S, Lin J, Yang G. Preventing venous thromboembolism in US hospitals: are surgical patients receiving appropriate prophylaxis? Thromb Haemost. 2008;99(4):796-797.

6. Geerts WH, Bergqvist D, Pineo GF, et al; American College of Chest Physicians. Prevention of venous thromboembolism: American College of Chest Physicians Evidence-Based Clinical Practice Guidelines (8th edition). Chest. 2008;133(6)(suppl):381S.

7. Parvizi J, Azzam K, Rothman RH. Deep venous thrombosis prophylaxis for total joint arthroplasty: American Academy of Orthopaedic Surgeons Guidelines. J Arthroplasty. 2008;23(7)(suppl):2-5.

8. Kanaan AO, Silva MA, Donovan JL, Roy T, Al-Homsi AS. Meta-analysis of venous thromboembolism prophylaxis in medically ill patients. Clin Ther. 2007;29(11):2395-2405.

9. Collen JF, Jackson JL, Shorr AF, Moores LK. Prevention of venous thromboembolism in neurosurgery: A metaanalysis. Chest. 2008;134(2):237-249.

10. Carlile MC, Yablon SA, Mysiw WJ, Frol AB, Lo D, Diaz-Arrastia R. Deep venous thrombosis management following traumatic brain injury: a practice survey of the traumatic brain injury model systems. J Head Trauma Rehabil. 2006;21(6):483-490.

11. Deep venous thrombosis and thromboembolism in patients with cervical spinal cord injuries. Neurosurgery. 2002;50(3)(suppl):S73-S80.

12. Green D, Sullivan S, Simpson J, Soltysik RC, Yarnold PR. Evolving risk for thromboembolism in spinal cord injury (SPIRATE study). Am J Phys Med Rehabil. 2005;84(6):420-422.

13. Khorana AA. The NCCN clinical practice guidelines on venous thromboembolic disease: strategies for improving VTE prophylaxis in hospitalized cancer patients. Oncologist. 2007;12(11):1361-1370.

14. Kakkos SK, Caprini JA, Geroulakos G, Nicolaides AN, Stansby GP, Reddy DJ. Combined intermittent pneumatic leg compression and pharmacological prophylaxis for prevention of venous thromboembolism in high-risk patients. Cochrane Database Syst Rev. 2008;(4):CD005258.

15. Mazzone C, Chiodo GF, Sandercock P, Miccio M, Salvi R. Physical methods for preventing deep vein thrombosis in stroke. Cochrane Database Syst Rev. 2004;(4):CD001922.

16. Austin MS, Parvizi J, Grossman S, Restrepo C, Klein GR, Rothman RH. The inferior vena cava filter is effective in preventing fatal pulmonary embolus after hip and knee arthroplasties. J Arthroplasty. 2007;22(3):343-348.

17. Mayer RS, Halpert DE, StreiffMB, Hobson DB, Berenholz SM. In:Implementation of evidence-based guidelines for venous thromboembolism prophylaxis leads to decreased incidence of venous thromboembolism among rehabilitation inpatients. Association of Academic Physiatrists; February; Colorado Springs, CO, USA; 2009.

18. Stein PD, Henry JW. Prevalence of acute pulmonary embolism among patients in a general hospital and at autopsy. Chest. 1995;108(4):978-981.

19. Michiels JJ, Gadisseur A, Van Der Planken M, et al. A critical appraisal of noninvasive diagnosis and exclusion of deep vein thrombosis and pulmonary embolism in outpatients with suspected deep vein thrombosis or pulmonary embolism: how many tests do we need? Int Angiol. 2005;24(1):27-39.

20. Kraaijenhagen RA, Piovella F, Bernardi E, et al. Simplification of the diagnostic management of suspected deep vein thrombosis. Arch Intern Med. 200222;162(8):907-911.

21. Rafee A, Herlikar D, Gilbert R, Stockwell RC, McLauchlan GJ. D-dimer in the diagnosis of deep vein thrombosis following total hip and knee replacement: a prospective study. Ann R Coll Surg Engl. 2008;90(2):123-126.

22. Schwarcz TH, Matthews MR, Hartford JM, et al. Surveillance venous duplex is not clinically useful after total joint arthro-plasty when effective deep venous thrombosis prophylaxis is used. Ann Vasc Surg. 2004;18(2): 193-198.

23. Muntz JE. Prevention of thromboembolic complications in the rehabilitation center: diagnostic and risk factor stratification tools. Am J Phys Med Rehabil. 2000;79(5)(suppl):S17-S21.

24. Gibson NS, Sohne M, Kruip MJ, et al. Further validation and simplification of the Wells clinical decision rule in pulmonary embolism. Thromb Haemost. 2008;99(1):229-234.

25. Sostman HD, Stein PD, Gottschalk A, Matta F, Hull R, Goodman L. Acute pulmonary embolism: sensitivity and specificity of ventilation-perfusion scintigraphy in PIOPED Ⅱ study. Radiology. 2008;246(3):941-946.

26. Fanikos J. Guidelines and performance measures for the prevention and treatment of venous thromboembolism. J Manag Care Pharm. 2008;14(6) (suppl A):14-23.

27. Snow V, Qaseem A, Barry P, et al. Management of venous thromboembolism: a clinical practice guideline from the American College of Physicians and the American Academy of Family Physicians. Ann Intern Med. 2007;146(3): 204-210.

28. Manganaro A, Ando G, Lembo D, Sutera Sardo L, Buda D. A retrospective analysis of hospitalized patients with documented deep-venous thrombosis and their risk of pulmonary embolism. Angiology. 2008;59(5):599-604.

29. Segal JB, Streiff MB, Hofmann LV, Thornton K, Bass EB. Management of venous thromboembolism: a systematic review for a practice guideline. Ann Intern Med. 2007;146(3):211-222.

30. Prandoni P, Lensing AW, Prins MH et al. Below-knee elastic compression stockings to prevent the post-thrombotic syn-drome: a randomized, controlled trial. Ann Intern Med. 2004;141(4):249-256.

（郑朝旭）

# *ASSISTIVE TECHNOLOGIES*

## ■ INTRODUCTION

Assistive technology (AT) has come to play a critically important role in the rehabilitation and functional self-sufficiency of persons with disability. With the aging of the population, there is a growing demographic trend toward improved longevity of individuals with chronic disease and associated disabilities and impairments. While the "gracefully graying" and disabled population often experiences challenges to their quality of life resulting from sensory, motor, and cognitive restrictions, AT has the capacity to substantially improve quality of life, bolster self-esteem, and enhance vocational potential. As the number of individuals with disabilities who use computers (both for vocational and recreational purposes) continues to grow, the importance of computer-related accessible technology solutions has concomitantly grown as well.

## ■ CHAPTER OVERVIEW

This chapter is intended as a primer and familiarization guide. Its goal is to enable the rehabilitation clinician to optimize care of patients with disability through educated selection of various empowering AT solutions aimed at computer-based vocational re-entry. The chapter will provide a birds-eye overview of the most common physical impairments encountered and specific AT solutions that can be applied.

Specific categories of impairments that affect computer use directly to be discussed include: Hearig impairments, visual impairments, motor and dexterity impairments.

For a more in-depth discussion of other forms of impairments including cognitive impairments and language and communication impairments, the reader is referred to other sources.

Although the scope of this chapter is a limited discussion of computer-associated and software-based assistive technologies, each section is preceded by a short discussion of general accessible technologies that are not necessarily computer related. In light of the vast number of technologies and fee-based add-on programs available, the authors have elected to limit their consideration of specific interventions to those that are complimentary and often freely bundled as part of existing versions of standard operating systems (OS). Since computers are an important tool for vocational re-entry and personal satisfaction, the central focus of this chapter is to highlight specific assistive technologies that increase the prognostic efficacy of vocational programs. Often times, the process may simply involve the clinician suggesting a specific "tweak and adjustment" made to standard OS to enable the activation of disability access utilities that are freely available on all computers.

## ■ NOMENCLATURE

AT is a general term referring to any assistive, adaptive, or rehabilitative device employed by persons with disabilities for the purpose of achieving independence. Assistive technology defined as "any item, piece of equipment or product (commercial or off the shelf), modified or customized used to increase or improve functional capabilities of people with disabilities," AT can improve both physical function as well as psychological status by promoting self-esteem and vocational independence [1].

AT can be a powerful tool to modify disablement and enable participation in activities of daily living, recreation, and vocational pursuits [2].

Individuals with disability are thought to benefit from AT in multiple dimensions: within their own body (eg, cochlear transplant to enhance hearing), in direct contact (scooter to improve mobility), and in the immediate environment (wheelchair lift adapted van) [3].

The term accessible technology has recently been introduced by the disability community as a "politically correct" more enabling alternative to AT, which emphasizes a person's abilities.

# ■ RELEVANCE TO PHYSIATRY

Since enhancing quality of life for people with disabilities is an overarching goal of physiatry, PM&R physicians must be well versed in AT options in order to better serve patients.

When physical limitations and impairments hamper basic activities of daily living and functional skill, the physiatrist must serve as a vital intermediary to suggest solutions.

## Health Condition, Impairment, Disability and Handicap, and the Enabling Role of AT

When considering the role of AT in enhancing quality of life among people with disabilities, it is important to review several fundamental definitions:

- A health condition is a disease, disorder, injury or trauma (eg, spinal cord injury, multiple sclerosis, or arthritis) that can result in some functional impairment.
- Impairment is an absence or abnormality of body structure or function (eg, reduced strength, amputation, or decreased range of motion).
- A disability is an activity limitation resulting from impairment [eg, reduced strength in an arm (impairment) can prevent a person from using a computer mouse and keyboard].
- A handicap is an activity limitation (social or otherwise) resulting from an underlying disability [eg, a woman who is unable to speak due to aphasia (disability from activity limitation in communication) and resulting in handicap (cannot meaningfully continue to work in a social setting that requires understanding and/or expressing speech) ].

# ■ HEARING IMPAIRMENTS

Hearing impairments constitute a wide range of conditions ranging from mild hearing loss to deafness, and are often serendipitously discovered on the rehabilitation unit or in the outpatient PM&R setting. The incidence and prevalence of hearing impairment rises dramatically with age and its presence can often interfere with the rehabilitation process. Hearing impairments within the occupational setting that are unaddressed can lead to reduced work productivity and decreased efficiency. People who have hearing impairments might be able to hear some sound, but might not be able to understand spoken words. Among adult computer users in the United States, it is estimated that 1 in 5 (21%) have a hearing difficulty.

# ■ GENERAL OVERVIEW OF HEARING

## Assistive Technology for People with Hearing Impairment

Amplification devices have long been the mainstay for people who are hard of hearing.

Amplification devices include hearing aides, amplification telephones and other technologies.

It is important for the clinician to remember that situations often arise in which hearing aides are incapable of providing adequate hearing assistance in noisy environments, hearing might be alternatively remedied by assistive listening devices such as induction loops, infrared, FM or personal amplification devices with directional microphones. With focused listening, these solutions often enhance the users' ability to optimize their experiences in movies, meetings, and seminars. An additional AT solution is TV monitor closed captioning. This device enables hearing impaired or deaf individuals to interact with computers by receiving information visually. With many of these add-on programs, it is possible to adjust sound options and volume.

## Assistive Technology for People Who are Deaf

### General Overview

Individuals who are deaf are often aided by flashing lights and vibrating signals to alert them about ringing phones, doorbells, smoke detectors, and alarm clocks. In addition, vibrating alarm watches and pagers exist. Teletypewriters (TTYs) or text telephones (TTs) also serve an important role. The standard communications protocol for the deaf or hard of hearing is called TT. TTYs or TTs provide the deaf person access to outsiders with normal hearing when used in conjunction with a relay service. With increasing frequency, individuals who are deaf are using text messaging capabilities, to communicate without the need for an intermediary.

## AT for People with Mixed Sensory Impairments (IE, Deafness and Blindness)

Individuals with significant loss of vision and hearing are sometimes referred to as persons who are deaf-blind. Many of the technologies are helpful to people with individual sensory impairments also apply to the deaf-blind population. Adaptations are often necessary. Telephone access can be optimized through the use of TTY's with large print capability. Refreshable Braille displays are another useful technology. People with even partial residual hearing ability can employ amplification phones equipped with Braille markings on large buttons.

To alert people about particular environmental sounds that might occur in the workplace, alerting devices that use vibration, scent, or fan-driven air provide an environmental signal that the phone is ringing or a smoke detector is activated. Alarm clocks equipped with crystal and tactile markings as well as pillow alarms are also available. Computer hardware coupled with software can successfully be deployed to translate television closed caption to TTY tones for reading on a Braille Output. Refreshable Braille displays for computers are an option for people who are blind and a necessity for people who are deaf blind.

# ■ TECHNOLOGY FOR PEOPLE WITH VISUAL IMPAIRMENT INCLUDING LOW VISION

## General Overview

### Technology solutions for people with low vision

For people with low vision, there are many magnification options including handheld optics, monocular glasses and binocular desks. For greater magnification, closed circuit TV (CCTV) may be employed to magnify and enhance images. CCTVs are readily available in a variety of formats including handheld cameras, self-contained units, and virtual reality style helmets.

Computer users with low vision may benefit from screen magnification programs, contrast enhancement applications, as well as cursor enhancement features. Screen color configurations can be altered to match the visual requirements of low vision patients. There are several screen magnification programs that offer an adjunctive speech component, which supplements the visible text with voice interpretation.

## Technology Solutions for the Blind

Blind people often benefit from provision of synthetic speech software that reads text aloud. There are a variety of "read aloud" devices including watches, clocks, thermostats, thermometers, scales, calculators, money identifiers, compasses, and dictionaries.

Additional solutions for the blind include items with Braille or tactile markings including thermostats, telephones, rulers, clocks, calendars, and ATM machines. Computer users can use screen reader programs. For people who prefer not to listen to computer synthesized voice output and would rather obtain Braille output, a refreshable Braille display offers an alternative. Refreshable Braille displays work by employing small retractable pins on a flat panel, which is sometimes attached to the keyboard. The message from the computer screen is sent to this Braille panel.

People who are blind can also benefit from books on tape and radio stations that broadcast aural readings of newspapers.

## The Low Vision and Blind Diabetic: Technologic Solutions

### Blindness: the detrimental effect of failing vision on employment

Failing or completely absent vision or blindness is frequently encountered among diabetics.

Often in the acute rehabilitation setting as well as in the sub-acute and outpatient arena, these diabetic related visual impairments become obvious to the clinician. For those diabetic patients identified in the rehabilitation setting who do not have visual disturbances or other forms of diabetic secondary complications, the rehabilitation team can actually play an essential preventive and educational role in averting the long-term consequences of the disease.

The blind diabetic poses a special rehabilitation challenge because of the critically important goal of balancing optimal management of glycemic control (maintaining sugars at a normal level) while addressing the goal of improving functional status through upgrade of essential activities of daily living.

Blind diabetics who live alone often encounter problems reading their standard glucose meters and drawing up insulin. Often this may lead to worsening of complications down the line.

### Rehabilitation of the blind diabetic: the role of the "talking glucometer"

The role of AT has evolved mightily in enhancing quality of life for people with disabilities, including those with visual deficits resulting from blindness. It is estimated that diabetic patients with visual impairment have approximately 75% reliability in monitoring and managing their sugars. For those who do not have access to helpers such as nurses, caregivers, relatives or volunteers to monitor sugars, a newly introduced "talking glucometer" can provide essential assistance.

The recent introduction of "talking glucometers"—a blood glucose monitoring device that "speaks out" the blood glucose levels, and which verbalizes other data such as the time, date, and historical sugar levels, has revolutionized the lives of people with disabilities.

## Technologic Solutions to Enable Blind & Low Vision Patient's to Use Computers

### Speech technology

The most recent version includes a text-to-speech (TTS) system, which is helpful to blind persons enabling natural intonation even when set at quick speaking rates. Its ability to analyze text one paragraph at a time and is thought to interpret the context more accurately.

### Make the keyboard easier to use

- Press keyboard shortcuts one key at a time.
- Hear a tone when you press CAPS LOCK, NUM LOCK, or SCROLL LOCK.
- Ignore or slow down brief or repeated keystrokes.
- Turn on bounce keys.
- Turn on repeat keys and slow keys.
- Underline keyboard shortcuts and access keys.
- Choose a Dvorak keyboard layout.
- Adjust cursor blink rate.
- Adjust character repeat rate.
- Find keyboard shortcuts.

### Make the mouse easier to use

- Change the color and size of mouse pointers.
- Control the mouse pointer with the keyboard (mouse keys).
- Activate a window by hovering over it with the mouse.
- Change what the mouse pointer looks like.
- A prosthesis for speech and motor impairment [4].

## Motor and Dexterity Impairments

### General Overview

A new and evolving generation of AT has facilitated the use of computers by people with motor disabilities. Modified keyboard size and mouse alternatives are available. To improve typing accuracy, word prediction software reduces keystroke errors by guessing the next word and presenting a list of alternatives. Artificial intelligence enables the software to learn the vocabulary most often uses.

Although voice recognition technology is often a viable alternative, many people with residual function prefer to use whatever residual function exists. Ergonomic configuration of the workstation can optimize access as well. Patients with quadriplegia, stoke, ALS, amputations or CP may benefit from environmental control units. Examples include doors that open with electronic openers and electronic locks. Other examples include coffee makers, lights, call buttons, and TV sets that can be controlled by switch control. Computer access can be optimized by simple switch access or by using on-screen keyboard. For people with NO hand use at all, a chin mouse, a radio signal generated by a headset, an eye gaze unit, or a mouth stick might represent reasonable alternatives.

## AT Solutions to Enhance Computer Use Among Persons with Motor and Dexterity Impairments

Persons in the workplace or newly disabled individuals with motor or dexterity impediments often encounter difficulty using a standard keyboard or mouse or trackpad. Among adult computer users in the United States, it is estimated that 1 in 4 (26%) have dexterity difficulties. Dexterity and coordination difficulty and impairment can be caused by a number of neurological and musculoskeletal conditions including stroke, carpal tunnel, arthritis, stroke, cerebral palsy, Parkinson's disease, multiple sclerosis, loss of limbs or digits, spinal cord injuries, and repetitive stress injury, among others[5].

Individuals with dexterity difficulties and impairments may benefit from the following AT solutions.

- Speech recognition systems, also called voice recognition programs, allow people to give commands and enter data using their voices rather than a mouse or keyboard.
- On-screen keyboard programs provide an image of a standard or modified keyboard on the computer screen. The user selects the keys with an alternative device such as a mouse, touch screen, trackball, joystick, switch, or eye gaze system.
- Keyboard filters can include typing aids, such as word prediction utilities and add-on spelling checkers. These products reduce the required number of keystrokes. Keyboard filters enable users to quickly access the letters they need and to avoid inadvertently selecting keys they don't want.
- Touch screens are devices placed on the computer monitor (or built into it) that allow direct selection or activation of the computer by touching the screen.
- Alternative input devices allow individuals to control their computers through means other than a standard keyboard or pointing device.

## Dexterity Impairments: Alternative Forms of Input

### Hands-on

- Keyboard
- Mouse
- Joystick
- Trackball
- Touch pads
- Touch screen

### Hands-free

- Sips and puffs
- Head movement
- Eye movement
- Touch screen
- Foot movement

## ■ SUMMARY

Assistive technology (AT) has come to play a critically important role in the rehabilitation and functional self-sufficiency of people with disability. With the aging of the population, there is a growing demographic trend toward improved longevity of individuals with chronic disease and associated disabilities and impairments. AT can improve both physical function and psychological status by promoting self-esteem and vocational independence. Amplification devices have long been the mainstay for people who are hard of hearing. Amplification devices include hearing aids, amplification telephones and other technologies. Many of the technologies helpful to people with individual sensory impairments also apply to the deaf-blind population. Adaptations are often necessary. Blind people often benefit from provision of synthetic speech software that reads text aloud. Additional solutions for the blind include items with Braille or tactile markings including thermostats, telephones, rulers, clocks, calendars, and ATM machines. A new and evolving generation of AT has facilitated the use of computers by people with motor disabilities. Modified keyboard size and mouse alternatives are available. Physiatrists can play an important role in taking care of people with disabilities by identifying particular disabilities likely to benefit from AT provision, and by forging collaborative partnerships with patients and by assisting patients in integrating AT into their lives.

## ■ IMPORTANT TERMINOLOGY

assistive technology　辅助技术
hearing impairment　听觉障碍
visual impairment　视觉障碍
motor and dexterity impairment　运动障碍
teletypewriter　电传打印机
text telephones　文字电话
CCTV　闭路电视

## ■ REVIEW QUESTIONS

1. Why assistive technology has come to play a critically important role in the rehabilitation and functional self-sufficiency of persons with disability?
2. What forms of impairments are discussed in this chapter?
3. List some of assistive technologies for people with Hearing Impairment.
4. What are the technology solutions for people with Low Vision?
5. How to enhance computer use among persons with motor and dexterity impairments?

## ■ REFERENCES

1. Young MA, Levi S, Tumanon RC, Desei M, Sokal JO. Independence for people with disabilities: a physician's primer on assistive technology. Md Med. Summer 2000;1(3):28-32.
2. Stiens SA. Personhood, disablement, and mobility technology. In: Gray DB, Quatrano LA, Lieberman M, eds. Designing and Using Assistive Technology: The Human Perspective; 1998:29-49.
3. Boninger ML, Choi H, Johnson K, Young MA, Stiens SA, Sears A. Assistive technologies: catalysts for adaptive function. In: O'Young BJ, Young MA, Stiens SA, eds. PM&R Secrets. 3rd ed. Philadelphia, PA: Mosby Elsevier Press;2008.
4. Chute DL, Quillen S. Computing applications to assist persons with disabilities, 1992. In: Proceedings of the Johns Hopkins National Search for. February 1-5, 1992:124-126. doi:10.1109/CAAPWD.1992.217426.
5. Sears A, Young M, Feng J. Physical Disabilities and Computing Techonologies: An Analysis of Impairments. In: The Human-Computer Interaction Handbook: Fundamentals, Evolving Technologies and Emerging Applications (2nd ed.). Sears A, Jacko J, eds. Florida: CRC Press, 2007:829-852.

（刘四海）

# *BLADDER MANAGEMENT*

## ■ INTRODUCTION

Voiding dysfunction is a common sequela following many neurologic processes. It can be classified based on presenting symptoms and confirmed using urodynamic testing. Untreated, a neurogenic bladder can lead to a variety of complications including urinary tract infections, renal calculi, renal failure, poor therapy participation, and poor reintegration into society. The proper diagnosis and management of a neurogenic bladder is paramount to rehabilitation.

## ■ ANATOMY OF THE URINARY TRACT

The urinary system is divided into an upper and lower urinary tract. The upper urinary tract consists of the kidneys and ureters. The lower urinary tract consists of the bladder and the urethra [1].

### Upper Urinary Tract

The kidney can be further subdivided into 2 portions: the renal parenchyma and the renal pelvis. The function of the renal parenchyma is to secrete, concentrate, and excrete urine into the renal pelvis. At the ureteropelvic junction, the renal pelvis narrows to become the ureter [1,2]. From here, the ureter functions as a conduit for urine to flow into the bladder. There are 3 areas of physiologic narrowing along the ureter: the ureteropelvic junction, the crossing point of the iliac artery, and the ureterovesical junction. These areas are of clinical importance when considering postrenal obstruction [1,2]. The ureteropelvic junction is the point where the ureter opens to the bladder. It allows urine to flow into the bladder while effectively creating a 1-way valve preventing urine reflux into the ureter. The ureteropelvic junction accomplishes this task by traversing obliquely between the muscular and submucosal layers of the bladder. In times of high intravesical pressures, these layers pinch the ureter, preventing urine reflux. Periods of sustained, high intravesical pressures can result in a physiologic postrenal obstruction [1-3].

### Lower Urinary Tract

The bladder can be divided into the detrusor and trigone [3,4]. The detrusor is a syncytium of smooth muscle fibers that interweave each other. As these fibers approach the bladder neck, they form 3 distinct layers arranged in a circular fashion. This arrangement allows them to act as a functional sphincter. The trigone extends from the ureteral orifices to the bladder neck on the inferior base of the bladder [1,2].

The urethra differs in both women and men. In women, the urethra is shorter and contains an inner longitudinal and outer semicircular layer of smooth muscle. In men, the urethra is surrounded by the corpus spongiosum [1].

## Urethral Sphincters

The urethra has 2 sphincters: the internal and the external sphincter. The internal sphincter is not a true anatomic sphincter. Rather, it is formed from the circular arrangement of bladder smooth muscle fibers. The voluntary, external sphincter differs in both men and women. In men, the striated muscle fibers run from the base of the bladder to the membranous urethra. In women, the striated muscle fibers circle the upper two-thirds of the urethra [2].

## Urine Transport

Urine is propelled from the kidneys to the bladder by the proximal tubular filtration pressure and the peristalsis of the calices, renal pelvis, and ureter. Ureteral dilation may impede efficient peristalsis which, overtime, may lead to hydronephrosis [3,4].

## ■ NEUROANATOMY AND NEUROPHYSIOLOGY OF THE URINARY SYSTEM

Urine retention and micturition is the result of a complex interplay of cerebral, parasympathetic, sympathetic, and somatic signals to the bladder, urinary sphincters, and urethra. It can be described in terms of an efferent and afferent system [2].

### Efferent System

The **parasympathetic** efferent nervous supply functions to promote micturition. Parasympathetic impulses begin in the intermediolateral grey matter of the second, third, and fourth sacral segments (S2-S4). They exit the cord as preganglionic fibers in the ventral roots and travel within the **pelvic nerve**. These preganglionic fibers synapse adjacent to or within the detrusor muscle stimulating muscle contraction by releasing acetylcholine [1-3].

The **sympathetic** efferent nervous supply functions to promote urine retention. Sympathetic impulses begin in the intermediolateral grey matter of the 11th thoracic segment extending to the second lumbar segment (T11-L2). They exit the cord and quickly synapse on the lumbar sympathetic paravertebral ganglia [5,6]. Postganglionic fibers travel within the hypogastric nerve and synapse on α- and b-adrenergic receptors within the bladder and urethra where they release norepinephrine [4-6]. α- and β-adrenergic receptors are strategically placed in the bladder and rethra [4]. Stimulation of β-receptors causes smooth muscle relaxation within the superior portion of the bladder. Stimulation of α-receptors in the base of the bladder and prostatic urethra causes smooth muscle contraction [4]. Together, this allows for increased bladder distention and sphincter constriction allowing for increased urine retention [5-8].

### Somatic

**Somatic** efferent nervous supply travels from the first through the fourth sacral segments (S1-S4) within the **pudendal nerve**, ultimately synapsing on the external sphincter. Activation of the external sphincter promotes contraction and thus, voluntary urine retention.

### Afferent System

The main function of afferent system is to receive sensory input from the bladder to stimulate a voiding response. There are 2 types of afferent fibers: myelinated AδA-fibers and unmyelinated C-fibers [4]. The myelinated Aδ-fibers are the predominant fibers involved in voiding and respond to bladder distention.

Unmyelinated C-fibers are activated by cold or chemical irritation of the bladder wall. Unmyelinated C-fibers are commonly termed "silent C-fibers" under normal circumstances because they do not respond to bladder distention [3,4,9].

### Central Nervous System Input

The central pontine micturition center modulates micturition. Through its connections with the spinal cord, it may send either excitatory or inhibitory impulses to coordinate detrusor contraction and sphincter relaxation. This enables normal urination.

# VOIDING PHYSIOLOGY

Micturition is completely under voluntary control. The detrusor response to stretch can be inhibited just as detrusor contraction can be voluntarily initiated. Micturition consists of 2 phases: a filling (storage) phase and an emptying (voiding) phase [3,4].

### Filling (Storage) Phase

The filling phase is predominantly controlled by the action of the sympathetic nervous system. During filling, there is very little rise in intravesical pressure due to bladder distention [4]. This is coupled with an increase in urethral sphincter contraction. Normal end filling pressures are between 0 and 6 cmH$_2$O [3,4]. When they reach levels greater than 15 cmH$_2$O, the elastic properties of detrusor are exceeded [3,4]. The resulting discomfort, under normal circumstances, cannot be tolerated [3,4].

### Emptying (Voiding) Phase

The emptying phase is predominately controlled by the action of the parasympathetic nervous system. The loss of sympathetic input to the urethral sphincter causes urethral relaxation. This is followed by the parasympathetically mediated detrusor contraction. The urethral sphincter remains open during voiding and there is no increase in intraabdominal pressure.

# BLADDER DYSFUNCTION AFTER NERVOUS SYSTEM DAMAGE

Neurogenic bladder dysfunction describes abnormal bladder and urethral function due to lesions affecting their innervation, either within the central nervous system or the lower urinary tract peripheral nerves.

Neurological conditions can alter bladder and urethral function by altering:

- detrusor function
- striated muscle sphincter activity
- smooth muscle sphincter activity
- bladder and urethral sensation

Specifically, Limin Liao proposed a more integrated classification system to better identify upper and lower urinary tract dysfunction [13].

# CAUSES AND MECHANISMS OF NEUROGENIC BLADDER DYSFUNCTION

Conditions that cause neurogenic bladder dysfunction include dementia, cerebrovascular accidents, Parkinson's disease, multiple sclerosis, spinal cord injuries, spina bifida, cauda equina syndrome and Fowler's syndrome.

Detrusor overactivity after suprapontine damage is different from that after spinal cord injury (SCI). Suprapontine damage leads to removal of tonic inhibition, resulting in involuntary detrusor contractions. SCI-related detrusor overactivity is caused by a segmental reflex at the level of the sacral cord mediated by capsaicin-sensitive C-fibre afferents. After an acute SCI, there is initially a period of spinal shock during which the detrusor is hypo- or hyper-contractile and associated with poor bladder emptying, followed by spontaneous contractions after about 6 weeks. Sensitisation of 'silent' C-fibres after SCI may involve changes in central synaptic connections and peripheral afferent receptors. For example, β-receptors in the upper bladder have been found to be reduced after SCI [4]. Injury to the suprasacral spinal pathway results in detrusor urethral sphincter dyssynergia (DSD), leading to voiding difficulties and incomplete emptying of the bladder. Incomplete emptying may also result from impaired parasympathetic drive due to descending bulbospinal tract injury. Lesions of the sacral or infrasacral pathways cause voiding dysfunction with poorly sustained or absent detrusor contractions and/or non-relaxation of the sphincter.

# ■ CLINICAL ASSESSMENT

Diagnosis of neuro-urological disorders should be based on a comprehensive assessment of neurological and non-neurological conditions. Initial assessment should include a detailed history, physical examination, and urinalysis.

## Neurologic History and Physical Exam

A thorough history is important to the diagnosis of a neurogenic bladder to differentiate between urinary retention and incontinence. Signs of retention include decreased stream, intermittent stream, sense of incomplete urination, and straining. Signs of urinary incontinence include frequency, urgency, and a feeling of wetness.

A thorough history also includes a complete review of systems as well as past medical history. Reversible causes of retention/incontinence in the elderly can be summarized by the mnemonic: DIAPPERS [10].

D-Delirium

I-Infection

A-Atrophic vaginitis, urethritis

P-Pharmaceuticals

P-Psychological

E-Endocrine

R-Reduced mobility

S-Stool impaction

Portions of the physiatric history of particular importance in the diagnosis and management of neurogenic bladder include: hand function, dressing skills, sitting balance, the ability to perform transfers, and the ability to ambulate [4].

A thorough neurologic exam must be completed with attention paid to motor or sensory deficits and signs of hyperreflexia.

## Urodynamic Tests

Bladder diaries are considered a valuable diagnostic tool in patients with neuro-urological disorders. A bladder diary should be recorded for at least two to three days.

Uroflowmetry and ultrasound assessment of post-void residual should be repeated at least two or three times in patients able to void.

Invasive urodynamic studies comprise mandatory assessment tools to determine the exact type of neuro-urological disorder. Video-urodynamics combines filling cystometry and pressure flow studies with radiological imaging. Currently, video-urodynamics is considered to provide the most comprehensive information for evaluating neuro-urological disorders. One commonly used method of urodynamic testing is the waterfill urodynamic study. It evaluates urine storage, transport, and voiding by examining intravesical, urethral sphincter, and intraabdominal pressures in addition to urine flow rate (Figure 12.1) [3].

Urodynamic investigations can characterize the nature of the detrusor and sphincteric abnormality to:

- identify those patients who are at risk of upper tract damage.
- formulate the best treatment strategies to achieve efficient bladder emptying and continence and reduce the incidence of urinary tract infections and autonomic dysreflexia.

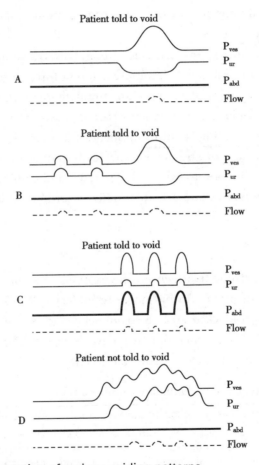

**Figure 12.1**  Schematic representation of various voiding patterns.
A. Normal. B. Uninhibited contractions occur with filling. The sphincter is attempting to inhibit contractions. Patient has a normal voiding phase. C. No bladder contractions. Rises in bladder pressure result from rises in abdominal pressure (ie, Valsalva voiding). D. Uninhibited contractions occur with simultaneous sphincter contractions (ie, detrusor sphincter dyssynergia).
$P_{abd}$-intraabdominal pressure; $P_{ur}$-urethral sphincter pressure; $P_{ves}$-intravesical pressure.

# ■ MANAGEMENT OF NEUROGENIC BLADDER DYSFUNCTION

In the management of neurogenic lower urinary tract function, there are two goals. The primary goal is to protect the upper urinary tract, ie, to achieve low intravesical pressure and to maintain minimal post-void residual urine. The secondary goal is to improve quality of life and/or achieve continence.

Further considerations are the patient's disability, cost-effectiveness, technical complexity, and possible complications.

## Conservative Treatment and Behavioral Modifications

Patients with urinary incontinence may benefit from a scheduled voiding regimen (timed voiding). Bladder training can be accomplished by progressively increasing the time between voids by 10 to 15 minutes every 2 to 5 days until a reasonable interval between voiding is obtained. In other cases, diapers may be used as a backup to other modifications[3].

The external urine collection device is mainly a condom type urine collection device for men, and the urine collection device for women is still far from ideal, and urine pads are often still needed. The urine collector is suitable for various types of urinary incontinence patients. The problem that needs to be solved is that it is not easy to fix and slip off, and improper use can cause complications such as infection, ulcer, necrosis and skin allergies.

Manual assisted voiding includes Crede manual voiding, Valsalva voiding, and trigger point voiding. Both the Crede maneuver and the Valsalva voiding use external force to squeeze the bladder to facilitate emptying. The essence of trigger point urination is to stimulate low-reflex urination, but the premise is to have a complete low-neural reflex arc, and patients with detrusor no reflex are not suitable for trigger point urination. Triggered reflex voiding is not recommended as there is a risk of pathologically elevated bladder pressures. Only in the case of absence, or surgically reduced outlet obstruction it may be an option. Bladder compression techniques to expel urine (Credé) and voiding by abdominal straining (Valsalva maneuvre) create high pressures and are potentially hazardous, and their use should be discouraged.

## Medical therapy

Antimuscarinic drugs are the first-line treatment for neurogenic detrusor overactivity, increasing bladder capacity and reducing episodes of urinary incontinence secondary to NDO by inhibiting parasympathetic pathways. For voiding symptoms, α-blockers are also recommended to reduce bladder outlet resistance. Moreover, avoid prescribing parasympathomimetics for underactive detrusor[11]. For a comprehensive list of important medications used in bladder management, refer to Table 12.1.

**TABLE 12.1** ▪ Pharmacologic interventions for bladder management

| Agent | Indication | Mechanism of Action | Starting Dose | Side Effects | Comments |
|---|---|---|---|---|---|
| Tolterodine | Urge incontinence | Anticholinergic Competitive antagonist of muscarinic receptors | Regular release: 2 mg PO q12 h Long acting: 2mg PO daily | Dry eyes, dry mouth, disorientation, headache, dizziness, constipation | Dose adjustment may be needed in pts. Taking CYP 3A4 inhibitors Contraindications: Gastric retention, urinary retention, angle closure glaucoma |
| Oxybutynin | Urge incontinence | Antispasmotic. Anticholinergic | Regular release: 5 mg PO 2-3 times/d Long acting: 5 mg PO daily Transdermal: 3. 9 mg/d patch q 3-4 days | Dry eyes, dry mouth, disorientation, headache, dizziness, constipation | Transdermal atch may contain conducting metal Contraindications: Gastric retention, urinary retention, angle closure glaucoma |

Continued

| Agent | Indication | Mechanism of Action | Starting Dose | Side Effects | Comments |
|-------|-----------|---------------------|---------------|--------------|----------|
| Imipramine | Urge Incontinence | Tricyclic antidepressant | 25 mg PO at bedtime | Agitation, anxiety, confusion, QT prolongation | Contraindications: Anticholinergic action Concurrent or recent use of MAO inhibitors |
| Tamsulosin | Sphincter spasticity | α1-adrenergic blocker | 0.4 mg PO daily | Hypotension, orthostasis dizziness, somnolence, weakness | Contraindications: Severe sulfonamide allergy |

## Minimal Invasive Treatment

Intermittent catheterization using aseptic technique is the preferred treatment for patients unable to void, requires thorough instruction and should be preferred to indwelling catheterization whenever possible. Indwelling urinary catheters are associated with a high risk of meatal ulceration and a high incidence of urinary tract infections (UTIs). Patients with urinary catheters may have asymptomatic bacteriuria that should not be treated unless a stone forming organism is identified (most commonly Proteus sp. but also Serratia sp. and Klebsiella sp.) [12]. See the next section for specifics on intermittent catheterization.

When antimuscarinic therapy is ineffective, botulinum toxin injection into the detrusor muscle is recommended to reduce neurogenic detrusor overactivity.

## Surgical Interventions

In adults with severe neurogenic bladder, surgical management is sometimes necessary. Indications for surgical intervention include severe detrusor hyperreflexia, bladder wall compliance, continued upper tract deterioration despite aggressive pharmacotherapy, behavioral treatment, or modalities. Surgical interventions include augmentation cystoplasty, artificial sphincter placement, subarachnoid block, sphincterotomy, cordectomy, and anterior or anteroposterior rhizotomy [3].

## ■ COMPLICATIONS

Complications of a neurogenic bladder include urinary tract infections, vesicoureteral reflux, hydronephrosis, renal calculi, renal deterioration, and bladder cancer. Since the renal failure is the main mortality factor in SCI patients who survive the trauma, impairment of upper urinary tract function requires particular attention. Detrusor overactivity in combination with DSD can result in high intravesical pressures, which in turn can lead to morphological changes in the bladder wall such as trabeculations and (pseudo-)diverticula, and increase the risk of upper urinary tract complications such as vesico-uretero-renal reflux, hydronephrosis, renal impairment, and eventually end-stage renal disease. Regular and proper bladder emptying through techniques like intermittent catheterization can reduce the risk of these complications.

## ■ REHABILITATION MANAGEMENT OF BLADDER DYSFUNCTION

Patients require bladder function rehabilitation once the primary cause of the neurogenic disorder has been controlled. As bladder dysfunction usually persists for a long time, in addition to behavioural therapy and bladder training, intermittent catheterization is also recommended for bladder management prior to resumption of voluntary voiding because of the minimal complications. However, patient satisfaction and compliance need to be considered and shared decision making is imperative. On the other hand, bladder rehabilitation techniques, such as electrical stimulation, biofeedback, rTMS (repetitive transcranial magnetic stimulation:), etc., will help to re-establish bladder function in patients with neuro-urological symptoms.

## Intermittent Catheterization

Intermittent catheterization (IC) is a technique used to regularly empty the bladder by inserting a catheter through the urethra. It was introduced as a safer alternative to continuous indwelling catheters, which destroy the aseptic state of the bladder and urethra and can easily lead to urinary tract infections. IC was first proposed in 1947 by Cuttmann for patients with spinal cord injuries, reducing infection risk and mimicking natural bladder function.

IC is typically started 1 to 2 weeks after spinal cord injury surgery, and patients are taught the procedure.

For patients with bladder detrusor weakness and higher residual urine volume, long-term intermittent catheterization is necessary. Family members can be taught to perform the procedure for regular use. IC is generally preferred over indwelling catheters due to its lower risk of complications, such as bladder stones and urinary tract infections. However, it may not be suitable for obese patients, women with adductor spasm, noncompliant patients, or patients who do not receive lasting help, requiring the use of an indwelling catheter.

## Electrical and Magnetic Stimulation Method

To date, bladder rehabilitation techniques are mainly based on electrical or magnetic stimulation. Strong contraction of the urethral sphincter and/or pelvic floor, as well as anal dilatation, manipulation of the genital region, and physical activity inhibit micturition in a reflex manner. The first mechanism is affected by activation of efferent nerve fibres, and the latter ones are produced by activation of afferent fibres. Electrical stimulation of the pudendal nerve afferents strongly and inhibits the micturition reflex and detrusor contraction. This stimulation might then support the restoration of the balance between excitatory and inhibitory inputs at the spinal or supraspinal level[11].

Peripheral temporary electrostimulation, including tibial nerve stimulation and transcutaneous electrical nerve stimulation (TENS), might be effective and safe for treating neurogenic LUT dysfunction, but more reliable evidence from well-designed RCTs is required to reach definitive conclusions. Combining active neuromuscular electrical stimulation with Pelvic Floor Muscle Training (PFMT) and EMG biofeedback can achieve a substantial reduction of neuro-urological symptoms in MS patients. Intravesical electrostimulation can increase bladder capacity and improve bladder filling sensation in patients with incomplete SCI or myelomeningocele (MMC). In patients with neurogenic detrusor underactivity, intravesical electrostimulation may also improve voiding and reduce residual volume. Repetitive transcranial magnetic stimulation: Although improvement of neuro-urological symptoms has been described in PD, SCI and MS patients, this technique is still under investigation.

## ■ SUMMARY

This section explores various aspects of the urinary system and neurogenic bladder dysfunction, including the anatomy and function of the upper and lower urinary tracts, and the mechanisms involved in urine retention and micturition. The dynamic interplay between various signaling pathways and the central nervous system that orchestrates the delicate balance in regulating bladder and urethral function. Going beyond the surface, this section explores the stages of micturition and the profound implications of neurogenic bladder dysfunction resulting from lesions within the central nervous system or peripheral nerves. By listing several conditions that can lead to neurogenic bladder dysfunction, this section emphasizes that the diagnosis of neuro-urological disorders requires a comprehensive assessment. The initial assessment includes a detailed history, physical examination, urinalysis and urodynamic studies such as bladder diaries, uroflowmetry and invasive urodynamic studies to determine the nature of the neuro-urological disorder and to guide appropriate management strategies. The management of neurogenic bladder dysfunction offers a plethora of options, ranging from conservative approaches to medical and surgical interventions. If the neurogenic bladder is not well managed, it leads to various complications including urinary tract infections, vesicoureteral reflux, hydronephrosis, renal calculi, renal deterioration and bladder cancer, with renal failure being a significant mortality factor in SCI patients. This section introduces us to the concept of intermittent catheterization, a safe and effective technique for emptying the bladder. Intermittent catheterization reduces upper urinary tract complications compared with indwelling catheters, but its applicability may vary depending on individual patient factors. Finally, this section highlights the potential of bladder rehabilitation techniques such as electrical and magnetic stimulation. However, it should be noted that further research is essential to fully validate the potential of these innovative methods.

## ■ IMPORTANT TERMINOLOGY

adrenergic receptors    肾上腺素能受体

catheter related infection    导管相关感染

clean intermittent catheterization    清洁间歇导尿

denervation hypersensitivity    去神经高敏状态

detrusor sphincter dyssynergia    逼尿肌括约肌协同失调

parasympathetic    副交感神经

pelvic nerve    盆腔神经

pudendal nerve    阴部神经

somatic    躯体的

urethral sphincter    尿道括约肌

urine flow rate    尿流率

urine retention    尿潴留

urodynamic    尿动力学

## ■ REVIEW QUESTIONS

1. What are the components of the urinary system and their functions?
2. Explain the two phases of micturition and the role of sympathetic and parasympathetic control.
3. What causes neurogenic bladder dysfunction, and how does it affect detrusor function and sphincter activity?
4. How is the diagnosis of neuro-urological disorders performed, and what assessment tools are used?
5. What are the primary goals in the management of neurogenic bladder dysfunction, and what treatment options are available?
6. What are the potential complications associated with a neurogenic bladder?
7. Describe the benefits and significance of intermittent catheterization compared to indwelling catheters.

# ■ REFERENCES

1.  Agur AMR, Lee MD, Grant JCB. Grant's Atlas of Anatomy. 10th ed. Baltimore, MD: Lippincott Williams & Wilkins; 1999: 184-188.

2.  Standring S. Grays Anatomy: The Anatomical Basis of Clinical Practice. 39th ed. Edinburgh, UK: Elsevier; 2005:1269-1294.

3.  Delisa J, Gans B. Rehabilitation Medicine: Principles and Practice. 3rd ed. Philadelphia, PA: Lippincott-Raven; 1999:1073-1094.

4.  Kirshblum S, Campagnolo D, DeLisa J. Spinal Cord Medicine. Philadelphia, PA: Lippincott Williams & Wilkins; 2002:181-203.

5.  Fletcher TF, Bradley WE. Neuroanatomy of the bladder-urethra. J Urol. 1978;119:153-160.

6.  Benson GS, McConnell JA, Wood JG. Adrenergic innervation of the human bladder body.J Urol. 1979;122:189-191.

7.  Elbadawi A. Autonomic muscular innervation of the vesical outlet and its role in micturation. In: Hinman F Jr, ed. Benign Prostatic Hypertrophy. New York: Springer-Verlag; 1983:330-348.

8.  Brunstock G. The changing face of autonomic neurotransmission. Acta Physiol Scand. 1986;126:67-91.

9.  De Groat WC. Mechanism underlying the recovery of lower urinary tract function following spinal cord injury. Paraplegia. 1995;33:493-505.

10. Resnick NM, Yalla SV. Management of urinary incontinence in the elderly. N Engl J Med. 1985;313:800-805.

11. Groen J, Pannek J, Castro DD. Summary of European Association of Urology (EAU) Guidelines on Neuro-Urology. European urology. 2016;69(2), 324-333.

12. Favazza T, Midha M, Martin J, Grob M. Factors influencing bladder stone formation in spinal cord injury.J Spinal Cord Med. 2004;27(3):252-254.

13. Liao Limin, Fan Zhang, Guoqing Chen. New grading system for upper urinary tract dilation using magnetic resonance urography in patients with neurogenic bladder. BMC urology. 2014;14.1: 1-7.

（袁　华）

# BOWEL MANAGEMENT (NEUROGENIC)

Neurogenic bowel (NBw) refers to the loss of normal bowel function due to the loss of direct somatic sensory or motor control with or without impaired sympathetic and parasympathetic innervation. Spinal cord injury (SCI) is most frequently associated with NBw, but there are multiple neurological conditions that can cause this impairment. These include stroke, amyotrophic lateral sclerosis, traumatic brain injury, multiple sclerosis, pelvic surgery, vaginal delivery, polyneuropathies, diabetes, conus or cauda equina lesions, muscular dystrophy, and even chronic straining. Patients can experience a variety of problems such as paralytic ileus, constipation, diarrhea, incontinence, gastric ulcers, gastroesophageal reflux disease, autonomic dysreflexia, and nausea to name a few. Bowel dysfunction can greatly affect a patient's quality of life as social incontinence is depressing and humiliating. After a complete work up and diagnosis, establishing an effective bowel program that prevents these complications can allow patients to be socially and vocationally active.

Normal defecation requires intact intrinsic enteric nervous system (ENS) and extrinsic somatic and autonomic innervation, which include sympathetic and parasympathetic systems. The ENS extends from esophagus to anus and coordinates colonic wall movement, which mixes and advances stool from segment to segment. It consists of 2 layers, the submucosal Meissner's plexus and the intramuscular myenteric Auerbach's plexus. Except in neuropathies, the ENS remains intact, even without autonomic and somatic innervation, and can be used for bowel habit training. The extrinsic colonic innervation consists of the autonomic and somatic systems. When stimulated, the sympathetic nervous system promotes fecal storage by enhancing anal tone and inhibiting colonic contractions via the superior and inferior mesenteric (T9-T12) and hypogastric (T12-L3) nerves. The parasympathetic system enhances colonic motility from the esophagus to colonic splenic flexure via the vagus nerve. The pelvic nerve (also called the nervi ergentes or inferior splanchnics) carries parasympathetic fibers from S2-S4 spinal cord levels to the descending colon and rectum. The vagus, pelvic, and hypogastric nerves carry the afferent and efferent fibers, which complete the reflex arcs and modulate peristalsis. Finally, the external anal sphincter (EAS) and pelvic floor are somatically innervated by the pudendal nerve (S2-S4) [1-3].

Normal colon physiology has 4 stages: storage, propulsion, continence, and defecation. Storage occurs as long as colonic pressure is less than that of the anal sphincter. Propulsion is coordinated by the ENS, chemically by neurotransmitters and hormones and myogenically. When the intestinal wall is stretched and dilated, the myenteric plexus causes the muscles above the dilation to constrict and muscles below to relax to allow propulsion. Vagal, gastrocolic, rectocolic, and spinal cord mediated reflexes via the pelvic nerve also increase motility and propulsive peristalsis. Continence is maintained by the anal sphincter mechanism. Sympathetically mediated tonic contraction of the internal anal sphincter (IAS) occurs while the puborectalis and EAS normal resting state is in tonic contraction. Of note, IAS tone is inhibited with rectal dilation by stool or digital stimulation. Defecation occurs by voluntary controlled contraction of abdominal musculature and relaxation of EAS and puborectalis muscles. The urge to defecate is due to stretching of the rectum and puborectalis, and one can retain stool by EAS voluntary contraction [1,2].

NBw diagnosis is done by physical exam and divided into reflexic, upper motor neuron (UMN), and areflexic, lower motor neuron (LMN) bowel. UMN bowel is typically due to neurological lesions in and above the conus medullaris, while LMN is due to lesions below conus, such as cauda equina syndrome. The key physical exam components include a rectal exam and all sacral reflexes such as anal tone and anocutaneous and bulbocavernosus reflexes. UMN diagnosis requires an intact reflex arc of the rectosigmoid and pelvic floor. These patients have normal or increased anal sphincter tone, intact anocutaneous reflexes (anal wink), and bulbocavernosus reflexes. LMN or areflexic bowel patients have reduced to no anal tone, absent anal wink, and bulbocavernosus reflexes, and the anus appears flattened due to tone loss [2]. These are important distinctions to make as the bowel program and treatment plans are very different.

Any patient who has risk factors for developing NBw and gastrointestinal (GI) complaints should have a comprehensive and systematic history, physical exam, and any additional diagnostic testing. The patient history should include the following elements: new and chronic medical conditions, recent surgeries or vaginal deliveries, premorbid and current bowel function, frequency, timing, stool consistency, medication use, accidents, and whether they have a current scheduled bowel program. What are the patient's symptoms such as abdominal distention, early satiety, nausea, difficult or unplanned evacuations, rectal bleeding, diarrhea, and pain? How does this affect patient's ability to perform activities of daily living, to do leisure activities, and carry out work responsibilities? What is their nutrition—daily fluid intake, constipating foods/meds, lactose intolerance, amount of daily fiber, calories, and meal frequency [1-3]?

A full functional history to evaluate the patient's activity level, knowledge, cognition, and ability to perform bowel care should be obtained to determine the individual's ability to complete care independently, at a modified independent level, or by directing a caregiver safely and effectively. This assessment should include the following elements: ability to learn and to direct others, sitting tolerance and balance, upper extremity strength and proprioception, coordination, spasticity, transfer skills, actual and potential risks to skin, anthropometric measurements, home accessibility, and equipment needs [1-3].

A physical examination should include the following: a thorough neurological exam, a complete abdominal assessment, including palpation along the course of the colon, a rectal exam, and all sacral reflexes (anal tone, anal wink, bulbocavernosus reflexes). An ASIA exam should be performed in traumatic SCI patients. Stool testing for occult blood should begin at age 50. After a complete physical exam, a UMN or LMN NBw diagnosis can be made [1,2].

After taking the history, conducting physical exam, diagnosing the type of NBw, and considering the patient's overall functional status, an individualized, patient-centered bowel program should be designed. The program should provide predictable and effective elimination to reduce evacuation problems and GI complaints and prevent medical complications, and it must be reviewed and revised as needed throughout the continuum of care [1]. Differences in bowel programs will be primarily due to the cause (reflexic UMN bowel vs areflexic LMN bowel) as well as patient preference. An effective program must include all of the following components: the type, dose, and timing of a rectal stimulant; goal consistency of stool; frequency of bowel care; optimal scheduling; optimal positioning; and appropriate fluid, fiber, and caloric intake. In LMN bowel, the reflex arcs are not intact. The goal stool consistency is firm formed, which can be manually evacuated easily. Patients are taught to assume side lying or upright position and perform gentle Valsalva with manual evacuation to be done once or twice daily [1-3]. UMN NBw care programs differ in that these patients have bowel reflex arcs, on which a chemical stimulant will work, and need to have soft-formed stools [1-3]. They assume the same position, place the stimulant on the rectal mucosa, and wait for it to activate. Some patients will need to use assistive techniques or repeat the stimulation until evacuation occurs.

NBw management in the home and community needs close attention as well. Appropriate bowel care adaptive equipment should be prescribed based on the patient's functional status, need for a caregiver, and environment. Adequate social and emotional support should be available to help individuals manage actual or potential disabilities and handicaps associated with NBw. All aspects of a patient's bowel program should be easily simulated in the patient's home and other common settings. Patient and caregiver knowledge of, performance of, and confidence in the NBw management program should also be assessed [3].

To evaluate effectiveness, the following variables should be documented with all NBw programs: GI symptoms, incontinence, evacuation frequency, time of day, position, stool color, consistency, amount, mechanical stimulation techniques, pharmacological regimen, any adverse side effects, time from rectal stimulation until completed defecation, total time for completion of bowel care, diet, fluid intake, and level of activity. When a patient reports strict adherence to one's bowel program but complains of continuing incontinence, GI symptoms, or other problems, one should consider all aspects of the program mentioned above for changes. Current guidelines recommend that a bowel regimen be completed 3 to 5 bowel care cycles before changes are made, unless the patient is having medical complications. Be sure to change only one element at a time to ensure effectiveness [3].

Finally, patient education on the rationale, goals, and techniques of bowel management is vital for adherence and independence. A formal education program must be comprehensive and well organized and involves the following topics: anatomy; basic bowel physiology and causes of NBw; long-term management of bowel dysfunction; safe use of assistive devices; the importance of timing, positioning, and regularity; and preventing complications such as diarrhea, impaction, hemorrhoids, rectal prolapse, obstruction and perforation, diverticula, colon cancer, and autonomic dysreflexia in SCI patients. The content and timing of such programs will depend on medical stability, readiness to learn, and other related factors [3].

## ■ SUMMARY

This section discusses neurogenic bowel (NBw), which is the loss of normal bowel function due to neurological conditions such as spinal cord injury, stroke, and multiple sclerosis. Patients with NBW can experience various problems, such as constipation, diarrhea, and incontinence, which significantly affect their quality of life. We also explain the anatomy and physiology of normal bowel function, including the intrinsic enteric nervous system and extrinsic somatic and autonomic innervation. Diagnosis of NBw is performed through physical examination and is divided into reflexic, upper motor neuron (UMN), and areflexic, lower motor neuron (LMN) bowel. An individualized, patient-centered bowel program should be designed to provide predictable and effective elimination, reduce evacuation problems and GI complaints, and prevent medical complications. The program must include the type, dose, and timing of a rectal stimulant, optimal scheduling and positioning, appropriate fluid, fiber, and caloric intake, and goal consistency of stool. Patient education on the rationale, goals, and techniques of bowel management is also vital for adherence and independence.

## ■ IMPORTANT TERMINOLOGY

neurogenic bowel　神经源性肠道
intrinsic nervous system　内在神经系统
enteric nervous system　肠神经系统
autonomic nervous system　自主神经系统
sympathetic nervous system　交感神经系统

parasympathetic nervous system　副交感神经系统
upper motor neuron bowel　上运动神经元肠道
lower motor neuron bowel　下运动神经元肠道

## ■ REVIEW QUESTIONS

1.  What is the role of nervous system in regulating normal defecation?
2.  What are the stages of normal colon function in defecation?
3.  What are the differences between reflexic UMN bowel and areflexic LMN bowel?
4.  What are the properties of a formal education program used in the treatment of NBw?

## ■ REFERENCES

1.  Braddom RL. Physical Medicine and Rehabilitation. 3rd ed.
2.  Delisa JA. Physical Medicine and Rehabilitation: Principles and Practice. 4th ed. Vol. 2. 2005:1641-1649.
3.  Paralyzed Veterans of America. Neurogenic Bowel Management in Adults with Spinal Cord Injury.

（廖维靖）

# BURN INJURIES REHABILITATION

## ■ INITIAL RESUSCITATION AND ASSESSMENT OF INJURY ACUTE MANAGEMENT

The primary survey of an individual with a major burn is carried out as soon as the patient is brought to a safe place. The cervical spine should be stabilized if there is any suspicion for a neck injury. The airway should be assessed and the presence of any singed facial hair or carbon particles in the nose or sputum should be noted, as these signs suggest an inhalation injury. Early intubation should be considered in those with likely inhalation injuries, as it may be difficult to intubate them later as airway edema develops. 100% oxygen should be administered with close monitoring of pulse oximetry. Two large-bore intravenous lines should be established, preferably at sites away from burned areas. If a patient is profoundly hypotensive on initial assessment, he/she should be assessed for cardiac abnormalities and for blood loss. The patient's level of responsiveness should be assessed using the Glasgow Coma Scale, and a thorough examination for concomitant injuries should be carried out. Environmental control is necessary to prevent hypothermia. Circumferential burns are usually treated with emergent escharotomies to prevent osteofascial compartment syndrome and, when involving the trunk, to allow adequate chest movement for breathing.

### Assessing the Severity of Burns

#### Burn Depth

Superficial burns, like most sunburns, involve only the epidermis. They may be quite painful but heal on their own. Partial-thickness burns involve both the epidermis and dermis. They may be superficial or deep. Superficial partial-thickness burns should blanch with pressure and should also heal on their own. Deep partial-thickness burns extend down to the subdermal tissue. They are associated with hypertrophic scarring and often require grafting. Lastly, full-thickness burns involve the epidermis, dermis, and subdermal tissue and may be less painful than more superficial burns due to damaged nerve endings. These burns also damage the sweat glands and can result in the impaired ability to regulate body temperature. Young children and the elderly are at risk for deeper burns due to their relatively thin dermal layers.

#### Total Body Surface Area

The percent of the total body surface area (TBSA) burned in adults can be determined using the Wallace rule of nines. The head and arm each represent 9% TBSA, and each leg represents 18% TBSA. The anterior and posterior trunk each represent 18% TBSA. The perineum represents the remaining 1%. The Lund and Browder chart is used to determine percent TBSA in children, as it is necessary to account for age-related differences in head and body proportions. Superficial burns are not included in the calculation of the percent of TBSA.

### Fluid Resuscitation

Fluid resuscitation is required in the initial management of major burns. The Parkland formula (4ml/kg per % TBSA) is commonly used to approximate the volume of lactated Ringer's required during the first 24 hours following a burn. The rate of fluid administration should be adjusted as needed to maintain a normal urine output of at least 30 ml/h.

### Concomitant Injuries

Peripheral nerve injuries are common after severe burns and will be further described later. Brain injuries may occur in patients who have had a period of hypoxia, which may occur due to smoke inhalation or a cardiac arrest. Brain and spinal cord injuries may result from electrical injuries, and such damage may not be apparent on imaging studies. Amputations may be seen following electrical injuries as well.

## ■ NUTRITION

Severe burn injuries are associated with a hypermetabolic state. Patients will have increased caloric needs, and consultation by a nutritionist is recommended to ensure these needs are met. High-protein diets are usually administered. Vitamin C and zinc supplementation may also be given to facilitate wound healing. Oxandrolone is an anabolic steroid that is sometimes used in the acute hospital to promote weight gain and improve muscle protein synthesis.

## ■ WOUND AND SKIN CARE TOPICAL ANTIMICROBIAL AGENTS

Topical antibacterial agents are applied after the burn wound is cleaned and dead tissue is debrided to prevent wound infection. Silver dressings are commonly used for this purpose.

### Debridement

Debridement refers to the removal of dead tissue and is performed to prevent infection and to allow for definitive wound coverage. Surgical debridement is often performed, but it can be accomplished by mechanical means as well. Hydrotherapy with a handheld shower sprayer is commonly used to help remove dressings and dead tissue. Enzymatic debriding agents may also be used for smaller areas.

### Grafting

Full-thickness and deep partial-thickness burns are unlikely to heal on their own and thus usually require excision and grafting. Temporary wound coverage with an allograft or xenograft may be performed, but these will eventually be rejected. Split-thickness autografts can be used to cover large areas. The grafted site is usually immobilized for 3 to 5 days postprocedure. Dermal replacement products, such as the Integra Dermal Regeneration Template, may be used for coverage in patients with large burns who lack sufficient donor sites. After placement of a dermal substitute, immobilization for 5 to 7 days is typical.

### Protection of the Skin

Vigilance is required to protect healing or healed skin after burn injury. Newly formed skin remains very fragile and vulnerable to even mild trauma. Healed burns may lack moisture, and the use of emollients is recommended to prevent cracks and skin breakdown. It is also recommended that healed or healing skin be protected from the sun. When avoidance of sun exposure is not possible, use of sunscreen should be encouraged.

## Pressure Ulcers

Patients with burn injuries are also at risk for pressure ulcers. The occiput is particularly vulnerable to skin breakdown in these patients. Caution is required with the use of bulky dressings and splints to prevent excessive pressure on the skin. The use of pressure-reducing devices may help prevent ulcers from developing and may be especially beneficial when used in the operating room during prolonged procedures.

# ■ POSITIONING AND RANGE OF MOTION POSITIONING

Following burn injuries, patients will often assume a flexed and adducted position, which is usually the most comfortable position for them, but it predisposes them to contracture. Patients' positioning needs will depend on the location of their burn(s), but the typical positions used to prevent contracture in patients with burns are listed below.

- Neck: neutral or slight extension
- Shoulders: 90° of abduction, 20° of forward flexion
- Elbows: extension and supination
- Wrists: slight extension
- Hands: MCP joints 60° to 90° of flexion; PIP and DIP joints in full extension, thumb in abduction and opposition
- Hips: extension, neutral rotation, 15° to 20° of abduction
- Knees: full extension
- Ankles: neutral to slight dorsiflexion

## Splinting

Splinting may be used to maintain the aforementioned positions in noncompliant patients, to reduce the potential for rupture of exposed tendons and to protect exposed joints. Oral devices that stretch the tissues around the mouth are commonly employed in facial burns to facilitate speech and eating. Resting hand splints are commonly used in hand burns to prevent claw hand deformity.

## Range Of Motion Exercises

Patients with burns should perform range of motion (ROM) exercises (Table 14.1). Stretching should be performed in the direction opposite the contractile force. When active ROM exercises cannot be performed by the patient, passive ROM should be performed for them. Consider applying a moisturizing cream to the involved skin prior to ROM exercises.

**TABLE 14.1** ▪ Recommended orders for burn patients in rehabilitation settings

Physical and occupational therapy for ROM, positioning, scar management, mobility, activities of daily living, etc.
Psychology consult for adjustment issues
Nutrition consult
Wound care, including dressing changes and the use of emollient several times daily
Pain medication, including a long-acting opioid for background pain control and short-acting opioid scheduled prior to dressing changes and therapy sessions and given prn for breakthrough pain

# ■ PAIN MANAGEMENT

## Background and Breakthrough Pain

Background pain is relatively constant pain that is present when the patient is at rest and not undergoing any procedures. This is best treated with the use of longer-acting regularly scheduled pain medications, such as long-acting oxycodone, methadone, or long-acting morphine. Patients may also experience breakthrough pain, which may occur spontaneously or be induced by movement, and which is usually treated with short-acting pain medications. If breakthrough pain tends to occur toward the end of a dosing interval for the agent being used for background pain, consider shortening that dosing interval.

## Procedural Pain

Procedural pain is often the most intense pain among patients with burns and is associated with significant anxiety and distress. Causes of such pain include wound debridement, dressing changes, and therapy sessions. The pain is often described as having a burning or stinging quality and can persist for hours following a procedure. Short-acting opioids are often used in the treatment of procedural pain and should be given a sufficient amount of time before a planned procedure to take effect. Benzodiazepines may help reduce pain and anxiety during dressing changes in patients with burns, but distraction and behavioral techniques may also be effective.

## Tingling And Itching

As patients' burns start to heal, they may experience an itching or tingling sensation. Pruritus can be very severe and may impair quality of life among burn survivors. Antihistamines and tricyclic antidepressants may be helpful in controlling itching. Massage and transcutaneous electrical nerve stimulation are also sometimes used to treat pruritus following burn injury.

# ■ COMPLICATIONS OF BURNS HYPERTROPHIC SCARRING

Hypertrophic scars are red, firm, raised areas within a healed burn that can result in poor cosmesis and in contractures when they cross a joint. They can take several months to develop following a burn injury. Children and individuals with heavily pigmented skin are at increased risk for scarring. Scar management may include compression, initially with elastic bandages or tubular elastic bandages. When burns are near healed, patients may be fitted with custom pressure garments, which they should be instructed to wear for 23 hours daily for up to 1 year. They should be refitted with new garments approximately every 3 months. Compression therapy in the form of pressure garments or a face mask may also be used for facial scars. Although compression therapy is commonly used following burn injuries, further research is required to determine its efficacy in scar management.

## Contractures

Contractures are also common following burn injuries, especially in those burns that cross a major joint. Other risk factors for contractures include larger burns, prolonged hospitalizations, and inhalation injury. The shoulder and elbow are commonly affected joints. Therapy and positioning techniques are employed to help prevent contractures, but when they do occur treatment may include surgical contracture release or serial casting.

## Heterotopic Ossification

Heterotopic ossification(HO) is uncommon following burn injuries but when present, can cause significant impairment. The elbow is the most commonly affected joint, and here, ectopic bone may cause compression of the ulnar nerve. Signs and symptoms include decreased range of motion and pain. Radiographs may appear normal initially. Surgical excision can be considered if HO severely impairs function. Surgery is usually not performed until the heterotopic bone has matured, which may take a year or longer following injury.

## Neuropathy

Neuropathy is a common complication following burn injury. Risk factors for polyneuropathy after a burn include age greater than 40 years, prolonged intensive care stays, and large burn size. Mononeuropathies are more common in patients with electrical injuries and those with a history of alcohol abuse. Careful attention to positioning should be given following burn injury to avoid pressure at common sites of nerve compression, including the fibular head.

# ■ PSYCHOLOGICAL ISSUES PREMORBID PSYCHOLOGICAL ISSUES

The incidence of mental illness and personality disorders is higher in burn patients than that in the general population. Preexisting depression and substance abuse are prevalent among these patients. Suicide attempts and assaults are not uncommon causes of burn injuries.

## Delirium

Delirium is common among patients hospitalized with burns and is associated with an increased risk of death. Causes may include metabolic disturbance, alcohol withdrawal, sensory deprivation, and infection. Male patients, patients with larger burns, and those with a history of substance abuse are at increased risk for delirium.

## Anxiety and Depression

The majority of burn survivors experience at least mild depression. Symptoms of anxiety and depression usually improve with time. Some have suggested that these symptoms are increased among those with facial and hand burns.

## Posttraumatic Stress Disorder

Posttraumatic stress disorder (PTSD) is common following burn injuries. Symptoms include hyperarousal and reexperiencing the trauma, as in flashbacks. Risk factors for PTSD after burn injury include severe pain and large burn size.

## Body Image

Disfigurement secondary to burns commonly affects one's body image, which may affect one's self-esteem and socialization. Body image may be more severely affected among women and those with larger burns.

# ■ SUMMARY

Burns are one of the most devastating forms of injury and a major global public health crisis. The survival rate of burn victims has risen to 92% for patients with more than 90% TBSA in the Chinese mainland. The most burn victims survive suffer from multiple disabilities, and the most common problems include the formation of hypertrophic scars, joint contractures, motor dysfunctions (such as loss of muscle strength, range of motion, coordination, and walking abilities), sensory disturbances (hypersensitivity, pain, itching, and loss of sensation), barriers to the activities of daily living (ADL), social problems, and psychological disturbances. Burn injury rehabilitation is an integrated management on the aforementioned disfunctions through the whole pathological course. Patients with burn injuries benefit from rehabilitation interventions through improvements in physical health, mental health, performance of ADL and quality of life.

## ■ IMPORTANT TERMINOLOGY

inhalation injury    吸入性损伤

burn depth    烧伤深度

total body surface area (TBSA)    总体表面积

concomitant injury    伴随损伤

debridement    清创术

grafting    移植

pressure ulcers    压疮

positioning    体位摆放

range of motion    关节活动范围

background pain    背景痛/基础痛

procedural pain    操作痛

hypertrophic scarring    增生性瘢痕

contracture    挛缩

heterotopic ossification    异位骨化

posttraumatic stress disorder (PTSD)    创伤后应激障碍

## ■ REVIEW QUESTIONS

1.  How to assess the severity of burn injury?

2.  Please illustrate some concomitant injuries after burns.

3.  How to protect the skin after burns?

4.  Describe the principle of position of patients with burn injury.

5.  What is the pain management following burns?

## ■ REFERENCES

1.  Edgar D, Brereton M. Rehabilitation after burn injury. BMJ. 2004; 329:343-345.

2.  Esselman PC. Burn rehabilitation: an overview. Arch Phys Med Rehabil. 2007;88(suppl 2):S3-S6.

3.  Esselman PC, Moore ML. Issues in burn rehabilitation. In: Braddom RL, ed.Physical Medicine and Rehabilitation. 3rd ed. Philadelphia, PA: Saunders Elsevier; 2007:1399-1413.

4.  Esselman PC, Thombs BD, Magyar-Russell G, et al. Burn rehabilitation state of the science. Am J Phys Med Rehabil. 2006; 85(4):383-413.

5.  Gordon MD, Gottschlich MM, Helvig EI, et al. Review of evidenced-based practice for the prevention of pressure ulcers in

burn patients. J Burn Care Rehabil. 2004;25(5):388-410.

6.  Helm PA, Kowalske K, Head M. Burn rehabilitation. In: DeLisa JA, Gans BM, Walsh NE, eds. Physical Medicine & Rehabilitation: Principles and Practice. 4th ed. Philadelphia, PA: Lippincott Williams & Wilkins; 2005: 1867-1889.

7.  Hettiaratchy S, Papini R. Initial management of major burn: Ⅰ —overview. BMJ. 2004;328:1555-1557.

8.  Hettiaratchy S, Papini R. Initial management of major burn: Ⅱ —assessment and resuscitation. BMJ. 2004;329:101-103.

9.  Kowalske K, Holavanahalli R, Helm P. Neuropathy after burn injury. J Burn Care Rehabil. 2001;22(5):353-357.

10. Patterson DR, Everett JJ, Bombardier CH, et al. Psychological effects of severe burn injuries. Psychol Bull. 1993;113(2):362-378.

11. Schneider JC. Burns. In: Frontera WR, Silver JK, Rizzo TD, eds. Essentials of Physical Medicine and Rehabilitation. 2nd ed. Philadelphia, PA: Saunders Elsevier; 2008:609-613.

12. Schneider JC, Holavanahalli R, Helm P, et al. Contractures in burn injury: defining the problem. J Burn Care Rehabil. 2006;27(4):508-514.

13. Summer GJ, Puntillo KA, Miaskowski C, et al. Burn injury pain: the continuing challenge. J Pain. 2007;8(7):533-548.

14. Thombs BD, Notes LD, Lawrence JW, et al. From survival to socialization: a longitudinal study of body image in survivors of severe burn injury. J Psychosom Res. 2008;64:205-212.

（殷　樱）

# CANCER REHABILITATION

## ■ INTRODUCTION

Rehabilitation is critical to improving quality of life for cancer survivors and maintaining dignity for those with terminal illness. Rehabilitation requires several components to be successful. Rehabilitation should be individualized to the patient's needs, desires, and situation. Rehabilitation that fails to respect a patient's wishes will fail altogether. Most problems in rehabilitation occur when there are differences in the team's goals and those of the patient. Goals should be meaningful, measurable, and achievable. Health care providers must balance realism with hope in counseling patients about their goals. Rehabilitation is not something done to an individual; it must be done with the individual. Rehabilitation is largely an educational process for the patient and family members.

## ■ INTERDISCIPLINARY TEAM APPROACH

Team members must demonstrate a high degree of communication skills, humility, and commitment.

### Active Participation of The Patient

Rehabilitation is not something done to an individual; it must be done with the individual. Rehabilitation is largely an educational process for the patient and family members.

### Disability

The World Health Organization has recently published an International Classification of Functioning, Disability and Health (ICF), which is meant to supplement the International Classification of Diseases (ICD-10). It lays out a series of definitions that are crucial to understanding the role of rehabilitation in improving quality of life [1].

## ■ EPIDEMIOLOGY OF CANCER DISABILITY

Due to the tremendous progress of prevention, early detection, and treatment of cancer in the last quarter century, there has been a decline in mortality rates from cancer. However, the number of cancer survivors continues to grow, as more people are living longer with cancer due to the new advances in surgery and medical and radiation oncology [1]. The result is that increasing numbers of patients face more years with cancer-related disability [2]. Data from the US National Health Interview Survey 2002 indicate that 11.3% of patients with cancer have difficulty with activities of daily living (ADLs) compared with 3.8% of people without cancer [3].

# ■ PHASES OF CANCER REHABILITATION

Cancer management requires vigilance and a comprehensive and preventive approach to illness and disability. To accomplish this, a systematic approach to patient evaluation throughout all the phases of the disease process is necessary.

## Initial Staging Phase

Anxiety and disruption of routines may present the greatest challenges. Education is a primary role for rehabilitation providers.

## Primary Treatment Phase

Symptoms of fatigue, nausea, pain, and sleep disruption may be the most significant problems. Acute supportive care and symptom management become the primary responsibilities.

## Posttreatment Recovery

At this phase, pain, anxiety, depression, and treatment side effects such as edema, neuropathy, and weakness may limit participation in work, leisure, and family activities. Care should focus on resumption of a normal, healthy lifestyle.

## Recurrence

At this stage, metastasis may cause significant neuromusculoskeletal, cardiopulmonary, or gastrointestinal impairments. Rehabilitation focuses on mobility, ADLs, endurance, bowel and bladder management, and education of both the patient and the family.

## End of Life

In terminal illness, focus should always be placed on quality-of-life issues. The patient may need to deal with issues of dependency, and caregiver burden is high. Symptom management is critical, as is psychosocial support.

# ■ IMPAIRMENTS

Cancer, even when localized to, or arising from, one organ system, causes the loss of bodily function across many organ systems in individuals. The physician must obtain a comprehensive review of systems when evaluating a cancer patient, as this will help identify impairments to be addressed by the treatment team. Delineating these impairments in individuals is the first step toward ameliorating them; this lies at the core of cancer rehabilitation [4].

## Pain

Virtually every cancer patient experiences pain during the course of the illness; it can often become debilitating [5,6]. The etiology of pain in cancer patients is myriad, frequently having multifactorial causation. The pain may be visceral (arising from internal organs), somatic (from soft tissue, muscles, and/or bones), or neuropathic (from the central or peripheral nervous system) [7]. Visceral pain tends to be poorly localized. It is often described as "deep" and "cramping." Somatic pain, on the other hand, is usually well localized. It is often characterized as "sharp" or "stabbing" and is frequently worsened by weight bearing or movement. There is often point tenderness on examination. Neuropathic pain tends to radiate along dermatomal or peripheral nerve distributions. Patients frequently describe "burning" or "pins and needles". The pain tends to be unrelenting. There may be associated with allodynia (pain with light stroking).

Sadly, pain is often inadequately treated in cancer patients. As many as 50% to 80% of nonhospice cancer patients receive inadequate analgesia. Yet pain can be well controlled in over three quarters of cancer patients using multimodal treatment, according to one study of 2 118 patients.

## Fatigue

Cancer-related fatigue (CRF) is defined as "overwhelming and sustained exhaustion and decreased capacity for physical and mental work. . . not relieved by rest". In addition, fatigue has been shown to impact negatively on one's economic, social, and emotional status. As many as 75% of cancer patients have CRF. Exercise has been shown to mitigate fatigue.

## Delirium and Cognitive Dysfunction

The incidence of delirium in studies of advanced cancer patients ranges from 20% to 86%. Delirium may be reversible in 50% of the cases with proper identification and management. Delirium in cancer usually has multifactorial etiology. Direct involvement of the central nervous system by primary or metastatic tumors, especially with resultant cerebral edema, is the most readily apparent cause. However, distant tumor cytokine production may also play a role. Medication side effects also contribute, and necessary modifications should be considered.

## Mood Disorders

Patients may experience a variety of normal fears throughout their treatment course, including fears of disability, loss of societal roles, loss of control, loss of desirability, abandonment, and death. Although most patients cope well, a significant number do experience serious mood disorders. The average estimates of the prevalence of depression among cancer patients are from 15% to 25%. The importance of correctly diagnosing and treating depression is underlined by research, which shows that depression is associated with poor compliance with medical care, longer hospitalizations, and higher mortality rates in patients with chronic illnesses.

## Hemiplegia

Tumors affecting brain tissue are either primary or metastatic in origin, with metastatic lesions comprising roughly 50% of all intracranial tumors. Brain tumors vary widely in aggressiveness and prognosis. To what extent tumor type or location has an impact on rehabilitation outcomes is not clear. However, one study found a tendency for greater gains for meningiomas and patients with left hemispheric lesions. Brain tumor patients receiving inpatient acute rehabilitation show similar gains between those with metastatic origin and primary brain tumor. Brain tumor patients have been found in some studies to have shorter lengths of stay on acute rehabilitation units as compared with other noncancerous brain disorders, possibly as a result of higher initial levels of functional independence on admission, fewer behavioral issues, better social support, and expedited discharge planning due to cancer-related prognostic factors. In a study of patients with brain tumor undergoing acute rehabilitation, the most common neurologic deficits included impaired cognition (80%), weakness (78%), and visual-perceptual dysfunction (53%).

## Paraplegia/Tetraplegia

Cancer-related spinal cord injury (SCI) incidence may actually exceed that from trauma and represents the most frequent type of nontraumatic SCI. Spinal metastases occur more commonly in the thoracic spine (70%), followed by the lumbosacral (20%) and cervical (10%) spine, and most often originate from primary tumors of breast (15%), lungs (10%), and prostate (10%). Lymphoma, myeloma, and primaries of unknown origin also metastasize to the spine, each accounting for around 10% of cases. Ninety-five percent of metastatic spine involvement is extradural, arising from a vertebral body. Primary tumors of the spinal cord such as meningiomas, neurofibromas, and gliomas are relatively rare. Spinal cord metastases produce a clinical syndrome characterized initially by pain in 90% of cases, followed by weakness, sensory loss, and sphincter dysfunction. Weakness is present in 74% to 76% of patients, autonomic dysfunction in 52% to 57%, and sensory loss in 51% to 53%. Positive results have been demonstrated following rehabilitation for individuals with disability from spinal cord tumors, with significant functional gains measured after inpatient rehabilitation.

## Bone Tumors, Amputation, Bony Metastases

Soft tissue and bony sarcomas are managed with amputation or limb-sparing procedures. Limb salvage procedures are increasing in frequency and are associated with long-term survival, local recurrence rates, and quality of life equivalent to those of amputations, largely made possible by improved surgical techniques that preserve unaffected tissue, advances in endoprosthetic design and durability, soft tissue reconstructive procedures, and radiation and chemotherapy effectiveness in controlling local and distal spread. Bone metastases are a frequent source of cancer-related physical impairment that requires the active involvement of the rehabilitation team. Challenges for the treating team arise when metastatic bone lesions produce severe pain that limits function or imposes risks of fracture during therapeutic exercise or mobility. Depending on the severity and location of the lesion, mobility restrictions can range from non-weight bearing to weight bearing as tolerated. Cancer patients suffering from pathological fractures and associated functional deficits have been shown to make significant gains when admitted to an inpatient rehabilitation hospital unit.

## Soft Tissue Impairments Associated with Cancer Diagnoses

Cancer and/or its treatments can cause significant soft-tissue abnormalities. One of the most frequently observed is lymphedema, extremity swelling that results from disruption of the lymphatics following axillary or groin dissection. The prevalence of this in breast cancer patients has been reported to be between 15% and 30%. Although the prevalence of limb edema is high following standard treatment, the treatment options for managing this have improved. The use of manual lymph drainage and compression garments is effective in controlling edema. When applied early in the course of treatment, before the development of significant volume increase (eg, 250 ml increase in the arm), lymphedema can almost be reversed. Radiation therapy can have long-term sequelae include fibrosis and contracture, eventually resulting in loss of muscle mass. The use of pentoxifylline in the treatment of this problem has shown promise. allogeneic bone marrow transplantation has prolonged life for many with hematologic malignancies. One of the complications of this procedure has been the rejection of the host by the transplanted, immuno-competent engrafted cells, called graft vs host disease. The immunological reaction is often quite brisk, resulting in organ damage (fibrosis) to lung, liver, and notably skin and soft tissue. In the chronic form of graft vs host disease, limb edema, peau d'orange, fasciitis, and enthesitis can occur resulting in significant loss of joint motion. There may be subsequent muscle atrophy secondary to disuse and associated loss of upper and lower extremity mobility.

## ■ ACTIVITY LIMITATIONS

With their multitudes of possible impairments, it is not surprising that many individuals with cancer have significant limitations in their activities. These limitations include reduced mobility and limited ability to perform ADLs.

## Activities of Daily Living

Basic ADLs include feeding, dressing, hygiene, and toileting. Impairments of upper limb function play an obvious role in limiting performance of ADLs, but other impairments also can impede these functions. Cognition is critical to sequencing, awareness, and carry over in the performance of ADLs. Pain and fatigue can also limit the individual's ability to complete these tasks. Lower limb impairments can limit standing and transferring, making dressing, hygiene, and toileting difficult. When individuals become disabled enough to require assistance with these skills, the burden generally falls on caregivers. In one study of 483 cancer patients at varying stages of their disease course, 18.9% had unmet needs in their ADLs due to lack of a suitable caregiver [8]. In advanced stage cancer patients, the percentage of caregivers with a high level of psychological distress varies from 41% to 62% directly depending upon the functional status of the patient [9]. Rehabilitation efforts, particularly with the involvement of occupational therapy, can significantly reduce this burden on caregivers and enhance the quality of life for cancer patients with disabling impairments. To improve feeding independence among cancer patients with upper limb neurologic dysfunction, Chinese researchers used positioning, feeding aid supports, and upper limb supports and significantly improved function over a 3-week treatment intervention [10].

## Exercise for Cancer Patients

Exercise is one of the most effective strategies for symptoms associated with cancer fatigue, sleep disruption, and abnormalities of mood, physical function, and quality of life [11]. A meta-analysis [12] suggests that for adults with a variety of cancer diagnoses and receiving a variety of exercise interventions, exercise improves physical function, quality of life(QoL), cardiorespiratory fitness and decreases CRF. Contraindications for exercise include:thrombocytopenia (<50 000 no resistive exercise; <20 000 only ADLs and light activity); anemia: Hb <8 g ADLs only, <10g light exercise as tolerated; bony metastatic disease: 25% to 50% cortical involvement in long bone, partial weight-bearing, avoid lifting, 0 to 25% full weight-bearing, but no high impact sports.

## ■ PARTICIPATION RESTRICTIONS

Participation is the role an individual plays in a society. These roles can include family and social relationships, vocational and avocational pursuits, and often require modes of transportation to accomplish. Cancer patients are often restricted in many of these functions.

## Family and Social Relationships

Cancer can often draw a family together; however, just as often it leads to significant distress for families. Support groups can be helpful, yet fewer than half of patients receive information about them, even in a large tertiary oncology center [13]. There are also significant economic burdens on families.

## Vocational Rehabilitation

Work disability following cancer diagnosis is a common occurrence. Short and colleagues conducted phone interviews of 1 433 cancer survivors at 1 to 5 years after diagnosis. More than half had quit work during their first year after cancer diagnosis, but fortunately 3 quarters of those returned to work subsequently. A projected 13% had indefinite work disability. Nevertheless, a great deal of barriers still stand in the way of gainful employment for cancer survivors with disability. These include ignorance of both employers and cancer survivors of their rights, discrimination, and limits on preexisting conditions in health insurance benefits.

## Participation in Recreation

Recreation is much more than fun and games; it is critical to physical and mental well-being. Fatigue, pain, weakness, depression, and other impairments will limit cancer survivors' participation in avocational pursuits. Health care providers and family members should encourage recreational activity for those with cancer. The benefits include improvements in fitness, musculoskeletal problems, immune system function, cognition, and sleep. One study looked at 97 European youngsters attending a summer camp for adolescents living with cancer and diabetes [14]. Significant improvements were seen in self-esteem, self-efficacy, and anxiety. Adults benefit as well. For example, Tai Chi Chuan, a Chinese mind-body practice, has been shown to have beneficial effects on cancer survivors in 11 small studies.

## Transportation

Cancer patients may be limited in their ability to drive, fly, or take public transportation. They may not have caregivers available to help with transporting them. This can become a major barrier to cancer treatment, which often involves frequent medical visits. Some patients forgo recommended treatments because of lack of adequate transportation[15]. Thus, it behooves physicians to explore with cancer patients any limits to their ability to get transportation.

## ■ OUTPATIENT MEN'S AND WOMEN'S HEALTH REHABILITATION FOR PELVIC FLOOR MUSCLE DYSFUNCTION

Therapy evaluation includes biomechanical and/or musculoskeletal assessment, education for client and/or caregiver, strengthening particularly of core muscles, myofascial and soft tissue techniques for pain relief abdominal, rectal, and vaginal, electrical stimulation and ultrasound, surface EMG for biofeedback to improve pelvic floor muscle functioning with and without the use of vaginal dilators and/or rectal probes.

### Goals

1. Maintain medical stability and prevent medical complications, including thromboembolism, pneumonia, seizures, urinary tract infections, uncontrolled pain, contractures, and skin breakdown.

2. Optimize nutritional status.

3. Attain bowel and bladder continence or independence with management of ostomy or nephrostomy systems and self-catheterization and/or bowel program.

4. Achieve safe and independent function including mobility and activities of daily living [feeding, grooming, bathing dressing, toileting, transfers, locomotion (wheelchair or gait with appropriate assistive device), bed mobility, household skills, functional cognition, and visual-perceptual skills].

5. Establish effective cognitive and communication strategies.

6. Patient and caregiver education, training, and discharge planning.

## ■ SUMMARY

Cancer rehabilitation has become increasingly important as the number of cancer survivors has dramatically increased in the last two decades. The central tenet of cancer rehabilitation is to help survivors to regain, improve and cope with physical, psychosocial and vocational functioning within the limitations imposed by their illness and treatment. There are a number of rehabilitation interventions that can help to mitigate the toxicities and complications of cancer and its treatment, such as cancer-related fatigue, lymphedema, and peripheral neuropathy. Cancer pain management is also a critical aspect of rehabilitation and requires physicians to take a comprehensive approach that considers the whole person. In addition, advising patients who seek complementary and alternative medical therapies for cancer is an important aspect of cancer rehabilitation. This review provides an overview of the role of rehabilitation in addressing these common cancer rehabilitation challenges and outlines approaches that can be taken to improve cancer survivors' quality of life, function, and well-being.

## ■ IMPORTANT TERMINOLOGY

pelvic floor muscle dysfunction    盆底肌功能障碍
cancer rehabilitation    癌症康复
psychosocial functioning    心理社交功能
vocational functioning    职业功能
cancer-related fatigue    癌症相关疲劳
lymphedema    淋巴水肿
neuromusculoskeletal    神经肌肉骨骼
cardiopulmonary    心肺
cancer pain management    癌症疼痛管理
comprehensive approach    综合治疗方法
rehabilitation interventions    康复干预

## ■ REVIEW QUESTIONS

1. What are the goals of cancer rehabilitation?
2. What are some common cancer rehabilitation challenges, and how can rehabilitation interventions mitigate them?
3. How can physicians evaluate impairments caused by cancer and its treatment in individual patients?
4. What complementary and alternative medical therapies are cancer patients likely to seek, and how can physicians advise them regarding these treatments?
5. What are the benefits of using a comprehensive approach to cancer pain management?

## ■ REFERENCES

1. National Cancer Policy board, Institute of Medicine. In: Hewitt M, Greenfield S, Stovall E. From Cancer Patient to Cancer survivor: Lost in Transition. Committee on cancer survivorship: Improving care and quality of life; November 15, 2005; Washington, DC: National Academies Press; 2006.
2. World Health Organization. 54th World Health Assembly. In: International Classification of Functioning, Disability and Health; Geneva, Switzerland: United Nations World Health Organization; May 22, 2001:1-25.
3. Boult C, Altmann M, Gilbertson D, Yu C, Kane RL. Decreasing disability in the 21st century: the future effects of controlling six fatal and non-fatal conditions. Am J Public Health. 1996;86(10):1388-1393.
4. Lethbridge-Cejku M, Schiller JS, Bernadel L. Summary health statistics for U.S. adults: National Health Interview Survey, 2002. Vital Health Stat 10. July 2004;(222):1-151.

5.  Cherney NI, Portenoy RK. The management of cancer pain. CA Cancer J Clin. 2000;44(5):262-303.

6.  Ventrafridda V, Ripamonti C, De Conno F. Symptom prevalence and control during cancer patients' last days of life. J Palliat Care. 1990;6:7-11.

7.  Chang HM. Pain and its management in patients with cancer. Cancer Invest. 2004;22(5):799-809.

8.  Siegel K, Raveis VH, Houts P, Mor V. Caregiver burden and unmet patient needs. Cancer. 1991;68(5):1131-1140.

9.  Dumont S, Turgeon J, Allard P, Gagnon P, Charbonneau C, Vezina L. Caring for a loved one with advanced cancer: determinants of psychological distress in family caregivers. J Palliat Med. 2006;9(4):912-921.

10. Lee WT, Chan HF, Wong E. Improvement of feeding independence in endstage cancer patients under palliative care—a prospective, uncontrolled study. Support Care Cancer. 2005;13(12):1051-1056.

11. Burnham TR, Wilcox A. Effects of exercise on physiological and psychological variables in cancer survivors. Med Sci Sports Exerc. 2002;34(12):1863-1867.

12. Holtzman J, Schmitz K, Babes G, Kane RL, Duval S, Wilt TJ, et al. Effectiveness of behavioral interventions to modify physical activity behaviors in general populations and cancer patients and survivors. Evid Rep Technol Assess (Summ). June 2004;(102):1-8.

13. Guidry JJ, Aday LA, Zhang D, Winn RJ. The role of informal and formal social support networks for patients with cancer. Cancer Pract. 1997;5(4):241-246.

14. Torok S, Kokonyei G, Karolyi L, Ittzes A, Tomcsanyi T. Outcome effectiveness of therapeutic recreation camping program for adolescents living with cancer and diabetes. J Adolesc Health. 2006;39(3):445-447.

15. Guidry JJ, Aday LA, Zhang D, Winn RJ. Transportation as a barrier to cancer treatment. Cancer Pract. 1997;5(6):361-366.

（刘元标）

# *CARDIAC REHABILITATION*

## ■ INTRODUCTION

Cardiac disease is the leading cause of mortality in men and women worldwide and accounts for 40% of deaths in the industrialized world. Cardiac rehabilitation reduces mortality by 28% [1] and improves quality of life including functional capacity, psychosocial function, exercise, and symptom tolerance. Multifactorial cardiac rehabilitation services are recommended in patients after a significant cardiac event. Unfortunately, only 25% to 30% and 10% to 20% of eligible men and women, respectively, participate in such programs [2].

## ■ ELIGIBILITY

The Centers for Medicare and Medicaid Services (CMS) of USA provide insurance coverage for cardiac rehabilitation of patients with 6 diagnoses:

1. myocardial infarction (MI) within the preceding 12 months.
2. stable angina pectoris.
3. coronary artery bypass surgery.
4. heart valve repair/replacement.
5. percutaneous transluminal coronary angioplasty or stenting.
6. heart (or heart-lung) transplant.

Appropriate indications for cardiac rehabilitation programs also include stable heart failure, but this diagnosis is not currently reimbursed by CMS. CMS guidelines allow 18 weeks in which to complete a maximum of 36 cardiac rehabilitation sessions. Additional sessions may be approved at the discretion of the local coverage determination contractor but may not exceed 72 sessions within 36 weeks. Although CMS is a dominant payer for cardiac rehabilitation and many other payers base their reimbursement on CMS rulings, the coverage parameters may vary by provider.

## ■ PROGRESSIVE EXERCISE TRAINING PRINCIPLES AND BENEFITS

Physiologic adaptation to exercise is known as the conditioning effect. Adaptation is triggered when the demands of an activity exceed that to which the body was previously conditioned, creating a state of overload. Overload triggers changes in the structure and function of specific bodily systems that were stressed, causing them to adapt to better perform that activity. This process occurs with a change in exercise parameters such as an increase in resistance, repetitions, or sets or a decrease in rest between exercises.

## Types of Exercise

Progressive exercise training in cardiac rehabilitation should include a combination of aerobic and resistance exercises to improve endurance and strength.

### Aerobic (Endurance) Training

This type of exercise forms the foundation of progressive exercise in cardiac rehabilitation because of its benefits on cardiovascular function and risk factors. It involves sustained activity of low to moderate intensity that increases the muscles' demand for oxygen. This results in a need for greater cardiac output. The primary conditioning effect of aerobic (endurance) training is an increase in muscle capacity to extract oxygen from blood. Thus, there is less need for cardiac output at any given workload. In addition, because of a decrease in the heart rate (HR) and a modest increase in stroke volume, the same amount of blood can be pumped more efficiently. Aerobic (endurance) training also decreases blood pressure (BP) at rest and during exercise. Functional benefits include being able to perform increasingly intense activities of daily living (ADLs) at the same cardiac workload.

### Resistance Training

This is an important supplement to aerobic (endurance) training in cardiac rehabilitation. It utilizes an opposing force to induce overload and trigger the conditioning effect. The conditioning effects of supervised prescribed resistance training (RT) include improved BP, endurance, and strength. Functional benefits include increased independence, functional capacity, disability, quality of life, and adherence, as it adds variety to the exercise prescription [3]. Common examples include conventional (strength) and circuit (endurance) RT.

### Conventional (Strength) RT

This utilizes higher resistance (ie, heavy weights), fewer repetitions, and longer rest periods to create a predominantly anaerobic overload to trigger adaptations that primarily increase muscular strength. Other conditioning effects include increases in lean body mass, basal metabolic rate, and quicker creation of adenosine triphosphate (ATP). This becomes increasingly important as exercise intensity increases, overwhelming the aerobic system's ability to create ATP fast enough to meet the demands of a task [4]. Conventional (strength) RT may also improve the efficiency of muscle contraction by increasing the number, size, and synchronicity of motor unit recruitment. Functional benefits include being able to perform increasingly heavy ADLs at the same cardiac workload, as they require a smaller proportion of the total available motor units. Angina may still be triggered at the same level of cardiac work; however, this threshold may not be reached until a higher level of activity by the peripheral muscles. Important additional considerations include the fact that strength is inversely associated with all-cause mortality [5] and metabolic syndrome [6,7]. Common examples of conventional (strength) RT include moderate-intensity weight lifting.

### Circuit (Endurance) RT

This utilizes lower resistance (ie, lighter weights), more repetitions, and shorter rest periods to create a predominantly aerobic overload to trigger adaptations that primarily increase muscular endurance as well as aerobic capacity. Other conditioning effects include modification of cardiovascular disease (CVD) risk factors, similar to aerobic (endurance) training and more effectively than conventional (strength) RT. Functional benefits include features of both aerobic (endurance) training and conventional (strength) RT.

# Exercise Prescription

Specific instructions from a health care provider may be more effective than a general instruction to "get more exercise". A physician's endorsement of the effectiveness of cardiac rehabilitation is the main predictor of referral. Patient participation is more likely when they are referred, educated, and married, have high self-efficacy and easily accessible programs[2]. Physiologic testing and monitoring should be used to determine appropriate exercise intensity levels. A balanced exercise prescription should include a combination of aerobic, resistance, and flexibility training.

## Physiologic Testing and Monitoring

An exercise stress test (EST) can be used to determine safe levels of metabolic activity. Exercise intensity levels can also be subjectively gauged by the patient using the rate of perceived exertion.

## Metabolic Equivalents of Task

The amount of energy required to perform an activity is measured in metabolic equivalents of task(METs). One MET is the energy requirement at rest. Increasingly strenuous activities require larger amounts of energy and higher MET levels, which correspond with increasing workload for the heart (Table 16.1). Guidelines for exercise and progressive return to activity are often quantified in terms of METs.

**TABLE 16.1** ▪ Energy requirements for daily activities

| Metabolic Equivalents of Task | Conditioning | Occupation | Recreation | Self-care/ Home Activity |
|---|---|---|---|---|
| <3 | Walk<3.2 kmh/level round | Vacuum/light effort | Vacation with walk and ride | Feed animal, sit as sport spectator |
| 3–5 | Water aerobics | Take out trash/moderate effort | Golf and carry clubs | Mow lawn, carry small child |
| 5–7 | Walk 4.8-6.4kmh/run, play with animals | Brush, groom, shear farm animals | Tennis doubles | Carry object 13.6–27.2 kg |
| 7–9 | Walk 8kmh | Dig ditch | Bicycling, general | Carry object 27.2–40.8 kg |
| >9 | Step aerobics, run 11.2kmh | Heavy labor | Track and field hurdles | Carry object >40.8 kg |

## Exercise Stress Test

Prognosis, risk stratification, and activity prescription are preferably guided by an EST. An initial EST should be conducted 6 to 8 weeks after hospital discharge. Patients who can perform at least 5 METs without ST depression or exercise-induced angina do not usually require further diagnostic testing. Treadmill testing is most common, though testing can also be done using a bicycle ergometer. The upper extremity ergometer can provide a viable alternative to treadmill testing for those unable to use the lower extremities, but HR will rise earlier at a lower workload.

## Rate of Perceived Exertion

The Borg RPE scale is a commonly used guide to exercise prescription[8], based on the subjective measure how hard the patient feels they are working. It is safe, effective, correlates well with MET levels, and is a practical means of prescribing and monitoring exercise intensity. The RPE scale is particularly useful for patients taking medications such as beta-blockers that attenuate the normal HR response to exercise. Most patients on cardiac rehabilitation should exercise "somewhat hard" to "hard" (level 13 or 14) on the RPE scale.

## Aerobic (Endurance) Prescription

Generally, patients beginning cardiac rehabilitation 7 to 10 days after discharge from hospital exercise at 70% to 85% of the HR level they achieved without signs or symptoms of myocardial ischemia during an EST (performed before cardiac rehabilitation). A typical aerobic workout plan is 45 to 60 minutes on 3 (preferably nonconsecutive) days per week. A 5- to 10-minute warm-up including stretching and range of motion (ROM) calisthenics helps prevent injuries and allows for gradual acceleration of the cardiovascular system. Next, a stimulus phase of 20 to 30 minutes at 70% (for beginners) or 85% (experienced patients) stresses the body to stimulate physiologic adaptation (conditioning effect). Lastly, a 5- to 10-minute cool-down (again including stretching and ROM calisthenics) limits the risk of postexercise hypotension caused by pooling of blood in muscles [9,10].

To determine a patient's target pulse rate range, identify the highest rate safely achieved during the most recent exercise test on the top line (maximum pulse line) and then locate the corresponding 10-second counts on the 85% and 70% lines directly below. These 2 values represent the limits of target rate range for exercise conditioning [10].

## Conventional (Strength) Rt Prescription

Conventional guidelines recommend a weight limit of 0.45-2.27kg for RT in the first 3 to 12 weeks after cardiac event or intervention [3]. Subsequent initial RT prescription in cardiac patients should consist of 1 set of 12 to 15 repetitions using 8 to 10 exercises to cover the major muscle groups 2 to 3 d/wk, using weights at 30% to 40% of the 1-repetition maximum (1-RM) for upper body and 50% to 60% of the 1-RM for the lower body [3]. Load-repetition relationship for resistance training [14], single set programs in the initial training period allow nearly the same relative increases in strength as multiple set programs and encourage adherence [3]. The initial RT prescription should use moderate weights, emphasize good technique, and allow recovery time to allow the full repetition range without straining, breath-holding, or Valsalva. This should facilitate musculoskeletal adaptation and minimize injury and muscle soreness [3]. Performing RT after the aerobic exercise will allow adequate warm-up. By 3 weeks after MI, many patients can safely perform moderate-intensity RT [11]. After the patient can comfortably perform 12 to 15 repetitions, the weight may then be increased approximately 5%. Similar to aerobic exercise, the RPE, HR, and BP should be monitored during RT [3] because the BP measured between sets may underestimate the pressor response during the actual lift [12]. The RPE should be 11 to 14.

## Circuit (Endurance) Rt Prescription

Typical programs use a variety of lightweight machines continuously to create an aerobic workout. They alternate between 30 seconds of weight lifting at 40% to 50% of 1-RM and 30 seconds of rest in between sets [9]. Weight machines may reduce the chances of injury by aiding in balance and acting as a spotter. Alternative exercises can use calisthenics, an elastic cord, pulley, dumb bell, or dowel [3]. During these exercises, the grip on the equipment should be secure but not overly tight so as to avoid excessive BP elevation [13].

### Flexibility Training Prescription

Stretching of major muscle and tendon groups should be conducted 2 to 3 times per week [3].

## ■ PHASES OF CARDIAC REHABILITATION

### PHASE I

This period consists of the acute inpatient hospitalization. It is subdivided into acute and subacute subsections. During the subacute period, particularly complicated patients may warrant admission to a comprehensive integrated inpatient rehabilitation program (CIIRP).

### Acute Period

During the first 3 days in the critical care unit, the workload may generally include exercise at 1 to 2 METs. This can include passive ROM, protective chair posture,  I bedside commode on day 1 (instead of a bedpan, which requires a higher MET level) and walking at ≤1 mile per hour (mph). It is necessary to avoid Valsalva, isometric exercises, and raising legs above the heart during this period as these activities may unduly stress the heart. Progressive activities may include initiation of ambulation and ADLs on days 2 to 4.

### Subacute Period

After discharge from the critical care unit, the workload may generally be advanced to 3 to 4 METs. This can include walking at 2 mph, light resistance exercise, and propelling a wheelchair [15].

### Comprehensive Integrated Inpatient Rehabilitation Program

During the subacute period of cardiac rehabilitation, patients with a complex cardiac event or significant comorbidities such as neuropathy, amputation, considerable arthritis, or a prior stroke may require admission to a CIIRP. CIIRP, formerly known as Acute Comprehensive Inpatient Rehabilitation, consists of an in-hospital rehabilitation unit in which patients reside 24 hours daily for an average of 13 days to benefit from coordinated, integrated interdisciplinary medical and rehabilitation services. To qualify for CIIRP under CMS guidelines, patients must have one of the eligible cardiac diagnoses listed above, in addition to the demonstrated need for and ability to safely benefit from a skilled multidisciplinary environment, which incorporates daily medical management by a physician, skilled rehabilitation nursing, and >3 hours of therapy daily (consisting of physical therapy, occupational therapy, speech language pathology or prosthetics and orthotics). Other services such as those that address nutrition and psychology are often beneficial, but do not count toward the 3-hour requirement. For non-CMS payers, the required admission diagnoses, therapy needs, and reimbursement requirements may vary.

### Hospital Discharge Planning

Before hospital discharge, patient education and family conferences should include information about cardiac symptoms such as angina, medications including sublingual nitroglycerin, coronary disease, modification of risk factors such as smoking and diet, and resumption of activities including work and sex.

### Follow-Up

Appointments should be scheduled with cardiology, primary care, or cardiac rehabilitation providers. These should include an opportunity to assess understanding of educational material after discharge. Where available, patient support groups lead by a cardiac rehabilitation professional in the first or second month may be quite informative and supportive for the patient. Supervised physical conditioning or patient-run heart clubs are often available in local communities. For a directory of comprehensive outpatient cardiac rehabilitation (secondary prevention) programs and education materials[9].

# PHASE II

This period consists of supervised electrocardiogram (EKG)-monitored outpatient therapy, usually lasting 2 to 3 sessions weekly for up to 12 weeks. It should ideally include participation in a comprehensive outpatient cardiac rehabilitation (secondary prevention) program and return to community ADLs. To improve accessibility, low-risk patients (ie, minimal risk of activity-induced angina or arrhythmia) may participate in home-based programs during phase II with equal safety and efficacy [16].

## Comprehensive Outpatient Cardiac Rehabilitation (Secondary Prevention) Program

These programs take place during phase II cardiac rehabilitation and should include a medical evaluation, prescribed exercise, a program to modify cardiac risk factors (ie, smoking, hyperlipidemia, hypertension, nutrition, obesity, and diabetes) and education and counseling on vocation, physical activity psychosocial factors, and proper use of prescribed medications. For most patients, important components of care after a myocardial event are easily remembered with the mnemonic ABCDE: Aspirin, Beta-blocker, Cholesterol-lowering medication (statin), Diet (for weight control, glycemic control, and improving the lipid profile) and Exercise training.

Comprehensive outpatient cardiac rehabilitation (secondary prevention) program facilities, under the supervision of a physician medical director, should be staffed by appropriately trained health care professionals (typically exercise physiologists, nurses, and physical therapists) and have continuous EKG, appropriate exercise, and resuscitative equipment. These providers should be trained in cardiopulmonary resuscitation and have readily accessible emergency care. Cardiac rehabilitation programs generally accept patients 1 to 2 weeks after hospital discharge.

## Return to Community ADLs

Consider the activities listed in Table 16.1 and similar references in combination with the results of an EST, clinical signs, and symptomatology to gauge readiness to engage in progressive activities. Angina, arrhythmia, or congestive heart failure warrants a cardiology consult and reconsideration of readiness to advance activity levels.

### Sex

Gradual return to sex can be recommended. If asymptomatic during ADLs, a patient may resume intercourse 4 to 6 weeks after MI. Foreplay and climax require 3 and 5 METs, respectively [17], approximately the same energy requirements as walking around the block briskly or climbing a flight of stairs [9]. Positions with sustained weight on the arms should be avoided as this may increase BP. It is advised that the patient wait 2 to 3 hours after a large meal before engaging in sexual activity. Sublingual nitroglycerin can be considered in otherwise stable patients with sex-induced angina. Caution should be exercised, however, in those taking sildenafil, tadalafil, and vardenafil (approved for erectile dysfunction) and especially in hypotension or aortic stenosis [9].

### Work

Most MI patients can return to work as most jobs require <6 METs. Initially, consider a trial of progressive part-time work.

# PHASE III

This period consists of supervised but non-EKG-monitored outpatient maintenance therapy. 7-8 METs of functional capacity and clinical stability are generally accepted criteria for transition to phase III. Repeat EST at the end of a few months of exercise training can help determine new target exercise levels.

# ■ SAFETY CONSIDERATIONS

Mild-to-moderate-intensity RT is considered safe as it generally causes a lower rate pressure product [RPP = HR × systolic BP (SBP) ] than maximal treadmill aerobic exercise [18] and does not exceed hemodynamic levels attained by patients with heart failure during standard exercise testing. Most cardiac patients can perform combined aerobic and resistance (circuit) weight training without orthopedic or cardiac complications. Cardiovascular risks are likely related to age, underlying CVD, fitness level, and intensity of RT. Lowrisk cardiac patients without evidence of myocardial ischemia with exercise or at rest, complex ventricular dysrhythmias, or severe left ventricular dysfunction have reported no major adverse cardiovascular events [3]. Supervised cardiac rehabilitation RT is considered safe in clinically stable women and men with CHD as it has been demonstrated to not induce angina, ischemic ST depression, complex ventricular arrhythmias, unusual hemodynamics, or cardiovascular complications in this population.

## CONTRAINDICATIONS

### Contraindications to Cardiac Rehabilitation

The following conditions disqualify the patient from participation in cardiac rehabilitation. Generally, participation may proceed when the condition has resolved:

1. resting SBP >160 or diastolic BP >110 mmHg
2. poorly controlled angina
3. atrial fibrillation with rapid ventricular response
4. heart block (second or third degree)
5. complex arrhythmias
6. significant congenital or valvular heart disease
7. recent acute mental or physical illness
8. severe dyspnea at low workloads
9. significant pulmonary, neurologic, or orthopedic limitations
10. acute endocarditis or pericarditis
11. severe aortic stenosis
12. unstable congestive heart failure or severe left ventricular dysfunction
13. serious noncardiac comorbidity

### Contraindications to RT

A list of absolute and relative contraindications to RT are listed in Table 16.2.

### Precautions

Cardiac rehabilitation is considered very safe and beneficial in most patients given the above exercise prescription parameters, proper patient selection, monitoring, precautions, and supervision [9]. However, the provider must remain vigilant in considering the following factors.

**TABLE 16.2** ▪ Absolute and relative contraindications to resistance training

**ABSOLUTE**
Unstable CHD
Decompensated heart failure
Uncontrolled arrhythmias
Severe pulmonary hypertension (mean pulmonary arterial pressure >55 mmHg)
Severe and symptomatic aortic stenosis
Acute myocarditis, endocarditis, or pericarditis
Uncontrolled hypertension (>180/110 mmHg)
Aortic dissection
Marfan syndrome
Uncontrolled diabetes
High-intensity RT (80%—100% of 1-RM) in patients with active proliferative retinopathy or moderate or worse nonproliferative diabetic retinopathy
**RELATIVE (SHOULD CONSULT A CARDIOLOGIST BEFORE ARTICIPATION)**
Major risk factors for CHD
Uncontrolled hypertension (>160/100 mmHg)
Low functional capacity (4 METs)
Musculoskeletal limitations
Individuals who have implanted pacemakers or defibrillators

## Cardiovascular Sequelae

The provider should monitor for common medical complications following a cardiovascular event including angina, arrhythmias, symptomatic congestive heart failure, Dressler syndrome (pericarditis), and arterial embolization.

## Environment

Conservative activity guidelines recommend avoidance of activities, which impose additional strain on the heart, especially during the first 3 months after MI. Thus, the patient should avoid working or exercising during very humid, hot, cold, or windy weather, taking very cold or hot baths or showers, exercising or walking on an inclined surface or hill, or engaging in any activity that creates worry or emotional stress[9].

## Medication Effects

Cardiovascular medications should be considered during EST interpretation and exercise prescription formulation. For instance, beta-blockers decrease peak HR, making RPE, symptoms, and EKG more useful parameters for EST and exercise prescription. Common antihypertensive medication effects on peak HR are as follows:

1. Decrease: beta-blockers, clonidine, methyldopa, verapamil;

2. No discernible effect: angiotensin-converting enzyme (ACE) inhibitors, angiotensin II receptor blockers, digitalis (in patients with CHF);

3. Increase: calcium channel blockers, hydralazine, minoxidil, nifedipine, nitrates, prazosin.

## Monitoring

EKG monitoring is recommended in patients at high risk for ischemia [left ventricular ejection fraction(LVEF)<35%, New York Heart Association Grade III or IV congestive heart failure, systolic BP decrease of >10mmHg during exercise, postoperative angina, ischemia during EST, or poor cognition leading to inability to reliably self-monitor and report symptoms of ischemia] or arrhythmia (LVEF <30%, history of atrial fibrillation/rapid ventricular rate, ventricular tachycardia, ventricular fibrillation, pacemaker, automatic implantable cardioverter defibrillator or ST elevation MI within 6 weeks). Excessive elevations of BP are generally not a concern with the recommended low- to moderate-intensity RT without Valsalva. BP during RT in cardiac patients was reported in a clinically acceptable range when lifting 40% to 60% of the 1-RM.

## Psychological Complications

Patients should be monitored for common psychological sequelae of cardiac disease including anxiety, depression, inappropriate fear of physical activity, denial of illness persisting beyond the first few days in hospital, and persistent or major depression. Depression and anhedonia occur in more than 25% of patients after MI. This correlates with mortality and recurrent coronary events. Selective serotonin reuptake inhibitors can be used safely in ischemic heart disease[19-22] and are preferred over tricyclic antidepressants [23].

## Screening

Low-risk patients warrant a graded approach to cardiac rehabilitation, but probably do not require an extensive cardiovascular screening before participation in RT. Moderate- to high-risk patients can safely participate in RT with appropriate preparation, surveillance, and guidance. Medical screening is not required for RT initiated at a low level. Patients with stable CVD are recommended for low- to moderate-intensity RT without further medical diagnostic testing if they have a functional capacity 2:4 METs [3]. This can be estimated by a questionnaire such as the Duke Activity Status Inventory.

## Technique

Avoid extended breath-holding while exercising, straining or lifting, working in a bent or stooped position or with arms held above head, doing work that requires continuous muscle tensing.

## Timing with Meals and Alcohol

Avoid exercising or working during the first hour after a meal, after consuming alcohol, or consuming excessive amounts of alcohol[9].

## When to Stop Exercise

If a patient's health status changes or they experience chest discomfort or undue shortness of breath during RT, they should stop RT and undergo further medical consultation [3]. Exercise should be ceased immediately if any adverse signs or symptoms arise such as chest pain, excessive shortness of breath, dizziness, or arrhythmias [12].

# Unique Patient Populations

## Arrhythmias

Most patients with a history of ventricular tachycardia will experience ventricular tachycardia or ectopy during cardiac rehabilitation. Intense exercise and exercising in a supine position should be avoided as they increase the likelihood of arrhythmias.

## Congestive Heart Failure

Isometric exercise should be avoided because of risk of arrhythmia. Exercise is beneficial because it can improve cardiac output and reduce plasma renin activity and sympathetic tone.

## Coronary Artery Bypass Graft

Cognitive deficits exist in 22.5% of patients 2 months after coronary artery bypass graft (CABG)[24]. These may dissipate by 1 to 3 years postoperatively when compared with nonsurgical controls with CAD[25].

## Elderly

Frailty may warrant a low-intensity exercise regimen. Elderly individuals who exercise can decrease by 25% the usual age-associated decrements in cardiac output, LVEF, and maximum HR and increase in end diastolic volume.

## Heart Transplant

### Atherosclerosis

Patients are at risk for accelerated atherosclerosis and cardiac disability. For instance, coronary artery disease can develop 5 to 10 years after transplant.

### Denervation

Without vagus nerve input, HR changes are based on circulating catecholamines, which are much slower than vagus nerve control. Therefore, HR increases with exercise and decrease to baseline after exercise will be delayed. The heart has increased resting HR [100 beats per minute(BPM) is normal] and decreased maximum effort (peak HR is 20% to 25% lower than age-matched controls, and many parameters are lower including work capacity, cardiac output, $VO_2$, and systolic BP). Ischemia and arrhythmia must be identified by EKG because sensations including angina are no longer reliable. (Fortunately, these occur less frequently than in other cardiac patients.) Therefore, exercise intensity should be based on RPE 11 to 14 or a percentage of $VO_2$ or maximum workload (not HR or angina since denervated)[15].

### Medication side effects

Posttransplant medication regimens may complicate medical management. For instance, immunosuppression may predispose to infection. Stroke risk is increased because of mycotic or embolic sources or sirolimus-induced vasculitis. Peripheral neuropathy or myopathy can arise from nerve impingement, critical illness, or posttransplantation medications including steroids and statins. Transplant medications may also cause tremor. Steroids can predispose to osteoporosis, especially given limited weight-bearing activity.

### Prognosis

Most patients increase exercise tolerance, work output, and return to community safely.

### Limited resources

If a cardiac rehabilitation program is not available, it is appropriate to follow guidelines such as those listed in the previous study in combination with a more complete list of MET demands for common activities[9,8]. The pace of these activities may be scaled up or down by results of early post-MI stress test when available. If no supervised program is available, patients' 2 months status after uncomplicated MI can use an EST to determine RPE and target HR.

## Neuropathy

This warrants special caution because of risks of orthostasis and injuries related to poor proprioception and pain perception[3].

## Pacemakers

Individuals with pacers should be carefully evaluated before RT, as pacer leads are prone to dislodgement or fracture during repetitive motion [26].

### Retinopathy

Vigorous exercise is contraindicated with retinopathy because of risk of retinal detachment and vitreous hemorrhage.

### Sternal Precautions

Sternal precautions are generally in place for 6 weeks postoperatively. Patients generally may not lift >45kg, reach overhead, or use arms to push up during transfers from sit to stand. Some studies have suggested that for the first 8 to 12 weeks after CABG, patients should avoid upper-body RT with >50% of maximum voluntary contraction to allow healing of the sternum. Restrictions should be specified on the discharge summary from the surgical team. During rehabilitation, pain at the surgical site must be considered during exercise prescription. The comprehensive outpatient cardiac rehabilitation (secondary prevention) program is generally delayed until sternal precautions are lifted.

### Stroke And Amputee

Patients commonly have comorbid cardiac disease. Hemiplegic ambulation has a much higher energy cost, as does gait with an amputation. Lower limb impairments may necessitate upper limb ergometry.

### Valve Surgery

Bio-prosthetic valves generally warrant aspirin, whereas artificial valves necessitate warfarin.

### Women

CVD is the most common cause of death in women worldwide, yet it is frequently unrecognized. Women most commonly present with typical signs and symptoms of myocardial ischemia, but frequently present with atypical symptoms including abdominal pains, nausea, or fatigue. They usually present with cardiac disease later in life and are half as likely as men to be referred to cardiac rehabilitation [27].

## ■ SUMMARY

Cardiac rehabilitation (CR) is a branch of rehabilitation medicine/physical therapy dealing with optimizing physical function in patients with cardiac disease or recent cardiac surgeries. CR services can be provided during hospitalization for the event or in an outpatient setting. While the "glue" of cardiac rehabilitation is exercise, programs are evolving to become comprehensive prevention centers where all aspects of preventive cardiology care are delivered. This includes nutritional therapies, weight loss programs, management of lipid abnormalities with diet and medication, blood pressure control, diabetes management, and stress management.

## ■ IMPORTANT TERMINOLOGY

cardiac rehabilitation   心脏康复
aerobic (endurance) training   有氧( 耐力 )训练
resistance training (RT)   抗阻训练
circuit RT   循环抗阻训练

exercise prescription 运动处方
exercise stress test (EST) 运动负荷试验
metabolic equivalents of task (MET) 代谢当量
rate of perceived exertion 主观用力程度分级
comprehensive integrated inpatient rehabilitation program (CIIRP) 综合住院康复项目
contraindication 禁忌证
denervation 失神经

# ■ REVIEW QUESTIONS

1. Describe the indication of cardiac rehabilitation.
2. What are the principles and benefits of cardiac rehabilitation?
3. Describe the phases in cardiac rehabilitation.
4. How to prevent the risks in cardiac rehabilitation?
5. What are the differences between endurance and resistance training?

# ■ REFERENCES

1. Taylor RS, Unal B, Critchley JA, Capewell S. Mortality reductions in patients receiving exercise-based cardiac rehabilitation: how much can be attributed to cardiovascular risk factor improvements? Eur J Cardiovasc Prev Rehabil. 2006;13(3):369-374.
2. Jackson L, Leclerc J, Erskine Y, Linden W. Getting the most out of cardiac rehabilitation: a review of referral and adherence predictors. *Heart* 2005;91(1):10-14.
3. Williams MA, Haskell WL, Ades PA, et al. Resistance Exercise in Individuals with and without cardiovascular disease: 2007 update. a scientific statement from the American Heart Association Council on Clinical Cardiology and Council on Nutrition, Physical Activity, and Metabolism. Circulation. 2007;116:572-584.
4. Pratley R, Nicklas B, Rubin M, et al. Strength training increases resting metabolic rate and norepinephrine levels in healthy 50 to 65-yr-old men. J Appl Physiol. 1994;76:133-137.
5. Fitzgerald SJ, Barlow CE, Kampert JB, et al. Muscular fitness and all-cause mortality: prospective observations. J Physical Activity Health. 2004;1:7-18.
6. Jurca R, Lamonte MJ, Barlow CE, Kampert JB, Church TS, Blair SN. Association of muscular strength with incidence of metabolic syndrome in men. Med Sci Sports Exerc. 2005; 37:1849-1855.
7. Jurca R, Lamonte JM, Church TS, et al. Associations of muscle strength and fitness with metabolic syndrome in men. Med Sci Sports Exerc. 2004;36:1301-1307.
8. Borg G. Subjective effort in relation to physical performance and working capacity. In: Pick HL, ed. Psychology: From Research to Practice. New York: Plenum; 1978:333.
9. Stewart KJ, Ziegelstein RC. Postmyocardial Infarction Care and Cardiac Rehabilitation. Principles of Ambulatory Medicine. Philadelphia, PA: Lippincott Williams and Wilkens, 2007:971-992.
10. Haskell WL. Design and implementation of cardiac conditioning programs. In: Wenger NK, Hellerstein HK, eds. Rehabilitation of the Coronary Patient. New York: Wiley; 1978:209.
11. Wilke NA, Sheldahl LM, Tristani FE, Hughes CV, Kalbfl eisch JH. The safety of static-dynamic effort soon after myocardial infarction. *Am Heart J.* 1985;110:542-545.
12. MacDougall JD, Tuxen D, Sale DG, Moroz JR, Sutton JR. Arterial blood pressure response to heavy resistance exercise. J Appl Physiol. 1985;58:785-790.
13. American College of Sports Medicine. ACSM's Guidelines for Exercise Testing and Prescription. 7th ed. Philadelphia, PA: Lippincott Williams and Wilkins; 2006.
14. Dingwall H, Ferrier K, Semple J. Exercise prescription in cardiac rehabilitation. In: Thow M, ed. Exercise Leadership in Cardiac Rehabilitation. West Sussex, England: Whurr Publishers Ltd; 2006:97-131.

15. Jafri, I. Cardiac rehabilitation. In: Cuccurullo SJ, ed. Physical Medicine and Rehabilitation Board Review. New York: Demos, 2004:610-628.

16. Dalal HM, Zawada A, Jolly K, Moxham T, Taylor RS. Home based versus centre based cardiac rehabilitation: cochrane systematic review and meta-analysis. BMJ. 2010 19;340:b5631. doi: 10.1136/bmj.b5631.

17. Hellerstein HK, Friedman EH. Sexual activity in the post-coronary patient. *Arch Intern Med*. 1970;125:987.

18. Featherstone JF, Holly RG, Amsterdam EA. Physiologic responses to weight lifting in coronary artery disease. Am J Cardiol. 1993;71:287-292.

19. 19. Shapiro PA, Lesperance F, Frasure-Smith N, et al. An open-label preliminary trial of sertraline for treatment of major depression after acute myocardial infarction (the SADHAT Trial). Sertraline Anti-Depressant Heart Attack Trial. Am Heart J. 1999;137:1100.

20. Roose SP, Laghrissi-Thode F, Kennedy JS, et al. Comparison of paroxetine and nortriptyline in depressed patients with ischemic heart disease. JAMA. 1998;279:287.

21. Strik JJ, Honig A, Lousberg R, et al. Efficacy and safety of fluoxetine in the treatment of patients with major depression after first myocardial infarction: findings from a double-blind, placebo-controlled trial. Psychosom Med. 2000;62:783.

22. Glassman AH, O'Connor CM, Califf RM, et al. Sertraline antidepressant heart attack randomized trial (SADHEART) group. Sertraline treatment of major depression in patients with acute MI or unstable angina. JAMA. 2002;288:701.

23. Roose SP, Glassman AH. Cardiovascular effects of tricyclic antidepressants in depressed patients with and without heart disease. J Clin Psychiatry. 1989;50(suppl):1.

24. van Dijk D, Keizer AM, Diephuis JC, Durand C, Vos LJ, Hijman R. Neurocognitive dysfunction after coronary artery bypass surgery: a systematic review. J Thorac Cardiovasc Surg. 2000;120(4):632-639.

25. Selnes OA, Grega MA, Borowicz LM Jr, et al. Cognitive outcomes three years after coronary artery bypass surgery: a comparison of on-pump coronary artery bypass graft surgery and nonsurgical controls. Ann Thorac Surg. 2005;79(4):1201-1209.

26. Lampert R, Cannom D, Olshansky B. Safety of sports participation in patients with implantable cardioverter defibrillators: a survey of Heart Rhythm Society members. J Cardiovasc Electrophysiol. 2006;17:11-15.

27. Jackson L, Leclerc J, Erskine Y, Linden W. Getting the most out of cardiac rehabilitation: a review of referral and adherence predictors. Heart. 2005;91:10-14.

（殷　樱）

# *GERIATRIC REHABILITATION*

## ■ SPECIAL CONSIDERATIONS WHEN CARING FOR GERIATRIC PATIENTS

### Physiologic Changes

Significant physiologic changes occur as people age, which may impact a patient's functional abilities and increase one's susceptibility to illness and injury. Loss of muscle mass and strength occurs with aging. Cardiovascular changes include a decline in maximal heart rate and maximum oxygen consumption, rise in blood pressure, and decreased baroreceptor sensitivity; the latter predisposes older patients to orthostatic hypotension. Creatinine clearance (Cr Cl), vital capacity, glucose tolerance, and peristalsis through the gastrointestinal tract also decrease with age. Older adults are also more susceptible to infections and may be less likely to mount a fever or leukocytosis in response to infection.

### Illnesses and Impairments

Older adults are more likely to have potentially disabling chronic illnesses, including osteoarthritis, osteoporosis, cerebrovascular disease, and Parkinson's disease. They may also have multiple medical comorbidities, cognitive impairment, visual and/or hearing impairments.

### Hospitalization, Bed Rest, and Deconditioning

Elderly patients often demonstrate impaired abilities to ambulate and to perform activities of daily living (ADLs) following an acute illness, making it essential to assess their mobility and independence with ADLs prior to discharge. Bed rest orders are often unnecessary and may have deleterious effects for older adults, including significant declines in lower extremity strength, power, and aerobic capacity. The use of mechanical restraints should be avoided as there is no evidence that they reduce the risk of falls in hospitalized patients, and they may be associated with an increased risk of injuries and agitation. Patients remain at risk for falls, pressure ulcers, delirium, and adverse drug reactions while hospitalized, which are further discussed below.

## ■ FALLS AND COMMON INJURIES

A number of factors increase the risk of falls among older adults, including lower limb weakness, impaired vision, cognitive impairment, orthostatic hypotension, and medications. Injuries commonly seen in older adults following falls are discussed in the following sections, but it should be noted that these injuries can also occur with minimal or no trauma.

### Hip Fractures

Hip fractures often result from falls among the elderly and should be suspected in patients reporting groin pain and in those who are unable to rise or bear weight on their injured leg following a fall. External rotation and a shortened appearance of the leg suggest a displaced femur fracture. Radiographs including an antero-posterior view of the pelvis and a lateral view of the proximal femur should be obtained as soon as possible. The presence of a fracture should prompt consultation with an orthopedic surgeon and preparation for surgery. Should radiographs fail to demonstrate a fracture but strong clinical suspicion for a fracture remains, additional imaging may be necessary. An older adult who sustains a hip fracture likely has osteoporosis, and as such, necessary precautions are required during physical activity to prevent further fractures.

## Pelvic Fractures

Pelvic fractures may result from forward or backward falls. Patients may initially complain of groin pain and subsequently of sacral pain. Radiographs may fail to reveal the fracture, necessitating bone scan or MRI for diagnosis. These fractures usually heal well, and bed rest should be avoided.

## Vertebral Compression Fractures

Vertebral compression fractures may result from falls as well. Patients may report the sudden onset of back pain, typically worse with standing or walking and may have tenderness to palpation over the fracture. Plain radiographs should be the initial imaging study performed and may demonstrate the classic wedge-shaped deformity. Compression fractures are usually stable fractures and can be treated conservatively with a short period of relative rest and pain medication.

## Subdural Hematomas

Subdural hematomas may occur in older adults who fall, especially those receiving anticoagulation. Symptoms may take time to emerge and may include headache, dizziness, and altered mental status. Head CT scan should be performed when a hematoma is suspected.

# ■ PRESSURE ULCERS

The elderly are predisposed to developing pressure ulcers, especially during periods of acute illness and immobility. Daily skin assessments should be performed while hospitalized. Patients should be repositioned every 2 hours, and the use of pressure-reducing devices should be considered to prevent ulcers. Nutritional consultation is beneficial in patients who develop pressure ulcers to determine if nutritional deficiencies are affecting healing.

# ■ DELIRIUM AND AGITATION

Delirium is an acute cognitive impairment with associated change in consciousness. It may have a fluctuating course with periods of lucidity. It is a clinical diagnosis, the differential for which is quite broad. The underlying cause(s) should be identified to allow for proper treatment and return to the patient's baseline mental status.

## The evaluation of delirium

### History

History taking should begin with obtaining information regarding the onset of symptoms, which is of the utmost importance given the difficulty discerning between delirium and dementia in older adults. All medications, and particularly any newly added medications, should be carefully reviewed.

## Physical examination

Vital signs including pulse oximetry should be obtained. A comprehensive examination should be performed, including a thorough neurological assessment and examination for signs of infection and other medical conditions.

## Labs

A bedside glucose reading should be taken. A complete blood count, comprehensive metabolic panel, and blood and urine cultures should be obtained. Coagulation studies should be obtained in patients receiving anticoagulants and in those with suspected liver dysfunction. Other lab work, such as blood alcohol levels or medication levels, may be clinically warranted. Lumbar puncture should be performed and cerebrospinal fluid sent for analysis when suspicion exists for meningitis or encephalitis.

## Imaging

A chest radiograph will help exclude pneumonia or congestive heart failure as the precipitating cause. A head CT should be performed in patients presenting with a significant change in mental status and in those with focal neurologic deficits.

## Sundowning

Sundowning refers to behavioral disturbances that occur in the late afternoon or evening among some older adults with dementia. Interventions may include structuring activities during usual times of agitation, redirection, reassurance, and meeting patients' physical needs, such as for pain control or toileting. Antipsychotic medications are most common used to treat the associated agitation, but must be used with caution as there is increased risk of mortality with these agents when used in individuals with dementia. When medication is required to manage the agitation, the lowest effective dose should be given.

# ■ MEDICATIONS AND ADVERSE DRUG REACTIONS

Adverse drug reactions (ADRs) are a significant cause of morbidity and mortality in the elderly.

## Factors Contributing to Increased Risk of ADRs among the Elderly

### Noncompliance with drug therapy

Reasons may include the cost of medication, inability to read instructions, and cognitive impairment. Compliance may be improved by patient education, use of a pill box or medication calendar, large type prescription labels, the use of less expensive generic medications, and the use of once-daily medications.

### Polypharmacy

The use of some combinations of medications may put a patient at higher risk for an ADR; for example, there is an increased risk of gastrointestinal bleeding with concomitant use of nonsteroidal anti-inflammatory drug and anticoagulants. One drug may also inhibit or increase the metabolism of another. Fluoxetine and paroxetine, for example, can inhibit the metabolism of other medications via the cytochrome P450 system, thereby prolonging their half-life. Thus, the use of alternative selective serotonin reuptake inhibitors is preferable in elderly adults with depression.

### Body weight and composition changes

Fat-soluble drugs, including benzodiazepines, tend to accumulate more in the fatty tissue of elderly patients, prolonging their half-life. Use of lorazepam is preferred over diazepam in older adults because of its more rapid pharmacokinetics.

### Decreased plasma protein binding capacity

This can lead to higher free drug plasma concentrations and may increase the risk of drug interactions. Consider checking free levels of medications that are highly protein-bound, including phenytoin.

### Altered hepatic clearance

Hepatic clearance of medications may be impaired in the elderly, though liver function tests may remain normal. The content of cytochrome P450 enzymes within the liver diminishes with age, affecting the phase I metabolism of some medications.

### Decreased renal excretion

Creatinine clearance (Cr Cl) declines significantly with age and cannot be determined solely on the basis of the serum creatinine. Dose adjustment of some medications, including gabapentin and allopurinol, is required when a patient's Cr Cl is less than 60 ml/min. Cr Cl calculators are available online and for personal digital assistant (PDA). Cr Cl can also be estimated using the Cockroft-Gault formula below:

$$Cr\ Cl = [(140 - age) \times weight\ in\ kg] / [72 \times serum\ creatinine\ (\times 0.85\ for\ women)]$$

### Increased sensitivity of the central nervous system

A number of changes occur in the central nervous system (CNS) pathways of the aging brain that predispose elderly patients to neurologic side effects of medications. Older adults with neurologic diseases, including Alzheimer's disease and Parkinson's disease, may especially be at high risk for ADRs. Anticholinergic medications, which include tricyclic antidepressants, tolterodine, oxybutynin, scopolamine, and trihexyphenidyl, may precipitate delirium. First generation antihistamines, including diphenhydramine, have anticholinergic properties and may cause confusion as well. Opioid medications and drugs used to treat Parkinson's disease, including levodopa, may also contribute to delirium.

## Potentially Inappropriate Medications in the Elderly

The Beers criteria, established by expert consensus, have identified medications that are potentially inappropriate for use in adults aged 65 and older. Medications included in the criteria that are commonly prescribed by physiatrists can be found in Table 17.1.

**TABLE 17.1** ▪ Medications prescribed by physiatrists that may be inappropriate for older adults

| | |
|---|---|
| Amitriptyline | Ketorolac |
| Barbiturates | Lorazepam |
| Bisacodyl | Meperidine |
| long-term use | |
| Carisoprodol | Metaxalone |
| Chlordiazepoxide | Methocarbamol |
| Cyclobenzaprine | Naproxen |
| Diazepam | Nitrofurantoin |
| Diphenhydramine | Oxybutynin |
| Doxepin | Propoxyphene |
| Fluoxetine | Promethazine |
| Hydroxyzine | Temazepam |
| Indomethacin | Triazolam |

## Strategies to Prevent ADRs in the Elderly

1. Patient education.

2. Consultation with pharmacist regarding proper drug dosages and potential interactions.

3. Use of nonpharmacologic treatments whenever possible.

4. Having patients bring with them all of their medications, including herbal supplements, to physician visits to allow for proper accounting of what they are taking.

5. Using the lowest efficacious dose of a medication available and increasing it gradually.

6. Avoidance of high-risk medications.

# ■ EXERCISE AND THE ELDERLY

## Recommendations for Older Adults Beginning an Exercise Program

There are many demonstrated benefits of regular exercise in older adults, but it remains important for patients to discuss their plans with their physician prior to beginning an exercise regimen. Elderly patients should first undergo a history and physical examination to identify physical limitations and cardiac risk factors. Exercise stress testing can be useful to determine the patient's fitness level and appropriate level of exercise intensity, as well as to identify patients who are at risk for a cardiac event during periods of increased metabolic demand. Older patients should be advised to gradually increase the intensity of their exercise and should not exceed the intensity at which they can no longer comfortably carry on a conversation.

## Exercise Precautions in Osteoporotic Patients

People with osteoporosis should avoid some forms of exercise, including high impact exercises such as jumping or running, and contact sports. They should also refrain from any exercise that vigorously or repeatedly flexes or rotates the spine, including sit-ups, toe touches, and the use of gym equipment with reciprocal arm movements. Such exercises may increase the risk of vertebral fractures.

# ■ PHYSICAL MODALITIES, TRACTION, AND MANIPULATION

Caution is required with the use of these treatments in older adults, as is summarized in the following sections.

## Heat and Cold Therapy

Heat and cold therapy are contraindicated in those with arterial insufficiency, impaired sensation, and in those who are unable to communicate or respond to pain. Older adults may have atrophic skin, increasing their risk of thermal damage with such therapies. Inquire about the presence of metal implants, including pacemakers and deep brain stimulators, prior to ordering deep heat modalities.

## Manual Traction

Caution is advised with use of manual traction in the elderly and is absolutely contraindicated in patients with osteoporosis.

## Spinal Manipulation

Spinal manipulation is also absolutely contraindicated in people with osteoporosis. Relative contraindications include severe spondylosis, osteopenia, and anticoagulation.

## ■ SUMMARY

Significant physiological changes occur with age, which may affect the function of the elderly and increase their susceptibility to disease and injury. Elderly patients often demonstrate impaired mobility and difficulties in activities of daily living. Elderly patients are at high risk of falls, pressure ulcers, delirium, and adverse drug reactions during hospitalization. Many factors increase the risk of falls in the elderly, including lower limb weakness, visual impairment, cognitive impairment, orthostatic hypotension, and medications. The common injuries caused by falls in the elderly include hip fracture, pelvic fracture, vertebral compression fracture and subdural hematoma. In addition, the elderly are also prone to delirium, an acute cognitive impairment with associated change in consciousness that requires detailed assessment. Due to the changes of physiological function of the elderly, the elderly need to be cautious in medication. Regular exercise has many benefits for the elderly. It is necessary to determine the intensity of exercise according to the health level of the elderly in order to reduce the risk of exercise. Therapist should be very careful when using physical modalities, traction, and manipulation in older adults.

## ■ IMPORTANT TERMINOLOGY

geriatric   老年的，老年病学

creatinine clearance   肌酐清除率

vital capacity   肺活量

osteoporosis   骨质疏松

cognitive impairment   认知障碍

delirium   精神异常、谵妄

orthostatic hypotension   直立性低血压

dementia   痴呆

compliance   依从性

anticoagulants   抗凝血药

benzodiazepines   苯二氮䓬类

atrophic   萎缩的

pacemaker   起搏器

## ■ REVIEW QUESTIONS

1. What are the most common fractures caused by falls in the elderly?
2. How to evaluate delirium in the elderly?
3. What factors should be considered in appropriate medications in the elderly?
4. How to make exercise plans for the elderly?
5. What should be paid attention to when applying physical therapy for the elderly?

## ■ REFERENCES

1. Bachman D, Rabins P. "Sundowning" and other temporally associated agitation states in dementia patients. Annu Rev Med.

2006; 57:499-511.

2. Brault JS, Kappler RE, Grogg BE. Manipulation, traction, and massage. In: Braddom RL, ed. Physical Medicine and Rehabilitation, 3rd ed. Philadelphia, PA: Saunders Elsevier; 2007;437-457.

3. Clark GS, Siebens HC. Geriatric Rehabilitation. In: DeLisa JA, Gans BM, Walsh NE, eds. Physical Medicine and Rehabilitation: Principles and Practice. 4th ed. Philadelphia, PA: Lippincott Williams & Wilkins; 2005;1531-1560.

4. Cornell CN, Sculco TP. Orthopedic disorders. In: Duthie EH Jr, Katz PR, Malone ML, eds. Duthie: Practice of Geriatrics. 4th ed. Philadelphia, PA: Saunders Elsevier; 2007:511-527.

5. Fick DM, Cooper JW, Wade WE, et al. Updating the beers criteria for potentially inappropriate medication use in older adults. Arch Int Med. 2003; 163:2716-2724.

6. Ginsberg G, Hattis D, Russ A, Sonawane B. Pharmacokinetic and pharmaco-dynamic factors that can affect sensitivity to neurotoxic sequelae in elderly individuals. Environ Health Perspect. 2005;113(9):1243-1249.

7. Gay RE, Bauer BA, Yang RK. Integrative medicine in rehabilitation. In: Braddom RL. Physical Medicine and Rehabilitation. 3rd ed. Philadelphia: Saunders Elsevier; 2007;511-513.

8. Graf C. Functional decline in hospitalized older adults. Am J Nurs. 2006;106(1):58-67.

9. Keefe KP, Sanson TG. Elderly patients with altered mental status. Emerg Med Clin North Am. 1998;16(4):701-715.

10. Kortebein P, Symons TB, Ferrando A, et al. Functional impact of 10 days of bed rest in healthy older adults. J Gerontol: Med Sci. 2008;63A (10):1076-1081.

11. Lyder CH, Preston J, Grady JN, et al. Quality of care for hospitalized medicare patients at risk for pressure ulcers. Arch Int Med. 2001; 161:1549-1554.

12. National Osteoporosis Foundation. Rehabilitation of patients with osteoporosis-related fractures. Osteoporos: Clin Updates. 2003;1-10.

13. Nied RJ, Franklin B. Promoting and prescribing exercise for the elderly. Am Fam Physician. 2002;65(3):419-426.

14. Pham CB, Dickman RL. Minimizing adverse drug events in older patients. Am Fam Physician. 2007;76(12):1837-1844.

15. Routledge PA, O'Mahony MS, Woodhouse KW. Adverse drug reactions in elderly patients. Br J Clin Pharmacol. 2003;57(2):121-126.

16. Weber DC, Hoppe KM. Physical agent modalities. In: Braddom RL. Physical Medicine and Rehabilitation. 3rd ed. Philadelphia, PA: Saunders Elsevier; 2007;459-477.

17. Williams CM. Using medications appropriately in older adults. Am Fam Physician. 2002;66(10):1917-1924.

（缪　萍）

# ORTHOPEDIC REHABILITATION

## ■ INTRODUCTION

Admission to inpatient orthopedic rehabilitation depends on the patient's degree of disability, their medical complexity, and social factors that would affect their functional independence in post hospital discharge such as availability of support and the accessibility of their home. According to the Centers for Medicaid and Medicare Services, recognized impairment categories include major multiple trauma, lower extremity fracture, lower extremity joint replacement, extremity amputation, and debilitating arthritides.

A multidisciplinary team consisting of physicians, nurses, and therapists create a structured rehabilitation program based on comprehensive medical and functional evaluations and the patient's goals. Goals of therapy focus on improving mobility, balance, strength, range of motion, gait, and activities of daily living (ADLs). Therapy goals should carryover to the outpatient setting. Due to the risk of developing complications in the acute postoperative period, physician monitoring and medical management in an inpatient setting are often a necessary first step to facilitate the patient's successful functional recovery.

## ■ ORTHOPEDIC REHABILITATION

### Pelvic Fractures

The pelvic ring or girdle is formed by the ilium, ischium, pubis, sacrum, and coccyx. It supports the spine and joins the trunk to the lower extremities. Any or all of these bones can be broken. It's about 3% of skeletal fractures involve the pelvis.

Pelvic fractures can result from low- to high-energy blunt trauma (eg, motor vehicle collisions 50%-60%, motorcycle collisions 10%-20%, motor vehicle vs pedestrian collision 10%-20%, and falls 8%-10%). In elderly women with osteoporosis, a fractured pelvis can result from a fall.

Determination of the stability of the fracture is paramount as it affects treatment and prognosis. The pelvic ring (alignment) is preserved and hence stable in a nondisplaced fracture. A displaced fracture is unstable as the pelvic alignment is compromised and is often associated with internal organ injury. The stability of the fracture is best determined by imaging.

### Diagnosis

Two classification systems for pelvic fractures are often used.

The Tile classification system is based on the integrity of the posterior sacroiliac complex.

■ In type A injuries, the sacroiliac complex is intact. The pelvic ring has a stable fracture that can be managed nonoperatively.

- Type B injuries result in partial disruption of the posterior sacroiliac complex. These are often rotationally unstable.
- Type C injuries are characterized by complete disruption of the posterior sacroiliac complex and are rotationally and vertically unstable.

The Young classification system is based on mechanism of injury: lateral compression (LC), anteroposterior compression (APC), vertical shear, or a combination of forces. LC fractures involve transverse fractures of the pubic rami, either ipsilateral or contralateral to a posterior injury.

- Grade I—Associated sacral compression on side of impact.
- Grade II—Associated posterior iliac ("crescent") fracture on side of impact.
- Grade III—Associated contralateral sacroiliac joint injury.

APC fractures involve symphyseal diastasis or longitudinal rami fractures.

In conjunction with the patient's mechanism of injury and symptoms, physical exam findings can be suggestive of pelvic fracture and associated internal organ trauma.

- Tenderness, laxity, or instability on palpation of the bony pelvis suggests fracture.
- Hematuria, vaginal, or rectal bleeding; a hematoma over the ipsilateral thigh, inguinal ligament, or in the perineum; neurovascular deficits in the lower extremities; and hemodynamic instability.
- Instability on hip adduction and pain on hip motion suggests an acetabular fracture, with or without an associated hip fracture.
- Signs of urethral injury in males include a high-riding or boggy prostate on rectal examination, scrotal hematoma, or blood at the urethral meatus.

Anteroposterior pelvic radiographs with inlet and outlet views are commonly used to detect pelvic fracture. CT scan and/or ultrasound of the pelvis and abdomen are important to survey for internal organ laceration and fluid collection.

If blood is found in the urine, urology consultation should be considered. Urethrography and cystography may be used to evaluate associated injuries to the urethra and bladder, respectively.

Arteriography might be necessary to evaluate vascular integrity and identify the source of intraabdominal blood loss if identified in previous studies.

Open reduction and internal fixation (ORIF) is preferred for definitive management of unstable fractures in hemodynamically stable patients with the goal of bone healing and prevention nonunion and malunion. Potential complications include the following:

- Infection
- Hemodynamic instability
- Deep vein thrombosis
- Pulmonary embolism
- Acute pain
- Sexual dysfunction
- Gait dysfunction
- Pelvic misalignment can result in chronic back pain.
- Fractures of the acetabulum include posttraumatic arthritis, femoral head osteonecrosis, neurovascular injury, and sciatic nerve palsy.

## Rehabilitation

Weight-bearing restrictions depend on the degree of fracture instability and are determined by the managing surgeon. Three months of non-weight bearing is usually recommended for vertically unstable fractures.

Physical therapy goals include protected weight-bearing with crutches or a walker in minimally displaced pelvic fractures until radiographic evidence of fracture healing is present. Once the fracture is stable (6-12 weeks), trunk and lower extremity strengthening and range of motion exercises may be introduced. Occupational therapy goals include upper extremity strengthening, transfer training, and instruction in use of adaptive equipment.

Full recovery from a pelvic fracture and resumption of normal activities may take 6 to 12 months.

## Hip Fractures

Hip fractures involve any aspect of the proximal femur from the femoral head to approximately 4 to 5 cm distal to the subtrochanteric area. Patients may complain of localized pain in their hip, groin, and/or knee that is aggravated by walking or an inability to walk.

A fracture of the hip can result from a low-velocity injury (ie, fall and running) or high-velocity injury (ie, motor vehicle collision). In the elderly, hip fracture risk factors include decreased bone mineralization (eg, osteoporosis), visual impairment, cognitive impairment, decreased depth perception, and decreased mobility. The disability resulting from a hip fracture in this population is associated with significant morbidity and mortality. Approximately 15% to 20% die within 1 year.

## Diagnosis

Hip fractures are classified as follows.
- Femoral neck (intrascapular): (45% of fractures)—proximal to greater and lesser trochanter.
- Intertrochanteric (extracapsular): (45% of fractures)—between the greater and lesser trochanter.
- Subtrochanteric: (10% of fractures)—distal to lesser trochanter.
  Physical examination findings include the following:
- Limb shortening and external rotation
- Limited passive range of motion
- Antalgic gait
- Inability to stand
- Tenderness in groin or proximal thigh
- Ecchymosis
  The following complications may occur after hip fracture:
- Avascular necrosis of the femoral head (femoral neck fractures)
- Hip osteoarthritis
- Deep vein thrombosis
- Pulmonary embolism
- Fat embolism
- Blood vessel injury
- Osteofascial compartment syndrome
- Internal bleeding
- Peripheral nerve injury
- Osteomyelitis
- Reflex sympathetic dystrophy

Femoral neck fractures compromise the tenuous blood supply to the proximal femur. The femoral head is at risk of avascular necrosis if the lateral and medial circumflex femoral arteries and the foveal artery are disrupted.

Diagnostic imaging should include radiographs of hip (AP/lateral) with 15° to 20° internal rotation. MRI should be considered if plain radiographs are negative and index of suspicion is high. Bone scan is more sensitive than plain radiographs and less specific than MRI.

## Management

Nonsurgical management includes casting and traction. Most of these fractures are treated surgically.

External fixation is indicated in cases involving severe soft tissue injuries or contamination. A frame around the leg is attached to the bone with pins. Early mobilization of the limb is an advantage of external fixation, but pin insertion sites are a nidus for infection requiring daily inspection and care. Pins may also interrupt arterial blood flow prolonging healing process.

Arthroplasty is indicated for treatment of femoral neck fractures. Advantages of arthroplasty include early mobilization, mechanical stability, and decreased pain. Range of motion restrictions is necessary for 12 weeks after surgery: no hip flexion greater than 90°, no internal rotation past neutral, and no adduction past neutral.

Open Reduction and Internal Fixation (ORIF) is the preferred treatment option for intertrochanteric fractures. Patients can be mobilized early after the procedure and there is no range of motion restrictions. Disadvantages of the procedure include infection and pain.

Intramedullary fixation is an alternative treatment method for intertrochanteric fractures. An intramedullary nail is inserted into the femur, spanning the fracture site. The nail is removed after the fracture heals. This procedure provides great fracture stability, but insertion of the nail can interrupt arterial blood flow prolonging healing process, femoral shaft fractures.

## Rehabilitation

Weight-bearing restrictions, determined by the surgeon, depend on the degree of fracture instability and method of surgical stabilization. The rehabilitation program can be introduced at the bedside level and advanced as appropriate.

If no weight-bearing restrictions are in place, rehabilitation can proceed as follows.

Postoperative day 1: bed or chair level exercises consisting of active range of motion of the quadriceps, and ankle dorsiflexors and plantar flexors. Instruction in performing activities of daily living safely to reduce pain and further injury and the proper use of adaptive equipment is introduced.

Postoperative day 2 to 5: bed to chair mobility and transfer training, gait training with assistive devices, and wheelchair mobility training.

Postoperative day 6 to 10: advanced transfer training (eg, car) and mobility training (eg, stairs).

Outpatient rehabilitation is recommended for progressive strengthening and endurance training 8 to 12 weeks post discharge.

## ■ HAND INJURY

Hand injuries comprise injuries to the upper limb distal to the carpal bones. These injuries are very common, including fractures, nerve injury, tendon injury, vascular damage, and the other soft tissue injury. The hand can assume almost countless positions and postures that allow it to perform numerous functions and manipulations. So the function of hand plays an very important part in daily life and work. The management of hand injuries should be directed in a proper and professional way, especially the rehabilitative treatment after surgery. To gain better function of the injured hand and develop the quality of life of these patients are the ultimate goals.

The functional position and the rest positionare the two important positions of hand. The functional position is defined: the wrist in extension of 20°-25°, the thumb in abduction with slight flexion of metacarpophalangeal joint and interphalangeal joint, and of the other fingers, metacarpophalangeal joint in flexion of 30°-45°, proximal interphalangeal joint in flexion of 60°-68°, distal interphalangeal joint in flexion of 10°-15°. The functional position of hand make it convenient to get into any movement quickly. And also, the rest position is defined: the wrist in extension of 10°-15° with slight bending into the ulnar direction, the fingers falling naturally into a cascade of increasing flexion from the radial to the ulnar side with the small finger the most flexed, the thumb in slight abduction with touching the radial side of distal interphalangeal joint of forefinger. The rest position of hand is the balanced state of all the hand muscles without motion. Better understanding of these two positions of hand is helpful to the rehabilitation of hand function when treating hand injuries.

## Diagnosis

Hand injuries usually have three major symptoms including pain at the site of injury, reduction or loss of function, and numbness distal to the injury. In addition, there are also many signs, such as swelling at the site of injury, bruising, reduction in the range of movement, lacerations and abrasions, bleeding, areas of numbness or reduced sensation, crepitus, deformity, pallor. Tendon injuries are difficult to detect and often missed. Examine the hand in the rest position. A finger out of the normal position suggests tendon, nerve, or bony injury. Examine lacerations when the affected finger is moved out of its range of movement. To test the function of the flexor digitorum superficialis tendon, make the patient flex the proximal interphalangeal joint with the other fingers in extension. Similarly, function of the flexor digitorum profundus tendon can be evaluated by holding the in proximal interphalangeal joint extension and having the patient flex the distal interphalangeal joint. Neurologic deficit is necessary to check out. Examine motor function of each nerve supplying the hand: ulnar nerve—check finger abduction and adduction; radial nerve—look for weakness of the wrist and finger extension; and median nerve—check flexion of the first three digits and thumb opposition. Check sensory function of all three nerves: ulnar nerve—test sensation at the tip of the small finger; radial nerve—check sensation of the dorsal aspect of the first web space; and median nerve—examine sensation at the tip of the second digit. Lacerations of the fingers can cause digital nerve damage and in these cases, examine sensation on each side of the affected fingers. Bone and joint injuries are important for surgeon to determine the therapeutic regimen. Check for any local tenderness, and look for pain on axial compression of each of the metacarpals and phalanges. Examine range of motion of each joint, and look for pain and swelling which can indicate intra-articular fracture. In theory, it is a better choice that all significant hand injuries must be radiographed. To avoid the chance of missing a fracture, three views of the injured part (anteroposterior, oblique, and lateral) are needed. Allen test can also be performed to assess viability of the blood supply to the hand. CT or MRI may be also performed when necessary.

## Management

In the treatment of hand injuries, the surgeon should develop a proper plan to achieve the goal of maximal restoration of the hand function. Although each patient presents aunique problem, and the management of these patients must be developed to suit that particular individual, in general the priorities of reconstruction are as follows: bone and joint stabilization, soft tissue coverage, nerve, and tendon. The stabilization of the bony skeleton should be achieved before nerve, joint, or tendon operations can be successfully performed. As the result of rigid bony stabilization, the soft tissue bed can also be stabilized, and the risk of secondary infection is lessened. Early in the reconstructive period, soft tissue coverage is not only to protect a wound from infection, but also to provide a protective cover beneath which the next surgical procedures can be done. And then early repair of nerves is very necessary and important. Because undue delay of the nerve surgery is likely to obstruct ultimate sensory recovery and the function recovery through reinnervation of specific muscles determines the future needs for specific tendon reconstruction. In addition, return of sensibility in the hand is essential for reasonable function and restoration of sensation may need more time to reach the ideal outcome. Before tendon transfers or grafting surgery, the joints being moved by those muscle-tendon units should be made as supple as possible. So the restoration of active motion of joints is accomplished by proper tendon transfers, grafts, or tenolysis. The main complication of hand injury is the nonfunctional hand. Deformity or impairment of grip, joint fibrosis or laxity, tendon fibrosis, osteomyelitis, limited range of useful motion of the joint, or nerve damage can all impair hand function and need to be taken seriously. So the rehabilitation of hand surgery after surgery plays a great role in hand function recovery.

## Rehabilitation

The postoperative rehabilitation of the patient play a more crucial role in hand surgery than that in other field of surgery. Every effort should be geared toward minimizing swelling, relieving pain, limiting immobilization of the hand to the minimal period according to the goals of the operation, and providing the patient with a specific postoperative exercise plan.

The general rehabilitation concepts are as follows:

Postoperative week 0 to 3: the major work is to keep the outcome of surgery and to avoid the second injury of hand, especially the repaired part.

Postoperative 3 weeks to 3 months: fracture non- or malunion with subsequent deformity should be prevented in this stage. The stabilization of the bony skeleton must be guaranteed which is the priority of hand function rehabilitation.

Postoperative 3 weeks to 6 months: it is the time to restore the range of useful motion of joints by different exercise program on the basis of details.

Postoperative 6 weeks to 6 months: in this period, training for strengthening the muscular power is very important to recover the hand function in daily life and work.

Postoperative 6 weeks to 12 months: return of sensation probably requires the longest time to reach the optimal end result.

As to tendon injuries in the hand, proper early motion has improved tendon healing, reduced complications and enhanced final outcomes. Rehabilitation-making should align with the phases of healing: inflammatory (0-5 days), fibroplasia (3-21 days) and remodeling (21 days to 3 months). After surgery, peritendinous adhesions become an obstacle to tendon excursion in some zones, with timely motion essential to regaining normal excursion. After flexor tendon injury, active motion should start at 4-5 days. But after extensor tendon injury, it is the best choice to start the early motion at 0-5 days without special circumstances. And also, recovery of sensibility in patients with injured never repaired depends on reestablishing the central analysis of input of new patterns, and much can be done to aid recovery by retraining that central perception. Training is started as soon as the patient can recognize stimuli at the fingertips, and it aims to improve function by improvement of the qualities of localization and recognition. In general, rehabilitation of a patient after hand surgery is frequently a complex problem and a long way to go.

## ■ KNEE ARTHROPLASTY

Knee arthroplasty is indicated for treatment of advanced degenerative joint disease (osteoarthritis, rheumatoid arthritis, and traumatic arthritis) that is unresponsive to conservative management.

### Diagnosis

Symptoms and signs include the following:

- Intractable pain
- Functional mobility impairment
- Knee instability
- Valgus, varus, and knee flexion deformities
  Common complications after knee arthroplasty include the following:
- Deep vein thrombosis
- Infection
- Patellofemoral instability, patellar fracture
- Arthrofibrosis
- Aseptic loosening
- Peroneal nerve palsy

Diagnostic imaging anteroposterior view, a lateral view, a 45° posteroanterior view of the knee, and a skyline view (or sunrise view) of the patella. Loss of joint space, cysts, subchondral sclerosis, and osteophytes confirm the diagnosis of osteoarthritis.

## Rehabilitation

Rehabilitation after knee arthroplasty usually progresses as follows.

Postoperative day 1: Bed or chair level exercises consisting of active range of motion of the quadriceps, gluteals, and ankle dorsiflexors and plantar flexors.

Postoperative day 2: Knee flexibility exercises introduced measuring the degree of active knee flexion, active assisted knee flexion, and terminal knee extension to reduce the risk of contracture and gait abnormality.

Strengthening exercises—ankle dorsiflexors and plantar flexors, quadriceps and gluteal sets, straight leg raises, and isometric hip adduction.

Gait training with an assistive device and functional transfer training (eg, sit-to-stand, toilet transfers, and bed mobility).

Postoperative days 3 to 5: Progression of ADL training, range of motion, strengthening exercises, and ambulation on level surface and stairs with assistive device.

## ■ SUMMARY

Goals of orthopedics rehabilitation are to restore range of motion (ROM), improve muscle strength, balance, gait and ADLs. To achieve objectives, a team which physiatrist, surgeon, and nurse should do their best to control pain, correct deformity, protect injured tissue, prevent complications, and guide exercise. Different patients have different situation. It is crucial to receive the knowledge of the mechanism of injury, type of fracture, orthopedic treatment received, normal course of healing for that type of fracture, complications, and expected outcomes. To analysis and evaluate, physiatrists should make different rehabilitation plans, including progression through various stages of ROM and strengthening exercises, ambulation training, bracing, home evaluation, adaptive equipment, vocational retraining, and coordination of care.

## ■ IMPORTANT TERMINOLOGY

activities of daily living (ADLs)　日常生活活动
range of motion (ROM)　活动范围
osteofascial compartment syndrome　骨筋膜隔室综合征

malunion   畸形愈合

nonunion   骨折不愈合

narcotics   麻醉剂

lateral compression (LC)   侧方压缩

anteroposterior compression (APC)   前后方向压缩

osteonecrosis   骨坏死

ecchymosis   瘀斑

arthroplasty   关节成形术

open reduction and internal fixation (ORIF)   切开复位内固定

metacarpophalangeal joint   掌指关节

interphalangeal joint   指间关节

continuous passive movement (CPM)   持续被动运动

nonsteroidal anti-inflammatories   非甾体抗炎药

active motion   主动运动

no known drug allergies (NKDA)   未知的药物过敏症

## ■ REVIEW QUESTIONS

1. What complications can occur after pelvic fractures?
2. What the symptoms and signs can indicate hip fracture?
3. What complications can occur after knee joint replacement?
4. Please describe the general rehabilitation concepts of hand fracture.

## ■ REFERENCES

1. Cifu D, Burnett, McGowan J. Rehabilitation after hip fracture. In: Grabois M, ed. Physical Medicine & Rehabilitation. Cambridge, MA: Blackwell Science, Inc.; 1997.

2. Dechert TA, Duane TM, Frykberg BP, Aboutanos MB, Malhotra AK, Ivatury RR. Elderly patients with pelvic fracture: interventions and outcomes. Am Surg. 2009;75(4):291-295.

3. Egan M, Jaglal S, Byrne K, Wells J, Stolee P. Factors associated with a second hip fracture: a systematic review. Clin Rehabil. 2008;22(3):272-282.

4. Flanagan SR, Ragnarsson KT, Ross MK, Wong DK. Rehabilitation of the geriatric orthopaedic patient. Clin Orthop Relat Res. 1995;316:80-92.

5. Lyons AR. Clinical outcomes and treatment of hip fractures. Am J Med. 1997;103(2A):51S-64S.

6. Schneider M, Kawahara I, Ballantyne G, et al. Predictive factors influencing fast track rehabilitation following primary total hip and knee arthroplasty. Arch Orthop Trauma Surg. 2009;129(12):1585-1591.

7. Howell JW, Peck F. Rehabilitation of flexor and extensor tendon injuries in the hand: Current updates. Injury. 2013;44(3):397-402.

8. Levanon Y.The advantages and disadvantages of using high technology in hand rehabilitation. J Hand Ther. 2013;26(2):179-83.

9. Wolfe SW, Hotchkiss RN, Pederson WC, et al. Green's Operative Hand Surgery. 6th ed. Philadelphia: Churchill Livingstone Publisher; 2011.

（藏　磊）

# 19

# OSTEOPATHIC MEDICINE IN MUSCULOSKELETAL CONDITIONS

## ■ INTRODUCTION

Osteopathic manipulative medicine (OMM) is a diagnostic and therapeutic tool used in many types of illness and disease. Hands-on treatment of musculoskeletal structures is used to reduce pain and normalize performance by reestablishing normal function of the body. This pragmatic approach to the neuromusculoskeletal system is ideally suited to address many complaints in physical medicine and rehabilitation. Osteopathic medicine has the goal of removing obstructions to the body's normal movement and fluid flow (vascular and lymphatic) to optimize function, given the patient's circumstances.

In this chapter, we will give examples of simple OMM (also known as osteopathic manipulative treatment, or OMT) for common bothersome syndromes seen by physiatrists. OMM has minimal side effects, and with an appropriate selection of techniques, it is safe to be used on the vast majority of patients. The suggested treatment schemes of this chapter are for both those trained in OMM and those without formal OMM training who are interested in understanding some very straightforward approaches to patient care. These options of treatment are not meant to be exhaustive, but rather a quick reference of initial treatment ideas for common syndromes. For further inquiry and or study, please see listed references. The American Academy of Osteopathy, an osteopathic medical specialty college, offers courses which are open to interested allopaths. Those who identify specific value of OMM for a patient but are not interested in doing this type of treatment may refer to a physician who practices OMM.

## ■ TYPES OF OMM

The sample treatments are based on 4 commonly taught OMM techniques: muscle energy (ME), counterstrain, myofascial release, and Still technique. Each of these is a system of diagnosis and treatment. OMM is based on analysis and treatment of the whole body, as biomechanical issues in one region affect all regions. The treatments presented, however, will often improve the patient's condition when used in isolation. If they do not, a more holistic analysis is warranted.

### Cervical Spondylotic Radiculopathy

#### Common findings

Pain, numbness, or weakness in the neck, shoulder, arm, or hand.

Tingling or pins and needles sensation in the affected area.

Limited range of motion in the neck.

Muscle weakness or atrophy.

Loss of reflexes in the affected area.

**Pain:** Neck pain, shoulder pain, and arm pain.

**Treatment:** Direct myofascial release

- patient in supine position.
- Physician standing on the side of the patient's head.
- The palm of the operator's hand is placed under the articular process (support point) at the level of the patient's dysfunction.
- Physician lifts the neck tissue of the patient.
- Control the strength only to press the skin and the superficial fascia under the skin.
- Ensure the hand does not slide on the skin.
- Physician pays attention to whether there is symmetrical or asymmetrical loose-tight obstacle when the joint rotates up and down, left and right and twists.
- After checking the loosening-tightening asymmetry, physician should also apply direct or indirect manipulation to the loosening-tightening area.
- The force should be very gentle and moderate.
- This technique should last for 20 to 60 seconds or continue until patient feel relaxed.

## Periarthritis of Shoulder

### Common findings

Shoulder joint pain and stiffness, especially in the morning or after rest.

Limited movement, especially in lifting and outward rotation.

Atrophy and weakness of shoulder muscles.

Possible neck and upper arm pain.

Patients may experience sleep disturbances and emotional problems.

**Pain:** Shoulder joint pain, neck pain, and upper arm pain.

**Treatment:** Muscle energy technique

Shoulder extension with elbow flexion

- Patient in the healthy side position.
- Physician standing opposite to the patient.
- Physician's near head side hand is placed on the patient's shoulder to fix any movement caused by any kind of debridement or fracture, the fingers are placed on the side of the splenial spine of the shoulder.
- The thumb is placed on the anterior aspect of the clavicular surface.
- Physician's proximal caudal hand grasps the patient's elbow.
- patient's shoulder is extended in the horizontal plane until the restrictive barrier is touched.
- At the end of the above movement, a slow, gentle tremor (arthroscopic, building and breaking) movement is applied.
- Muscle energy activation method: The patient attempts to contract the shoulder against the resistance applied by the operator. This contraction lasts for 3 to 5 seconds.
- After a period of rest, the shoulder is extended again until a new obstacle is touched and cannot be moved.
- Repeat 3 to 5 times and then assess the patient's degree of extension.
- Apply a resistance force to the patient's extension (mutual inhibition), which will improve the treatment effect.

**Goal:** strengthen the rotator cuff muscles, while stretching the pectoralis muscles to improve positioning of the humeral head in the glenoid fossa, and decrease internal rotation of the humerus. Strengthening of rhomboids, lower trapezius and serratus anterior was undertaken to improve scapula control.

## Epicondylitis

### Common findings

Radial head somatic dysfunction

Restricted forearm pronation

Restricted forearm supination

Tenderness of epicondyle to palpation

**Pain:** Elbow pain and wrist pain.

### Treatment

- Patient seated.
- Physician facing patient.
- Have the patient flex the forearm.
- Support the proximal forearm with one hand, placing your index finger laterally and posteriorly behind the radial head.
- Restricted supination:
  - With your other hand, grasp the distal forearm and introduce supination to the initial point of restriction.
  - Have the patient attempt and maintain pronation against physician resistance for 3 to 5 seconds.
  - After contraction, wait 2 seconds in the same position, then gently reengage forearm supination restriction.
  - Repeat the procedure 3 to 5 times, slightly increasing the range of supination each time.
- Restricted pronation:
  - Start as above. With your other hand, grasp the distal forearm and introduce pronation to the initial point of restriction.
  - Have the patient attempt and maintain supination against physician resistance for 3 to 5 seconds.
  - After contraction, wait 2 seconds in the same position, then gently reengage forearm pronation restriction.
  - Repeat the procedure 3 to 5 times, slightly increasing the range of pronation each time.

## ■ CARPAL TUNNEL SYNDROME (MEDIAN NEUROPATHY AT THE WRIST)

### Common findings

Tight transverse retinaculum

Tinel test

Weakness of affected hand

Pronator teres syndrome (proximal median nerve impingement)

### Pain

Tingling and numbness in digits on affected side

Radiating pain into hand

Radiating pain proximally in forearm

**Treatment:** Direct myofascial release

- Patient in seated position.
- Physician facing the patient.
- Grasp the patient's affected wrist with both hands.
- Position thumbs over the transverse retinaculum.
- Apply deep and lateral pressure for 1 to 2 minutes to patient tolerance, stretching the soft tissue by slowly moving your thumbs outward as the tissue relaxes.
- Repeat on several visits as needed for symptoms to resolve.
- Can be done prophylactically on unaffected side.

### Self-Treatment

Teach the patient to stretch the transverse retinaculum by pulling the tendons deeper into the carpal tunnel.
- Have the patient place the affected hand palm down, with the middle and distal phalanges of the long and ring fingers against a flat surface.
- Place downward pressure on the long and ring fingers, while using the other hand to pull the thumb posteriorly for about 30 seconds.
- This can be done several times a day.

## LOW BACK PAIN

### Possible Diagnoses

Idiopathic low back pain (LBP)

Musculoskeletal LBP

Non-radiating LBP Low back strain

Iliolumbar ligament syndrome

Psoas syndrome

Lumbar somatic dysfunction

### Common findings

Tenderness to palpation of lumbar paravertebral musculature

Accentuated or diminished normal spinal curves

Compensatory postural or gait patterns

Functional leg length discrepancy

### Pain

Lumbar myofascial pain

Abdominal pain

Groin pain

**Treatment:** Modified Still technique

First, rule out ruptured disk, bony, neurologic, or soft tissue pathology. Then rule out serious diagnoses, if a functional musculoskeletal condition still remains, the musculoskeletal dysfunction treatment is required.

The treatment given is for the very common L5 somatic dysfunction; however, the same principle can be applied at superior lumbar segments after treating L5. LBP can come from many different causes and somatic dysfunctions, and the scope of this publication does not permit a full analysis. The sample below is for articulatory dysfunction at L5/S1 and multifidus/myofascial soft tissue texture abnormalities.

■ Position patient supine on the exam table with space for the examiner to move freely.

■ Place the fingers of your most cephalad hand under the patient at L5 to monitor the segment; check for tenderness lateral to the spinous process (if treating at superior levels, at the transverse processes).

■ Flex hip and knee toward the abdomen with most caudal hand on the patient's knee of side nearest the examiner.

■ Continue to slowly flex hip to point where you feel motion at your finger behind the vertebra.

■ Adduct the thigh slightly, noting whether abnormal tissue texture decreases at your palpating finger (if so, this is a flexion somatic dysfunction of L5).

   ■ The patient should feel some degree of pain or tension resolution.

   ■ If no resolution is noticed, slowly abduct the hip to about 60° while retaining flexion to L5, This should be accompanied by a palpable release of tissue tension (if so, this is an extension somatic dysfunction of L5).

■ Ideally, complete resolution of the tenderness is noticed when the area is re-palpated; however, significant improvement without complete resolution may yield success.

   Once the position of greatest resolution is found:

   ■ Apply a slight compressive force through the knee toward the lumbar spine.

   ■ While maintaining this compression, slowly move the knee laterally (for a flexion dysfunction, medially across the midline for an extension dysfunction), then extend it and the hip in a smooth arc, ending up with the leg fully extended on the table.

### Additional LBP OMM Treatments

Virtually, any form of OMM can be selected and used to treat LBP, depending on the training of the physician, the condition of the patient, and the application of good clinical judgment.

   Lumbar spine, pelvis, or sacral somatic dysfunctions are often treated with the following:

   ME

   Counterstrain

   Myofascial release

   High velocity low amplitude

   Still technique

   Craniosacral

## Osteoporosis

### Common findings

Fractures: including spinal fractures, hip fractures, and wrist fractures, these fractures often occur with minor trauma.

   Decreased height: due to the occurrence of spinal fractures, patients' height may be shortened.

   Lower back pain: due to spinal fractures or disc herniation, patients may experience lower back pain.

   Bone density loss: bone density loss can be seen through X-ray examination.

   **Pain:** Lower back pain and joint pain.

   **Treatment:** Muscle energy technique

■ Patient seated.

■ Physician stand opposite to the side of the rotational disorder.

■ Patient's right hand is placed behind the neck.

- Patient's left hand is placed on the right elbow.
- Physician's left arm is extended under the patient's left arm and grasps the patient's right forearm.
- The right hand monitors the L2, L3 spinous process or L2, L3 intervertebral space while the left arm and left hand flex and extend the patient's torso until L2 and L3 are in a straight line.
- The right hand monitors the localized flexion and rotation of the L2, L3 transverse process while the left arm and left hand bend the patient's torso to the right and then rotate it to the left.
- Patient rotates or pushes the right shoulder to the right, while the Physician's left hand applies a vertical counterforce.
- The isometric contraction is held for 3 to 5 seconds and the patient is instructed to relax.
- After the patient is completely relaxed, physician maintains the L2 neutral position to maximize the patient's right bend and left bend.
- Repeat 3 to 5 times or until there is maximum improvement in the movement of the dysfunctional area.
- Reassess the movement of the dysfunctional area to determine the efficacy of the technique.

## Osteoarthritis

### Common findings

Pain: Affected joints might be hurt during or after movement.

Stiffness: Joint stiffness might be most noticeable upon awakening or after being inactive.

Tenderness: Your joint might feel tender when you apply light pressure to or near it.

Loss of flexibility: You might not be able to move your joint through its full range of motion.

Grating sensation: You might feel a grating sensation when you use the joint, and you might hear popping or crackling.

Bone spurs: These extra bits of bone, which feel like hard lumps, can form around the affected joint.

Swelling: This might be caused by soft tissue inflammation around the joint.

**Pain:** Back pain, pelvic pain and knee pain.

**Treatment:** Direct myofascial release

Lumbosacral area

- Patient in prone position.
- Physician standing next to the patient.
- Physician places one hand below the patient's lumbar region (eg, 4th and 5th lumbar vertebrae) and the other hand above the lumbar region (eg, 1st and 2nd lumbar vertebrae).
- Physician should note whether there is symmetrical or asymmetrical loose-tight impairment of joint up-down, left-right rotation and counterclockwise and clockwise movement function.
- After identifying the site of the asymmetric loose-tight disorder, physician applies direct or indirect manipulation to the disorder, respectively.
- The force should be very gentle and moderate.
- The technique should last for 20-60 seconds or until a sensation of relaxation is felt.

Limbs

- Patient lies supine on the consultation bed.
- Physician stands on the side of the patient's foot.
- Physician holds the patient's heel cuff and heel bone from below with both hands (manual study upward).
- patient's legs are lifted upwards by 20° to 30°.
- patient's calves are gently stretched backwards to produce a stretching effect on the calf and skeletal joints.

- Physician applies rotation and traction toward the inside and/or outside and/or along the leg to confirm whether there is an asymmetric loose-tightness disorder during movement and which is more pronounced in the pelvis, medullary knee, and other tissues.
- After determining the site of the asymmetric loose-tight disorder, the operator applied direct and indirect manipulation to the disorder.
- The force should be very gentle and moderate.
- The technique should last for 20-60 seconds or until a sensation of relaxation is felt.

## PSOAS SYNDROME

### Possible diagnoses

Lumbar sprain/strain

LBP

Acute iliopsoas strain

Hypertonic Iliopsoas

### Common findings

Patient is unable to straighten up, and is leaning toward affected side

Tenderness in the iliac fossa

Thomas test (functional)

### Pain

Deep LBP

Leg, groin or pelvic pain

Sacroiliac joint pain

**Treatment:** Counterstrain technique

- Patient in supine position.
- Physician on the side of the dysfunction.
- Find the tender point about 5 cm medial to the anterior superior iliac spine (ASIS) and deep in the iliac fossa.
- Maintain a monitoring finger on the tender point.
- Have the patient flex the hips and knees to about 90°, placing your thigh under the distal legs.
- Have the patient spread the knees apart, so that the thighs are abducted and in external rotation.
- Fine tune the position by passively flexing the patient's hips farther, or inducing further external rotation on the affected side by moving the affected thigh into further abduction.
- Hold for 90 seconds in this position.
- Slowly and passively return the patient's hips, thighs, and legs to neutral position.
- Retest the tender point.

**Goal:** Achievement of at least 70% reduction of tenderness after the patient is returned to neutral position.

## FUNCTIONAL LEG LENGTH DISCREPANCY

### Possible diagnoses

Short leg syndrome

Runner's short leg syndrome

Pelvic somatic dysfunction

## Common findings

Limp

Functional scoliosis

Foot arch asymmetry

Pelvic asymmetry

## Pain

LBP—secondary to compensatory scoliosis

Sacroiliac pain

Pelvic pain

Knee pain

Foot arch pain

**Treatment:** ME technique

Pelvic asymmetry

Short leg treatment—posterior rotation of ipsilateral pelvis

- Patient in prone position.
- Physician on side opposite to the dysfunction.
- With your caudad hand, grasp the flexed knee of affected side.
- Place your cephalad hand over the posterior superior iliac spine (PSIS) on the side of dysfunction.
- Passively extend the hip until you feel motion at the PSIS.
- Have the patient pull the knee down toward the table.
- Have the patient maintain this muscle contraction for 3 to 5 seconds.
- Have the patient relax, then wait 2 seconds in same position; gently reengage the hip extension barrier.
- Repeat patient contraction 3 to 5 times, resetting to the barrier after each contraction.

Long leg treatment—anterior rotation of contralateral pelvis

- Patient in supine position.
- Physician on the side of the dysfunction.
- With your caudad hand, grasp the thigh under the ipsilateral flexed knee.
- Place your cephalad hand on the ASIS on the side of the dysfunction.
- Passively flex the hip until motion is sensed at the ASIS.
- Have the patient push the thigh against your hand, and maintain the contraction for 3 to 5 seconds.
- Have the patient relax, then wait 2 seconds in the same position; gently reengage the hip flexion barrier.
- Repeat patient contraction 3 to 5 times, resetting to the barrier after each contraction.

## PIRIFORMIS SYNDROME

## Common findings

History of fall on buttocks

Postpartum

Pelvic asymmetry

## Pain

Buttock pain

Hip pain/greater trochanteric pain

LBP

Pelvic pain

## Tender point location

- Find while patient is in the prone position.
- The tender point is located half to two-thirds of the way on a line between the inferior lateral angle (ILA) of the sacrum and the greater trochanter (muscle body/musculotendinous junction of the piriformis).
  **Treatment:** Counterstrain technique
- Patient in supine position. This technique can also be done in the prone position with affected leg over side of table, accompanied by hip flexion, external rotation, and abduction.
- Physician on the affected side.
- Find the tender point and monitor it with one finger.
- Flex the hip (90° or more) and knee on the affected side.
- Shorten the muscle further by adding hip abduction and external rotation until tenderness is decreased by 70% or more.
- Hold for 90 seconds in this position of least tension.
- Slowly and passively return the lower extremity to neutral.
- Reassess the tender point by palpating it with your monitoring finger.
  **Goal:** Achievement of at least 70% reduction of tenderness after the patient is returned to neutral position.

# PROXIMAL TIBIOFIBULAR JOINT PAIN

## Common findings

Decreased range of ankle motion

Tenderness of fibular head to palpation

Pain with running or walking

## Pain

Fibular head glide restriction with malalignment

Impingement of deep peroneal nerve

**Treatment:** Modified Still technique

- Patient in seated position.
- Find ankle direction of least movement.
  - Decreased ankle plantar flexion—fibular head has restricted posterior glide.
  - Decreased ankle dorsiflexion—fibular head has restricted anterior glide.
- Place the affected knee into about 15° of flexion; place the ankle in the direction opposite to its restriction.
- Have the patient relax the leg.
- Apply a small axial force through the ankle with one hand while resisting force with the other hand at the fibular head.
- With hand at the knee, apply translational force to the fibular head.
  - Decreased ankle plantar flexion—apply an anterior to posterior force on the fibular head.
  - Decreased ankle dorsiflexion—apply a posterior to anterior force on the fibular head.
- While continuing to apply axial force and translational force on fibular head, start with the ankle in the

most relaxed position and place it through the range of motion toward the direction of the restriction.

■ Retest the proximal fibular head glide.

# INVERSION ANKLE SPRAIN

## Possible diagnoses

Lateral ankle sprain

Recurrent ankle sprain

Chronic ankle pain

First- and second-degree acute ankle sprains

## Common findings

Weak tibialis anterior

Weak fibularis (peroneal) musculature

Restricted dorsiflexion

Ankle instability

## Pain

Lateral ankle pain

Knee pain

Low back pain

Proximal tibiofibular pain

**Treatment:** Counterstrain technique

■ Patient in lateral recumbent position with affected side down on table.

■ Have the patient flex the knee, placing the affected foot and lateral malleolus over the edge of the table.

■ Place a rolled towel under the distal fibula to provide padding for comfort.

■ With monitoring hand, grasp the affected ankle proximal to the malleolus.

■ Find the diagnostic tender point in a depression about 3 cm anterior to and inferior to the posterior portion of the lateral malleolus.

■ With operating hand, grasp the planter aspect of the mid-foot.

■ Place the foot in eversion.

■ Apply up to 15 kg of pressure (promoting eversion) through the thenar eminence of the operating hand, focused at a point approximately 3 cm distal to the medial malleolus.

■ Adjust the position and patient comfort with external rotation and plantar flexion, until tenderness is reduced by at least 70%.

■ Hold in this position for 90 seconds.

■ Slowly and without patient assistance, return ankle to neutral.

■ Retest tender point.

**Goal:** Achievement of at least 70% reduction of tenderness after the patient is returned to neutral position.

# PLANTAR FASCIITIS

## Common findings:

Tenderness to palpation of plantar fascia

Tight gastrocnemius and Achilles tendon

Flat arches

High arches

**Pain**

Plantar fascia

■ Inflammation

■ Muscle hypertonicity

Heel pain

Calf pain

**Treatment:** Counterstrain technique

■ Patient in prone position.

■ Physician on the affected side.

■ Find the tender point on the plantar surface at the most distal aspect of the calcaneus where the plantar fascia attaches.

■ Flex the knee on the affected side to about 70°.

■ Place your foot on the table, and the dorsal surface of the patient's foot on your thigh.

■ With your cephalad hand, push the calcaneus toward your thigh, shortening the plantar fascia.

■ At the same time, use your other hand to push the distal foot toward the tender point, shortening the plantar fascia from the distal end until the tenderness is decreased by at least 70%.

■ Hold for 90 seconds in this position of least tension.

■ Slowly and without patient assistance return ankle back to neutral.

■ Reassess the tender point by palpating it with your monitoring finger.

**Goal:** Achievement of at least 70% reduction of tenderness after the patient is returned to neutral position.

## ■ SUMMARY

Osteopathic manipulative medicine (OMM) is also known as osteopathic manipulative treatment (OMT). This hands-on treatment of musculoskeletal structures is based on analysis and treatment of the whole body, as biomechanical issues in one region affect all regions. OMM is ideally suited to address many complaints in physical medicine and rehabilitation. It is aimed to remove obstructions to the body's normal movement and fluid flow (vascular and lymphatic), thus reducing pain and normalizing performance by reestablishing normal function of the body. There are 4 common OMM techniques, muscle energy, counterstrain, myofascial release, and Still technique, each of which is a system of diagnosis and treatment. These techniques often improve the patient's condition when used in isolation. In addition, they have minimal side effects, and are safe to be used on the vast majority of patients. Examples of simple OMM are given for common bothersome syndromes seen by physiatrists, including epicondylitis, carpal tunnel syndrome, low back pain, psoas syndrome, functional leg length discrepancy, piriformis syndrome, proximal tibiofibular joint pain, inversion ankle sprain, and plantar fasciitis. For each syndrome, common characteristic is introduced, and possible diagnoses are provided when necessary. Subsequently, one type of technique is chosen with a detailed description of how to perform it.

## ■ IMPORTANT TERMINOLOGY

osteopathic manipulative medicine　整骨疗法医学

neuromusculoskeletal system   神经肌肉骨骼系统

muscle energy   肌肉能量

counterstrain   拮抗松弛术

myofascial release   筋膜放松

Still technique   Still 技术

restricted pronation   旋前受限

restricted supination   旋后受限

carpal tunnel syndrome   腕管综合征

cephalad hand   近端手

caudal hand   远端手

anterior superior iliac spine   髂前上棘

posterior superior iliac spine   髂后上棘

plantar flexion   跖屈

dorsiflexion   背屈

thenar eminence   鱼际

## ■ REVIEW POINTS

1. Please describe the advantage of OMM.

2. Please describe OMM techniques.

3. Please describe the self-treatment of carpal tunnel syndrome.

4. Please describe the common findings of LBP.

5. Please compare the treatment between flexion and extension somatic dysfunction of L5 in LBP.

（倪国新）

# PAIN MANAGEMENT

## ■ EPIDEMIOLOGY

According to the National Center for Health Statistics of the USA, 76.2 million people had pain issue or were treated for pain during 2006 at an estimated cost of approximately 100 billion dollars, in health care expenses, lost income, and lost productivity. In the same report it was noted that 37% of Americans aged 20 years or more and almost 60% of those aged 65 years or more reported pain. For comparison, there are 23.6 million people with diabetes or 23.3 million people with coronary artery diseases in the United States.

Of the 40 million visits for new pain to primary care physicians (PCPs), 41% was for musculoskeletal pain issues. Acute pain issues made up 15% to 20% of those complaints, subacute pain 50% to 60%, and chronic pain 25% to 30%. Of all complaints, low back pain was the most common diagnosis and cause for missed workdays with an annual incidence of 15% to 20% of the adult population and a lifetime incidence of 60% to 85% of the population. Approximately 14% of U.S. adults have serious chronic back conditions.

## ■ PAIN EVALUATION

Pain is a subjective experience. Currently, there is no system that definitively provides independent data to determine a patient's degree of pain. There are tools that help determine how a patient's pain is affecting or impairing their function, but these are for the most part subjective. They rely on patients being sincere and honest in their answers, but they have good reliability. A list of some common questionnaires is noted below (Table 20.1). Refer to Table 20.2 for the Functional Pain Scale.

**TABLE 20.1** ▪ Scales used for evaluating pain

| Questionnaire | Description |
| --- | --- |
| McGill Pain Questionnaire | Developed in 1971 by Melzack and Torgerson, these 20 questions group various descriptive words together and patients are to pick 1-2 words that describe their pain. |
| Pain Disability Index | Developed 1987 by Tait et al, it is designed to measure the impact of chronic pain on various daily activities. |
| Cancer Total Quality Pain Management Patient Assessment Tool (TQPM) | Developed by Paice et al, in 1998, it measures pain management outcomes, expectations, barriers, and satisfaction of inpatients as well as outpatients. |
| Profile Fitness Mapping (PFM) | This was developed between 1992 and 1994 at the Alfta Rehabilitation Center in Sweden as a clinical-based back-specific questionnaire that incorporates both functional limitation and a symptom scale along with subclassification of severity and temporal aspects of symptomatology [1]. |

Continued

| Questionnaire | Description |
|---|---|
| Becks Depression Inventory- II | Originally developed in 1961 and revised and republished in 1996 by Dr. Aaron T. Beck, it includes 21 multiple-choice questions. The score (0-63) is reliable for measuring the severity of depression. No depression (0-9); mild to moderate (10-18); moderate to severe (19-29); and severe (30-63) [2] 1996. |
| Functional Pain Scale (FPS) | This scale was developed specifically to incorporate both subjective and objective components and reliably assess pain in older adults [3]. |

**TABLE 20.2 ▪ Functional pain scale (Adult)**

| Functional Pain Scale | Simple | Description |
|---|---|---|
| 0 | No pain | No functional impairment |
| 1 | Tolerable | Does not interfere with activities |
| 2 | Tolerable | Interferes with some activities |
| 3 | Intolerable | Able to use phone, TV, or read |
| 4 | Intolerable | Unable to use phone, TV, or read, ambulate |
| 5 | Intolerable | Unable to verbally communicate |

Treating pain like most other areas of medicine requires skills in the evaluation, observation, and interpretation of diagnostic, radiologic, and interventional techniques to determine the cause of a patient's pain as well as to evaluate their response to medications and other treatments.

## Pain Management Guidelines

There are several basic approaches to the treatment of pain, and clinical guidelines also vary depending on the group's point of view. There are 4 societies whose mission is primarily pain management that have very different perspectives on treatment and different algorithms for the treatment of pain (Table 20.3).

As an example, some physicians question the validity of discography (for discogenic pain) based on a single randomized controlled trial[4] in 2000 concluding that discography was affected by somatization. Other studies challenge this conclusion. A study by Manchikanti et al in 2001 reported that when properly performed[5], discography is not affected by somatization disorder at all[6]. Other studies by Derby et al[7,8] and Bogduk[9] showed that when properly performed by a trained interventional pain physician, the technique was approximately 80% specific. This is one example of how conflicting evidence can affect clinical practice and the development of practice guidelines. Because of this, we recommended that all practitioners involved in pain management be familiar with guidelines from the groups mentioned in Table 20.3 and that in areas of conflicting evidence, practitioners review the primary literature to draw conclusions.

**TABLE 20.3 ▪ Source and focus of available pain management guidelines**

| Society | Focus |
|---|---|
| American Pain Society | Noninvasive focus—medications and physical therapy |
| American Society of Interventional Pain Physicians | Combination of medications and interventional therapy |
| North American Spine Society | Surgical focus |
| International Spine Interventional Society | Interventional focus |

## Physical Examination

The physical examination is a very important component of any evaluation. Pain patterns are suggestive but not always consistent with the origin of a pain. The goal of the physical examination is to help narrow the differential diagnosis, as it pertains to the potential causes of a patient's pain.

The spine is the most common source of pain. The intricacy of spinal anatomy complicates diagnosis because any of the multiple parts of the spine can refer pain to the same area or cause pain focally. Nerve compression, nerve root irritation, and facet joints can all cause pain both in the spinal area and pain referred to the extremities. It is important to understand that facet joints and nerve root irritation can result in pain in the extremities. Intervertebral disc issues can cause both axial back pain and pain in the extremity by causing nerve root irritation.

The spine is commonly divided into 3 columns to describe stability and the need for surgical intervention.

The 3-column principle can be used for localizing common spinal pathologies or causes of spinal pain, which is again the most prevalent source of back pain. The 3-column primary reference point is the spinal canal, thus, dividing the spine into anterior canal, intraspinal canal, and posterior spinal canal areas (Table 20.4). Thinking about the spine in this context provides a framework to systematically evaluate spinal sources of pain and to determine appropriate treatment. Figure 20.1 illustrates how to apply this approach in the case of lumbar pain.

The usual general physical evaluation of the patient with a painful complaint should include inspection, palpation, range of motion (ROM), sensation, and strength. Below are some physical signs or symptoms that are useful when evaluating these patients.

**TABLE 20.4** ▪ The 3-column division of the spine

| Anterior Spinal Column or Anterior Spine | Middle Spinal Column or Intraspinal Canal | Posterior Column or Posterior Spine |
| --- | --- | --- |
| Posterior longitudinal ligament | Spinal cord | Lamina |
| Vertebral body | Nerve roots | Facet joints |
| Intravertebral disc | Pedicles | Intraspinal ligament |
| Anterior longitudinal ligament | Epidural space Contents of spinal canal | Spinous process Paraspinal muscles |

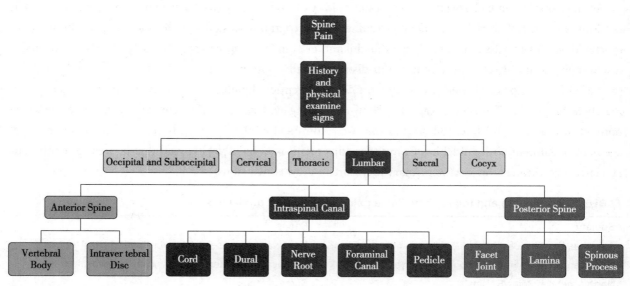

**Figure 20.1** Example of using the 3-column approach for lumbar spinal pain. Using this approach, all the potential sources of pain are evaluated systematically.

## General Appearance

Overall appearance can give some insights as to the presence and severity of pain. These nonspecific signs cannot be correlated to pain severity objectively.

## Provocative Maneuvers

Physical examination maneuvers can help the diagnostician to narrow down the possible areas of pathology (Table 20.5).

A study has shown that a positive response to interventional facet joint therapy or diagnostic medial branch block (which if confirmed twice will respond to radiofrequency ablation of the medial branch nerve) is likely if 5 or more of the facet joint maneuvers detailed in Table 20.5 are positive (92% positive predictive value) [10].

**TABLE 20.5 ▪ Provocative maneuvers and physical examination signs to determine site of spinal pathology**

| Location | Methods of Evaluation | Description and Findings |
|---|---|---|
| Facet joints | Facet loading | Rotation and extension focal at suspected level of pathology results in pain being produced at the involved level |
| | Extension/ hyperextension | Pain will be noted during the extension phase as the problematic level of the facets is activated |
| | Rising from a flexed position | From a seated position the patient arises. Patient reports pain focally in the back at the levels involved |
| | Focal palpation | In patients where soft tissue allows, palpation occurs lateral to the spinous process over the region of the facets. Pressure to the facet capsule will result in pain. In some cases, muscle spasms will prevent this palpation |
| | Decreased or impaired range of motion in suspected spinal segment not otherwise expected | Instructions: Palpate over each spinal segment as the individual segment is activated in the movement of extension, flexion, or rotation. Alteration in normal movement, a halt to the movement process, or pain noted by the patient as an individual segment is activated will suggest that the segment is involved in the pain process |
| | Blot maneuver | Posterior to anterior load performed by placing the palm across the area of the 1-2 individual spinous levels while the patients is lying flat on his/her stomach and then applying a light to moderate light load briefly. This should produce pain at the involved segment |
| Vertebral body or disc | Spinal loading | Produces pain |
| | Prolonged sitting | Produces pain |
| | Blot maneuver | Palm over only 1 segment with moderate load will result in pain |
| | Prolonged standing | Produces pain |
| Vertebral body or disc | Movement avoidance | Patient may prefer to stay still with no rotation, extension, or flexion |
| | Flexion or extension | Pain on flexion is suggestive |
| | Blot maneuver | Produces pain (as described above but with moderate to heavy pressure) |

## Pain Timeline

Pain duration should be described in every case. Commonly accepted terminology is described in Table 20.6.

**TABLE 20.6** ▪ Pain duration descriptors

| Pain Type | Duration/Time |
|---|---|
| Acute pain | 0-4 weeks |
| Subacute pain | 1-6 weeks |
| Chronic pain | 6 months or more |

## Specific Pain Conditions

### Acute Pain

Acute pain makes up 15% to 20% of all pain issues or 40 million visits a year to PCPs. The approach for treating acute pain differs between different health care professionals. For a physiatrist, the primary goal is to determine and treat risk factors, biomechanical imbalances, and pathologies that result in acute pain. Once the aforementioned problems are determined, a treatment program will be developed to educate, adapt, or fix biomechanical imbalances and treat the primary pathology causing the patients pain (Figure 20.2).

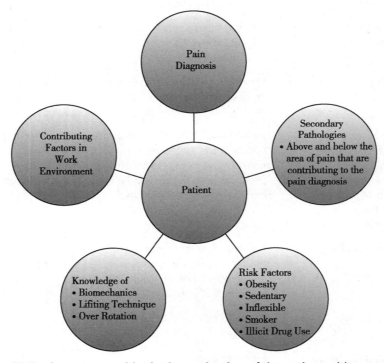

**Figure 20.2** Areas to consider in the evaluation of the patient with acute pain.

### Subacute Pain

Subacute pain is the most prevalent type of pain that requires evaluation and treatment according to initial visit to both the emergency room and PCPs [11]. In this setting, most patients have had the pain for a minimum of 4 weeks and as long as 6 months. In these cases, an initial diagnosis may have already been given.

The primary components of a subacute pain evaluation are the following:

1. Ensure that all the underlying pathologies or disease processes have been halted if possible.

2. Ensure all related pathologies and diagnoses have been determined and treated.

3. Ensure that the pain is not referred from other areas or undiagnosed biomechanical dysfunction.

4. Ensure appropriate adherence to initial medical recommendations or other recommendations.

## Subacute Pain Sample Case

The patient is a 65-year-old female former factory worker with a known diagnosis of cervical radicular pain and a C5 disc herniation with continued pain despite 6 weeks of physical therapy. She reported 60% pain relief with the initial treatment plan and has undergone 2 epidural steroid injections.

Repeat epidural steroid injection or surgical referral for possible cervical discectomy and fusion are considerations; however, it would be reasonable to reevaluate this patient and ensure that there is no residual pain secondary to other spinal pathology such as facet-mediated pain or shoulder pathology. For example, a previous otherwise stable partial rotator cuff tear could be aggravated by altered mechanics because of severe radicular pain. These concomitant painful pathology overlaps can be missed. Ensuring early pain control and adherence to treatment are also necessary to prevent the development of a chronic pain syndrome. Educating the patient regarding all factors that contribute to their pain is crucial. These include comorbid diseases, social behaviors (smoking, inactivity, or others), poor body mechanics, and work environment. Important factors to consider for the patient with subacute pain are summarized in Figure 20.3. Creating a treatment program that focuses on the multiple factors that may be contributing to continued pain is extremely important and can help minimize the conversion of a patient from subacute to chronic pain issues.

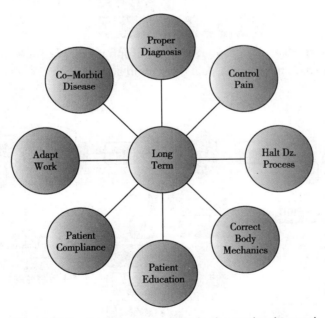

**Figure 20.3** Factors to consider in the evaluation and treatment of patients with subacute pain.

## Diagnostic Testing

As time goes by and painful complaints remain unresolved, the decision on further diagnostic testing should be based on the initial impression while considering other contributing factors as described above.

An important consideration is the patient's age. With increased age, the number of intraspinal or general pathologies that can be present on imaging evaluation increase without necessarily contributing to their pain issues. The multitude of spinal pathologies in the older population complicates evaluation and make more difficult to determine which is the primary pain generator. In those cases, diagnostic injections become increasingly important to aid in making an accurate diagnosis. The diagnostic tests in a particular case should be based on the most likely pain generator (ie, bone, joint, muscle, nerve, spine, or soft tissues). The decision-making process is described in Figure 20.4. In the case of joint pain, the decision process for ordering diagnostic testing is described in Figure 20.5.

**Figure 20.4** Determination of appropriate diagnostic testing based on the primary pain generating system.

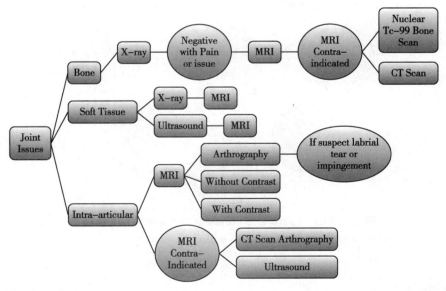

**Figure 20.5** Decision-making algorithm in cases of joint pain.

## Opioid Pain Medications

Opioids can be useful in managing pain in selected cases. The most common delivery routes are oral, intravenous, intramuscular, and transdermal. Opioids can have both short and long duration of effect from 15 to 20 minutes to 72 hours and are metabolized by either the liver or kidney or both.

The choice to start a patient on opioids varies depending on the physician's background, education, and experience level with opioid medication. The comfort level and experience a physician has prescribing opioids can affect their choices and use of these drugs.

Physicians should consider the following factors when deciding whether opioid pain medications are appropriate for a patient:

1. Patients respond to opioids differently. Some studies suggest that there might be genetic polymorphism for human opioid sensitivity[12]. Patients with decreased opioid sensitivity may require higher doses of medication for appropriate pain relief and demonstrate drug-seeking or addictive behaviors that resolve when the pain is appropriately treated (also known as pseudoaddiction).

2. The purpose of any medication is to improve the quality of life, improve function, and when reasonable to return to normal function without resulting in additional damage to the injured region or another region.

## Chronic Pain

The factors noted in Figure 20.2 and Figure 20.3 are involved and contribute in the process of acute and sub-acute pain progressing into chronic long- term pain. When comorbidities and precipitating factors are not treated and pain is not controlled, early pain worsens. Multimodal approaches as noted in Figure 20.6 can help minimize or halt pain progression.

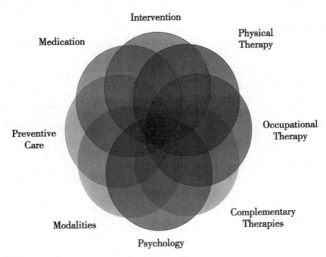

**Figure 20.6**   Multimodal approach for pain management.

Common issues that can preclude improvement if unnoticed include:

1. Obesity
2. Lack of flexibility of hips and legs, increasing stress across the spine, or general lack of flexibility
3. Depression
4. Sleep dysfunction
5. Obstructive sleep apnea
6. Poor posture
7. Poor body mechanics
8. Poor core and proximal strength
9. Smoking or drug abuse
10. Psychological issues or psychiatric disease

11. Poor understanding and knowledge of condition
12. Poor nutrition
13. Work ergonomics
14. Home ergonomics
15. Social stressors

Proper management of the patient as a whole addressing physical, emotional, and social stressors can help prevent pain from becoming chronic.

## Facts About Injections And Injection Agents

Most injections will use a combination of an anesthetic and a corticosteroid.

## Anesthetics

The faster the onset, the shorter the medication half-life. Fast agents should be considered when immediate local anesthesia is desired. Slow-acting anesthetics should be considered when a longer duration of analgesia is needed.

The 2 most common anesthetics used are lidocaine and bupivicaine.

a. Lidocaine is supplied in concentrations of 1% to 5%. It has one of the fastest onsets (depending on the tissue onset, it is usually between 30 and 120 seconds). Duration of effect is approximately 1 to 2 hours.

b. Bupivicaine is supplied in concentrations of 0.25%, 0.50%, and 0.75% and has a slower onset but the duration can be between 2 and 6 hours.

## Steroids

Common steroids used and their relative potency are listed below.

| Generic | Potency |
| --- | --- |
| Cortisone | 1 |
| Hydrocortisone | 1.25 |
| Triamcinolone | 6 |
| Prednisone | 5 |
| Methylprednisolone | 6 |
| Dexamethasone | 33 |
| Betamethasone | 41 |

## ■ SUMMARY

Pain is a leading public problem in modern society. Pain management, is a promising branch of medicine depending on an interdisciplinary approach for easing the suffering and improving the quality of life of those living with pain. The typical pain management team includes medical practitioners, pharmacists, clinical psychologists, physiotherapists, occupational therapists, physician assistants, and nurses. Effective management of chronic pain, however, frequently requires the coordinated efforts of the management team. Treatment approaches to chronic pain include pharmacological measures, such as analgesics, antidepressants and anticonvulsants, interventional procedures, physical therapy, physical exercise, application of ice and/or heat, and psychological measures, such as biofeedback and cognitive behavioral therapy.

# ■ IMPORTANT TERMINOLOGY

provocative maneuvers   刺激性操作/检查

intravertebral disc   椎间盘

nerve root   神经根

positive response   阳性反应

focal palpation   病灶触诊

opioid pain medications   阿片类镇痛药

anesthetics   麻醉药

patient education   患者教育

# ■ REVIEW QUESTIONS

1. How to exam a patient with pain?
2. Describe the 3-column approach for lumbar spinal pain.
3. Can you tell the differences in acute, subacute and chronic pain?
4. How to choose an optimized method on pain management?

# ■ REFERENCES

1. Bjorklund M, Hamberg J, Heiden M, Barnekow-Bergkvist M. The assessment of symptoms and functional limitations in low back pain patients: validity and reliability of a new questionnaire. Eur Spine J. 2007;16(11):1799-1811.

2. Beck AT, Steer RA, Ball R, Ranieri W. Comparison of beck depression inventories Ⅰ A and Ⅱ in psychiatric outpatients. J Pers Assess. 67(3):588-597.

3. Gloth FM Ⅲ, Scheve AA, Stober CV, Chow S, Prosser J. The Functional Pain Scale: reliability, validity, and responsiveness in an elderly population. J Am Med Dir Assoc. 2001;2(3):110-114.

4. Carragee EJ, Chen Y, Tanner CM, Truong T, Lau E, Brito JL. Provocative discography in patients after limited lumbar discectomy: a controlled, randomized study of pain response in symptomatic and asymptomatic subjects. Spine. 2000;25(23):3065-3071.

5. Manchikanti L, Singh V, Pampati V, et al. Provocative discography in low back pain patients with or without somatization disorder: a randomized prospective evaluation. Pain Physician. 2001;4:227-239.

6. Manchikanti L, Singh V, eds. Interventional Techniques in Chronic Spinal Pain. Paducah, KY: ASIPP publishing; 2007.

7. Derby R., Howard M, Grant JM, Lettice JJ, Van Peteghem PK, Ryan DP. The ability of pressure controlled discography to predict surgical and non-surgical outcomes. Spine. 1999;24:364-371.

8. Derby R, Kim BJ, Lee SH, Chen Y, Seo KS, Aprill C. Comparison of discographic findings in asymptomatic subject discs and the negative disc and chronic LBP patients: can discography distinguish asymptomatic discs among morphologically abnormal discs? Spine. 2005;5:389-394.

9. Bogduk N. Lumbar disc stimulation (provocation discography) in: practice Guidelines for Spinal Diagnostic and Treatment Procedures. ISIS 2004, 20-46.

10. Schwarzer AC, Aprill CN, Derby R, et al. Clinical features of patients with pain stemming from the lumbar zygapophyseal joints. Spine. 1994;19:1132-1137.

11. Manchikanti L, Singh V, eds. Interventional Techniques in Chronic Spinal Pain. Paducah, KY: ASIPP publishing; 2007.

12. Rathmell JP. Atlas of image-guided interventional in Regional Anesthesia and Pain Medicine. Philadelphia, PA: Lippincott; 2006:26-27.

（虞乐华）

# PROSTHETICS, ORTHOTICS, AND AMPUTEE CARE

## ■ ORTHOTISTS AND PROSTHETISTS AND THE MULTIDISCIPLINARY REHABILITATION TEAM

The complete multidisciplinary rehabilitation team should include the prosthetist, orthotist, and pedorthist. These health care professionals are uniquely trained to provide orthoses, prostheses, and pedorthic services. Prosthetists, orthotists, or prosthetist/orthotists (CP, CO, CPO) are health care professionals with the education and clinical training to evaluate, design, fit, and fabricate prostheses and/or orthoses. Pedorthics is the design, manufacture, and modification of pedorthic devices to prevent or alleviate foot problems caused by disease, congenital defect, overuse, or injury.

### Materials and Fabrication Considerations

Three primary issues are to be considered in the fabrication of an orthotic or prosthetic device: (1) the detailed selection of components and materials, (2) the level of customization, and (3) the process of evaluation and provision of the device. There are a wide array of fabrication materials available including plastics, leather, metals and elastomeric gels. All have properties that make them suitable for use as a part of an external appliance. Customization generally involves the selection of either a custom fabricated or a prefabricated device. The decision for custom fabricated or prefabricated involves questions about pathology, clinical outcomes, the need for a total contact fit vs a limited contact fit, body type, acute vs chronic use, cost, practitioner preference, patient prior use, and market availability.

## ■ PROSTHESES

External limb prostheses ie, replacement limbs.

### Lower Limb Prostheses

Evaluating a patient for and prescribing a prosthesis begins with a functional assessment. Specifically, assessing the potential of the client to use a prosthesis and thereby determine the appropriate prosthesis design necessary to achieve the goal of maximizing pain-free functional independence. Functional prosthesis use includes safe basic mobility as well as a normalized gait pattern for those clients with the ability to achieve it. Prosthesis design and prescription are based on (1) the durability of the residual limb; length, strength, skin integrity, sensation, proximal joint health, and so on; (2) the assessed functional ambulatory potential of the client; (3) prior prosthesis use; and (4) the patient's goals and lifestyle. Preparatory prostheses are valuable in making these assessments as they allow the user time to integrate the prosthesis into their daily routine. The individual's medical history, physical presentation, and current function are used to establish their functional potential. There are many standardized tests available to assist with this assessment. The most widely utilized system in the United States has been provided by The Centers for Medicare and Medicaid Services (CMS) to assist with lower limb prosthesis knee and foot/ankle selection. Functional categories labeled 0 through 4 describe progressively increasing potential ambulatory function with a prosthesis (Figure 21.1). The Amputee Mobility Predictor (AMP) is another particularly useful performance assessment tool[1].

| MFCL Level | Foot/Ankle Assembly | Knee Units |
|---|---|---|
| 0  No functional potential with prosthesis | Not eligible for a prosthesis | Not eligible for a prosthesis |
| 1  Transfers and limited household distances | SACH or single axis only | No fluid control allowed |
| 2  Household and limited community distances | Flexible keel or multi–axis allowed | No fluid control allowed |
| 3  Community distances; variable cadence; traverse environmental barriers | Any foot/ankle assembly; including energy storage and multi–axial dynamic response | Most knee units; includes fluid, micro–processor fluid control; No High Activity Knee Frames |
| 4  High activity, impact and stress; active adult, athlete or child. | Any foot/ankle assembly | Any knee unit |

**Figure 21.1**   CMS components and functional levels chart.

Prosthesis design in general reflects the level of limb loss (Figure 21.2) and the intended functional use of the prosthesis. General types of prostheses are immediate and early post operative prostheses (IPOP/EPOP), preparatory prostheses, definitive prostheses, and specialty or activity-specific prostheses. Immediate and early postoperative prostheses are provided shortly after amputation, often in the operating room, with the goals of preventing edema, protecting the incision line and limb to relieve pain and promote healing, and facilitating early functional independence. Preparatory prostheses are provided as soon as the limb can tolerate the forces of the removable socket and are intended for the achievement of 3 primary goals: limb maturation (volume reduction, shaping, strengthening, and desensitization), maximizing early functional independence, and assessing for the definitive prosthesis. The definitive prosthesis is provided when the aforementioned goals are achieved and is intended to be used for a longer period of time with the option of a more cosmetic restoration. The definitive prosthesis is modified or replaced when there are significant changes in limb size or volume, significant changes in function, and/or due to wear and tear. Specialty or activity-specific prostheses may be provided for vocational or avocational activities wherein the primary prosthesis is not appropriate such as aquatics, sprinting, or use in extreme environments.

The basic components of lower limb prostheses are the user and machine interface (socket + suspension), construction,

**Figure 21.2**   Lower limb amputation levels.

replacement functional units (foot/ankle, knee, hip), and socks, liners, and accoutrements.

The prosthesis interface includes concepts of the socket (stance or weight-bearing control) and suspension (swing or non-weight-bearing control) as a system. The specifics of the interface vary based on level/type of residual limb and the details of the potential user.

Construction considerations that apply for all lower limb prostheses include materials, connectors and the alignment of the various functional segments. The general construction techniques used in lower limb prostheses are Exoskeletal; composed of a rigid external shell as the supporting structure and Endoskeletal; composed of a rigid internal, modular (pylon and connectors) supporting structure. Exoskeletal construction remains an option primarily for prior users and has been replaced by endoskeletal systems in most cases. Modular endoskeletal components and fabrication have become the predominant construction technique primarily due to the reduction in weight and the relative ease of adjustments and repairs when compared to exoskeletal construction. Dynamic endoskeletal pylons are available that allow for shock and torque attenuation through spring loaded pistoning and rotation action or as flexible pylons that absorb force via bending. These functions would be in addition to the function of the selected foot/ankle. The alignment of the prosthesis refers to the spatial relationship of the major functional segments of the prosthesis in all 3 planes so that the interface, and thereby the user, is located over the functional segments (foot/ankle, knee, hip) to create a balance of stability and mobility. An even roll over shape and control of torque in the frontal plane (varus/valgus), sagittal plane (flexion/extension), and transverse plane (internal/external rotational) during stance phase allows for comfortable and efficient gait. Mal-alignment of the prosthesis can lead to safety issues such as knee buckling, limb pain and skin problems from uncontrolled shear and pressure, gait deviations and inefficiencies, and premature wearing of mechanical components.

Prosthetic foot/ankle systems remain largely passive devices using dynamic materials to accommodate but not actively adapt to the ground surface. They can be categorized into 2 main groups with a few subgroupings (Figure 21.3). The solid ankle cushion heel (SACH) nonarticulated foot uses a compressible foam heel to simulate plantarflexion and a rigid shortened anterior keel to allow for stance phase roll over or third rocker. The anterior support of the SACH foot is often insufficient for active users creating a drop-off effect at the end of stance. The flexible keel foot allows for a longer and more accommodating toe lever which improves control on uneven terrain and with variable cadence. The energy storing foot is designed with a long and dynamic anterior lever arm which allows for greater simulated push off and control at the end of stance due to the leaf

| Foot Category | Foot Sub–Category | Foot Function | CMS level |
| --- | --- | --- | --- |
| Non–Articulated | SACH | Soft compressible heel, short rigid keel simulates PF and DF | 1 |
| | Flexible Keel | Soft compressible heel, longer flexible keel simulates limited tri–planar motion | 2 |
| | Energy Storing | Long elastic keel to maximize simulated push off effect | 3 |
| Articulated | Single Axis | Sagittal plane motion only; PF at heel strike and DF stop at heel off | 1 |
| | Multi–Axis | Tri–planar motion with rigid keel | 2 |
| | MultipAxis, Dynamic Response | Tri–planar motion with long elastic keel to maximize simulated push off effect | 3 |

**Figure 21.3** Prosthesis foot chart.

spring effect of the keel. The energy storing foot is appropriate for users with the functional potential to walk at variable speeds and manage environmental obstacles such as stairs, ramps, and uneven terrain. Articulated feet with either a single axis or multiple axes allow for greater accommodation to the ground surface. The multiaxis, dynamic response foot provides this ground accommodation with the additional feature of an energy storing anterior lever arm or keel for users with the ability to vary their cadence. Stand alone modular ankle units are available and are designed to allow multiaxial motion or patient adjustable heel height. Microprocessor-controlled ankles are available. They provide a greater degree of adaptation to the ground surface instead of simple accommodation and are a new design focus.

Prosthetic knee mechanisms can be categorized based on the function of the knee during the stance and swing phases of gait and by the number of mechanical axes, single axis or polycentric (Figure 21.4). Polycentric knee joints allow for shortening of the shank section during flexion and are therefore often provided for users with long residual limbs. The polycentric knee joint configuration is also designed for stability and maximizes the use of the ground reaction force as an extension bias during stance. Alignment of the major components of the prosthesis and the management of the ground reaction force are commonly used to create an extension torque bias at the knee for weight-bearing stability and to reduce the risk of buckling. In addition to this alignment technique, many prosthetic knee joints have flexion resistance mechanisms such as weight-activated brakes or hydraulic damping units to further stabilize the knee against inadvertent knee flexion or buckling and the risk of a fall. Manual locking knees are often provided to prosthesis users who are unable to control the knee. They provide the maximum resistance to buckling as they are locked in extension during standing and walking. Fluid controlled knees provide a flexion damping under load during stance phase and also assist with the control of the knee during swing under variable speed conditions. Knee mechanisms without this fluid control allow for only single speed swing phase movement. This single speed knee swing creates gait deviations such as terminal impact or excessive heel rise if the user changes their pace. Microprocessor-

| | Common Terminology | Prescription Notes |
|---|---|---|
| **Stance Control** (Stance or Weight bearing control) | Knee Joint Alignment | Ground reaction force at knee axis is biased towards extension under a weight bearing load |
| | Weight Activated Stance Control | Mechanical breaking mechanism supports user within a small range of flexion (0–25) under a weight bearing load |
| | Fluid Control | Hydraulic stance control for flexion damping |
| | Fluid Control with Micro–processor | Hydraulic stance control for flexion damping wider and automated resistance range adjustment; hydraulic only |
| **Swing Control** (Swing or Non–weight bearing control) | Friction | Constant rabe, not cadence responsive |
| | Extension Assist | Promotes knee extension at end of swing |
| | Fluid Control | Variable cadence responsive; pneumatic and/or hydraulic |
| | Fluid Control with micro–processor | Variable cadence responsive with wider and automated resistance range adjustment; pneumatic and/or hydraulic |
| **Single Axis Construction** | One axis of rotation | Most common design for stance fluid control with or without micro–processor |
| **Multi–Axis/ Poly–Centric Construction** | Multiple axes allows for shortening of shank during swing phase and sitting flexion | Inherently stable by design; limited stance fluid control options |

**Figure 21.4** Prosthesis knee chart.

and fluid-controlled prosthetic knee units provide automated control of the hydraulic damping mechanism through a broad range of force and speed. They rely on sensors built into the knee and/or pylon to determine position and torque. The potential for variable cadence (swing control) and need for advanced stability (stance control) for both stumble recovery and flexion damping (down ramps, stairs, and curbs) are indications for swing and stance phase hydraulics. Knee and foot/ankle components should be considered one integrated system to maximize the balance of stability and mobility. Knee units with powered extension force are limited at this time, but are a new design focus.

## Partial Foot Prostheses

General considerations in the design of partial foot prostheses are based on the level of amputation and function of the remaining foot (Figure 21.5). Common amputations levels are Toe, the hallux being the most disruptive of function, ray resection, Lisfranc, Chopart, and Boyd and Pirogoff. The biomechanical goals of the partial foot prostheses are to support the residual foot structure, control the distribution of forces, replace the lost anterior lever arm, and allow for shoe fit. The prosthesis structure and lever arm control are determined by the height of the device and the materials selected therefore; typically the shorter the residual limb the higher the device. Three general designs based on the height of the prosthesis are submalleolar, supramalleolar, and tibial tubercle height. The residual limb length, available ankle and foot ROM, strength, sensation, and weight-bearing stability all help to determine the required prosthetic leverage to achieve a normalized gait pattern. Drop off at the end of stance phase, and subsequent compensations, due to an insufficient anterior lever are common gait deviations. Selection of the height of the prosthesis, the materials, socks, or other interface additions, as well as, the appropriate footwear make up the basic prescription.

**Figure 21.5** Partial foot amputation.

## Syme Ankle Disarticulation Prostheses

The basic components of the Syme's prosthesis are the interface (socket + suspension), the construction, the foot/ankle, and socks, liners, and accoutrements (Figure 21.6).

Syme ankle disarticulation prostheses are designed to maximize the advantages of this amputation level. These advantages are distal weight bearing allowing for reduced proximal loading, a bulbous distal shape allowing for reduced proximal suspension, and a long lever arm and surface area for distribution of force and greater control of the prosthesis. The disadvantages of the Syme ankle disarticulation prosthesis are the limited space distal to the socket for prosthetic foot and ankle mechanisms and the difficulty achieving satisfactory cosmetic restoration for many clients. With the Syme ankle disarticulation prosthesis, the interface is commonly designed for full distal weight bearing and for self-suspension. Due to limits on space distal to the end of the limb, the socket is generally mounted directly onto the foot with a short modular connector. The socket either has a window or door (medially or posteriorly) to allow donning or is created in a cylindrical shape with a soft foam insert. Socks or gel liners are used as additional interface materials. Foot selection is limited due to the available space (approximately 5-8cm for adults) and requires the use of a lower profile ankle/foot design. Despite this limited space, energy storage feet remain an option.

## Transtibial Prostheses

The basic components of the transtibial prosthesis are the interface (socket + suspension), the construction, the foot/ankle, and socks, liners, and accoutrements (Figure 21.7).

**Figure 21.6**  Syme's prosthesis.

**Figure 21.7**  Transtibial prosthesis.

The design of the transtibial prosthesis reflects the anatomy of the residual limb creating an interface that optimizes weight-bearing and swing-phase forces over a relatively small surface area. By definition the transtibial region extends from the distal Syme ankle disarticulation to the proximal knee disarticulation level; however, there are surgical considerations which determine optimal length. Leverage and surface area increase with longer limbs, but at the distal levels of the shank, soft tissue coverage may be limited and may predispose the limb to skin problems. Proximally the extensor mechanism must be maintained to allow for knee control, and the short leverage and surface area would generally indicate socket designs that extend above the knee joint such as supracondylar/suprapatellar or joints and corset resulting in a more cumbersome fitting. Midshank lengths approximating the musculoskeletal junction of the gastrocnemius/soleus muscle group are considered the ideal length region providing for reasonable distal soft tissue coverage and leverage for control. Full distal end loading is not generally tolerated without specialized osteoplastic procedures so that weight is borne over the entire limb with considerations for pressure sensitive areas. Many design options are available for the transtibial interface with the ultimate goal of comfort and control (Figure 21.8). The use of gel liners have become common practice. Gel liners are intended to provide for improved suspension; control for variances in sheer and pressure; and loading of the residual limb in a more uniform, reliable pattern. Gel liners can be used with mechanical locks or with sealing sleeves to create a suction or elevated vacuum fitting which significantly reduces pistoning thereby improving swing phase control. With more room for prosthetic components distal to the end of the residual limb, all foot/ankle designs are an option including the longer "J" shaped energy storage feet with leaf spring levers extending to the shank, multiaxial dynamic response feet, as well as integrated shock, and torque attenuation pylon systems.

| | Common Terminology | Prescription Notes |
|---|---|---|
| **Socket** (Stance or weight bearing control) | Patella Tendon Bearing (PTB) | Specific weight beaning on pressure tolerant areas and relief of pressure sensitive areas |
| | Patella Tendon Bearing, Supra–condylar & Supre–patellar (PTBSCSP)l | Variance of PTB that encapsulates the knee for suspension or control |
| | Joints and Corset | Variance of PTB that encapsulates the knee for suspension or control Medial and lateral metal knee joints and thigh lacer for residual limb weight bearing reduction and knee support |
| | Total Surface Weight Bearing | Designed for use with gel liners to more evenly distribute forces and allows for improved suction and vacuum |
| **Suspension** (Swing or non–weight bearing control) | Supra–Condylar Cuff, Fork Strap and Waist Belt | Strap suspension above knee and extended to the waist; simple |
| | Supra–Condylar and Supra–patellar | Solf suspension over femoral condyles |
| | Suspension Sleeve | May be primary or secondary suspension; used for sealing suction or vacuum sockets |
| | Silicone Suction Socket | Use of gel liners with a pin and locking mechanism or without(with sleeve) |
| | Elevated Vacuum Socket | Mechanical or electro–mechanical pump and sealed socket with gel liner creates elevated vacuum12–20 in Hg |

**Figure 21.8**   Transtibial interface chart.

## Knee Disarticulation Prostheses

The basic components of the knee disarticulation prosthesis are the interface, which is the combination of the socket and suspension as a system, the construction and materials, the prosthetic knee mechanism, the foot/ankle mechanism, and the required socks or liners.

Knee disarticulation prostheses are designed to maximize the advantages of this level of amputation. The advantages of the knee disarticulation or through knee amputation limb are distal weight bearing allowing for reduced proximal loading, full hip motor power available allowing for improved control and gait efficiency, a bulbous distal shape allowing for reduced proximal suspension, and long lever arm and surface area for control of prosthesis. The disadvantages of the knee disarticulation limb and prosthesis are the limited space distal to the socket for prosthetic knee mechanisms and the difficulty achieving satisfactory cosmetic restoration for many clients. Socket design for the knee disarticulation level prosthesis is often relatively simple when compared to the transfemoral prosthesis. In particular, the availability of distal limb weight bearing may eliminate or significantly reduce the need for pelvic (ischial tuberosity) weight bearing and the use of aggressive proximal socket brim designs for control. Self-suspension also reduces the need for proximal suspension systems such as belts (Figure 21.9). These advantages make the interface of the knee disarticulation prosthesis less cumbersome for the user and allow for improved comfort in both walking and sitting. As with transtibial prostheses, endoskeletal construction is common. Polycentric knee joint mechanisms are commonly prescribed as they allow for the shortest possible thigh length and sitting comfort. Foot and ankle selection is based on the functional potential of the user and is determined along with the function of the knee unit for an integrated foot/ankle and knee system.

| | Common Terminology | Prescription Notes |
|---|---|---|
| **Socket** (Stance or weight bearing control) | Quadrilateral | Pelvic weight bearing on the ischial tuberosity which is outside of the socket |
| | Ischial Containment | Pelvic weight bearing on the ischial tuberosity which is captured in the socket for greater limb control |
| **Suspension** (Swing or non–weight bearing control) | Silesian Belt | Flexible belt that attaches to the lateral proximal socket and wraps over the contralateral illiac crest |
| | Hip joint, pelvic band and belt | Rigid metal hip joint and band creates improved frontal plane control |
| | Full Suction | Socket and limb in direct contact creating a suction effect; commonly used with a "pull in" stocking and an auto–expulsion air valve |
| | Silicone Suction Socket | Use of gel liners with a pin and locking mechanism or without(with sleeve) |
| | Elevated Vacuum Socket | Mechanical or electro–mechanical pump and sealed socket with gel liner creates elevated vacuum 12–20 in Hg |

**Figure 21.9**   Transfemoral/KD interface chart.

## Transfemoral Prostheses

The basic components of the transfemoral prosthesis are the interface (socket + suspension), the construction and materials, prosthetic knee mechanism, the foot, ankle and pylon system, and associated socks, liners, and accoutrements (Figure 21.10).

At the transfemoral level, residual length becomes a primary consideration. The shorter levels of amputation create significantly reduced surface area and leverage for controlling forces. This is of particular concern for prosthetic knee control. In the frontal plane, the balance between hip abductors and adductors and the desired adducted position of the femur in the prosthetic socket become difficult to maintain. The imbalance can lead to gait deviations such as Trendelenburg's gait or the gluteus medius lurch compensation which compromise gait efficiency and user comfort. Accommodations for short limbs must be made in the design of the prosthesis often leading to a more cumbersome fitting with aggressive socket brims and pelvic suspension straps for stance and swing phase control, respectively. Very short transfemoral limbs may be fit with a hip disarticulation style prosthesis. While long residual limbs are desirable for leverage and control, there may be limited room for some knee units with very long limbs approaching the femoral condyles.

**Figure 21.10**   Transfemoral prosthesis.

The primary transfemoral socket shapes are Quadrilateral and Ischial Containment (Figure 21.9). Both require pelvic weight bearing on the ischial tuberosity and thereby unload the distal end of the residual limb. The quadrilateral socket shape relies on a narrowed anterior-posterior socket dimension to maintain the ischial position, and the user sits on the posterior-medial aspect of the top of the socket when bearing weight on the prosthesis. The ischial containment socket relies on a narrowed medial-lateral dimension and an extended capture of the medial aspect of the tuberosity and descending ramus for weight bearing and frontal plane control. The ischial containment socket design is intended to provide greater control of the femur and thereby reduce socket instabilities leading to gait deviations such as lateral trunk lean. The primary goal for the transfemoral socket remains user comfort and control.

Knee selection is based on the functional potential of the user and the available residual limb leverage among other factors as mentioned previously (Figure 21.4). With loss of the knee and the foot/ankle complex, shock and torque attenuation become concerns. Dynamic pylons with shock and torque absorbing mechanisms may be provided. Foot/ankle selection should be considered with the knee as a system (Figure 21.3).

## Hip Disarticulation and Trans-Pelvic Prostheses

The basic components of the hip disarticulation or trans-pelvic prosthesis are interface (socket + suspension), construction, hip joint, knee joint, foot/ankle, and socks, liners, and accoutrements (Figure 21.11).

General considerations in the design of the hip disarticulation and trans-pelvic prosthesis are based on the residual pelvic structure and, in particular, the availability of the ischial tuberosity for weight bearing and the iliac crest for suspension. Without these 2 boney anchors, socket control is reliant on soft tissue compression and may be less stable. The socket interface is most commonly fabricated as a single piece with a rigid attachment to the hip joint and a flexible closure wrapping around and encapsulating the entire residual pelvis for weight bearing, suspension, and rotational control. Pelvic motions (posterior pelvic tilt) are used to initiate swing phase. Weight-bearing stability is built into the alignment with extension biased at the knee and hip joints under load. Hip joints are largely single axis joints with extension assist mechanisms and are aligned with the axis placed on the distal anterior aspect of the socket for maximal extension bias and for sitting comfort. Without active control of the hip joint, knee and foot/ankle component selection is largely based on the need for stance stability and safety.

**Figure 21.11** Hip disarticulation prosthesis.

## Trans-Lumbar Prostheses

General considerations are based primarily on the client's general health and on upright positioning potential. If the client is medically stable and can tolerate an upright position, a custom seating socket can be fabricated to allow for sitting and for wheelchair mobility. The custom socket is made from a casting of the residual body and extends to at least mid-thoracic level. Custom air chambers are commonly used to maintain support and even pressure distribution. Ambulation with prosthetic legs is not currently an option. Selection of materials and the connection of the custom seating socket with an appropriately prescribed wheelchair are essential for successful functional outcome. The details of this prescription are best left as a multidisciplinary task with input from all members of the team.

## Upper Limb Prostheses

The population of upper limb prosthesis users is quite different than lower limb prosthesis users representing a very small minority of the limb loss population. This is primarily due to the limited number of upper limb amputations and to the much higher prosthesis rejection rate. Unilateral upper limb amputees will quickly become ADL proficient with the remaining limb. There is generally considered to be a 3 to 6 months critical period for upper limb amputees to be successfully fitted with a prosthesis after which time they are much more likely to reject a prosthesis. Bilateral upper limb amputees can become independent in the majority of the essential ADLs with appropriate training. The description of upper limb prostheses mirrors the level of amputation (Figure 21.12). Long, medium, short and very short level descriptions as percentages of the intact limb are used as guidelines. There are 6 basic options for clients with upper limb loss: no prosthesis, passive or static terminal device, body powered, externally powered, hybrid, or specialty prostheses.

**Figure 21.12**  Upper limb amputation levels.

## Partial Hand Limb Prostheses

General considerations are based on the level of amputation, the function of the remaining hand with potential prehension abilities being critical, and unilateral or bilateral involvement. Levels of amputation include-partial or complete digit(s) disarticulation, ray resection, trans-metacarpal, and trans-carpal. Partial hand prostheses are more likely to be rejected than any other level of prosthesis due to their limited function and poor aesthetics. The device provided may be considered more an orthosis than a prosthesis depending on the functional intent. Occupational therapists are critical to successful prosthesis prescription and should be involved as early as possible. As the function of the hand is so complex and the function of most partial hand prostheses so inadequate, more than one device may be required to provide necessary functional restoration. Three design concepts should be considered: aesthetic restoration, protection, and prehension; static or dynamic prehension designs are possible.

## Wrist Disarticulation and Transradial Prostheses

The basic parts of the wrist disarticulation or transradial prosthesis are interface (socket + suspension), control system, wrist unit, terminal device, and associated socks, liners and accoutrements (Figure 21.13). The design of the wrist disarticulation and transradial prosthesis are based on the length of the residual limb and the available forearm rotation (pronation and supination). With the wrist disarticulation level, full forearm length and an intact radius and ulna allow for improved control, distal pressure tolerance, and full pronation and supination. However, there is limited space at the end of the socket for a wrist and terminal device so that the prosthetic limb may be longer than the intact contralateral limb. At the transradial level, the length of the lever arm determines the control system, component, and interface (socket and suspension) selection. A short residual limb length requires a prosthetic interface that captures more of the limb and may extend above the elbow joint. The self-suspending supraepicondylar Muenster socket is a common design. The use of silicone liners and sleeves as used with lower limb prostheses has become more prevalent. Control system options are passive, body power, or external power. The term passive refers solely to the terminal device which may not be activated to open or close however; the prosthesis is functional as an extension of the residual limb for bi-manual activities and for manipulating objects in space. Passive systems are often more cosmetically acceptable. Body powered systems are cable and harness operated and require the user to provide tension to the cable via biscapular abduction or gleno-humeral flexion or abduction. Externally powered systems at this level are largely myo-electrically controlled through electro-myographic (EMG) signals from the residual wrist/hand flexors and extensors. Terminal device options are hook or hand. Hook ter-

**Figure 21.13** Transradial prosthesis.

minal devices can be body powered and are either voluntary opening or voluntary closing. They are available in a wide range of shapes and sizes. Externally powered hooks are available as well. The prescription of more than one hook and the combination of a hook and a hand is common to allow the user to interchange terminal devices based on desired function. The most common wrist unit is the friction wrist which allows passive rotational positioning of the terminal device. Mechanical flexion wrist units are available to assist with midline activities. Powered, myoelectric wrist rotators are also available.

## Elbow Disarticulation and Transhumeral Prostheses

The basic components of the elbow disarticulation or transhumeral prosthesis are interface (socket + suspension), control system, elbow unit, wrist unit, terminal device, and associated socks, liners, and accoutrements (Figure 21.14). Residual limb length and control of the prosthesis are primary concerns in the design of the elbow disarticulation and transhumeral prosthesis. At the elbow disarticulation level, full humeral length, broad and tolerant distal humeral end, and full leverage allow for improved control of the prosthesis. However, there is limited room for a prosthetic elbow mechanism often requiring the use of external hinges or an elbow unit which is positioned much lower than the contralateral/nonamputated limb. At the transhumeral level, the length of the lever arm determines the control system, component, and interface (socket and suspension) selection. Longer limbs allow the socket trimlines to remain relatively low and end distal to the shoulder joint. At mid length levels, socket extensions onto the pectoralis area anteriorly and the scapular area posteriorly for rotational control are common. At higher levels with shorter lever arms, the socket may extend over the acromion process as a shoulder cap; and at very proximal levels, clients are fit with a shoulder disarticulation level prosthesis as the residual humerus does not provide sufficient leverage for control. The use of silicone liners and sleeves as used with lower limb prostheses

**Figure 21.14** Transhumeral prosthesis.

has become more prevalent. Control system options are passive, body power, external power, or hybrid, a combination of body and external power. Body powered systems are cable and harness operated and require the user to provide tension to the cable via biscapular abduction or gleno-humeral flexion or abduction. For a fully body powered transhumeral prosthesis, a single cable controls both elbow movement and terminal device open/close. A separate cable locks and unlocks the prepositioned elbow. This requires a sequential control pattern: preposition the elbow and terminal device in space, lock the elbow in position, and operate the terminal device. Externally powered systems at this level are largely myoelectrically controlled through EMG signals from the residual elbow flexors and extensors. Selection of the elbow unit is based on the control system selected. Terminal device and wrist unit selection is then made based on the control system and elbow unit selected. A common hybrid control system is a body powered elbow unit and an externally powered hand terminal device.

## Shoulder Disarticulation and Intra-Scapular/Thoracic Prostheses

The basic parts of the shoulder disarticulation or intra-scapular/thoracic prosthesis are interface (socket + suspension), control system, shoulder unit, elbow unit, wrist unit, terminal device, and associated socks, liners, and accoutrements. General considerations in the design of prostheses at these proximal levels involve the availability of the shoulder girdle for control of both the interface (suspension and force control) and for potential myoelectric sites at the pectoralis, upper trapezius, and scapular muscles. Without the shoulder girdle, control is diminished, and, most clients choose to forgo prosthesis fitting and may be fit with a shoulder cap only which allows for proper fitting of clothing and protection of the body segment. Passive systems are common at this level and often have manual locking elbow units operated and prepositioned with the contralateral limb. Full body powered systems are possible at this level but often require the use of inguinal control straps and chin nudge switches which are cumbersome and make the prosthesis likely to be rejected. Hybrid systems with body power and external power combinations are more common. Full externally powered systems are the current design focus. Efforts at expanding myoelectric sites through surgical intervention such as targeted reinnervation as well as the use of powered shoulders, elbows, wrists, and hand for increased movement and sequential control are now possible and have demonstrated significant functional gains[2].

## ■ ORTHOSES

An orthosis is a device, applied to the exterior of the body, for the purpose of supporting, correcting, aligning, or improving the function of moveable parts of the body or reducing pain of the head, spine, or extremities. General terminology for orthoses may be organized into the following: lower limb, upper limb, and spinal categories. Further subcategories are based on the joints affected by the orthosis. Standardized terminology includes the use of simple initialisms describing the joints affected and ending with "orthosis". For example, ankle foot orthosis (AFO), wrist hand orthosis (WHO), and thoracic lumbar sacral orthosis (TLSO) are standardized terms that allow for quick communication of the basic device. Further descriptors may be added to specify the desired function, materials, or design criteria. For example, articulated, dorsiflexion (DF) assist AFO; or wrist powered tenodesis WHO; or rigid, tri-planar control, custom molded TLSO. These standardized terms allow quick communication, although still commonly used terms such as splints, braces, and supports are nonstandard and nonspecific and should be avoided in favor of the aforementioned terminology.

Orthosis users are a heterogeneous group and not easily categorized by diagnosis alone. Therefore, in many cases the focus of orthotic prescription is on orthosis design and function, and less on the underlying etiology and diagnosis. Evaluation for orthoses involves a functional assessment and the establishment of reasonable functional goals, anticipated outcomes, and duration of use. Selecting materials for the construction of the orthosis includes the decision on custom fabricated or prefabricated. This decision involves questions about pathology, clinical outcomes, the need for a total contact fit vs a limited contact fit, body type, acute vs chronic use, cost, practitioner preference, patient prior use, and market availability.

## Lower Lime Orthoses

The prescription and design of a lower limb orthosis begins with a clear diagnosis and physical exam including functional assessment and gait analysis and involves the selection of the joint control (ankle/foot, knee, and/or hip), construction and materials (custom fabricated vs prefabricated; metal, plastic, and hybrid), straps and fitting modifications for control, and recommendations for appropriate footwear.

### Shoes

The shoe is considered part of the lower limb orthosis system and should be prescribed with the orthosis (Figure 21.15). In the case of traditional double upright metal orthosis systems, the orthosis is physically attached to the shoe. Shoes may be custom molded and are often modified to improve fit or create a specific biomechanical effect. Common shoe modifications are heel lift to accommodate a plantar-flexion (PF) contracture, heel and sole lift to accommodate a leg length discrepancy, rocker sole to simulate ankle PF and DF, extended rigid shank to limit forefoot extension, cushioned heel to simulate PF, heel flares (medial and/or lateral) to control for frontal plane instability (varus or valgus), Thomas and reverse Thomas heel to support the medial and lateral longitudinal arches, respectively, and heel and sole wedge to accommodate inversion/varus or eversion/valgus deformity.

A. Inner sole
B. Tongue
C. Vamp
D. Closure
E. Toe box
F. Counter
G. Heel
H. Outsole
I. Midsole
J. Throat

**Figure 21.15**   Shoe.

These can be combined to address a wide variety of lower limb problems. Shoes to be used with plastic orthoses generally have removable innersoles and are often fit 1/2 size larger for extra depth, width, and length. Shoes to be used with metal systems must have a firm sole for attachment of the stirrup or caliper box.

### Foot Orthoses

Foot orthoses (FOs) are employed to directly support and align the foot to prevent or correct foot deformities and, thereby, imp rove the function of the foot and lower limb. FOs can reduce stress on the foot, ankle, knee, hip, pelvis, and spine by correcting faulty alignments and properly controlling the motion within the foot, support the longitudinal and transverse arches of the foot, provide relief for painful areas, provide an even distribution of the weight-bearing stresses over the entire plantar surface of the foot, and equalize leg length discrepancy. FOs can be either prefabricated or custom and are made with a wide range of materials that span an almost unlimited spectrum of durometer. FOs can be generally described as either accommodative or corrective/ functional with further classification into soft, semi-rigid, or rigid subcategories. The detailed design of the foot orthosis includes posting or wedging under the rearfoot, forefoot, or both, metatarsal arch support, reliefs or cut outs for painful areas, and forefoot extension modifications.

### Ankle Foot Orthoses

The general indications for an AFO are (1) motor control deficits of the lower limb and resultant functional deficits (safety, mobility limitations, and gait inefficiency), (2) foot, ankle or knee instability causing pain, deformity, or limited function, (3) immobilization required for pain control, fracture stabilization, burns, trauma, or wound management, and (4) foot/ankle joint contracture management. The orthosis includes the foot and ankle and therefore has lever arms extending proximal and distal to the ankle joint. The length of the lever arms, the ankle joint control, and the materials used to fabricate the AFO determine the control.

Traditional AFOs (Figure 21.16) are made of 2 metal side bars and joints connected proximally by a leather covered calf band and attached distally to the shoe. Molded plastic AFOs (Figure 21.17) are intended to be in contact with the limb for more control, are lighter weight, and allow for easier use with more than one shoe. The ankle joint control provided by an AFO can be considered to either limit or assist motion and can be constructed either with or without an ankle joint (Figure 21.18). Common nonarticulated versions are solid ankle which significantly limits motion and posterior leaf spring (PLS) which assists DF during swing phase and creates only limited restriction of stance phase motion. Common articulated designs include free motion in the sagittal plane for frontal plane control only, DF assist, and limited motion. A very common limited motion adjustable ankle joint is the bichannel adjustable ankle locking (BiCAAL) joint, also known as the dual channel joint. The BiCAAL joint allows for control of both plantar flexion and DF with either springs for assist or

**Figure 21.16**   AFO metal.

**Figure 21.17**   AFO plastic.

| Joint Type | Function | Construction |
|---|---|---|
| Free Motion | Free sagittal motion, limited frontal and transverse plane motion | Articulated; metal or plastic joints are available |
| Limited Motion | Plantar–flexion and/or dorsi–flexion stops | Articulated; metal or plastic joints are available |
| | | Non–articulated, sold ankle creates both PF and DF stops |
| Dorsi–flexion Assist | Spring assisted dorsi–flexion during swing phase | Articulated; metal or plastic joints are available |
| | | Non–articulated, posterior leaf spring construction creates this effect |

**Figure 21.18**   Orthotic ankle joints.

rigid pins for stops. The addition of straps and padding to the orthosis allows for more aggressive control of instability either due to weakness or due to ROM limitations from spasticity or contracture.

Many variations on the concept of the AFO are available. The supramalleolar ankle foot orthosis with a short proximal lever arm is used for frontal and transverse plane control of the subtalar, midtarsal, and forefoot. The patellar tendon bearing orthosis is commonly prescribed without an ankle joint for a rigid solid ankle restriction and a rigid attachment to an orthopedic shoe with extended rigid shank for axial unloading and immobilization of the ankle joint following major trauma or reconstruction. The floor reaction AFO (Figure 21.19) uses a DF stop and a molded pretibial shell to create a knee extension stabilizing force for patients with knee buckling from quadriceps weakness or other pathology. The Charcot Reducing Orthosis Walker (CROW) is a removable

**Figure 21.19** AFO floor reaction.

custom molded walking boot and alternative to total contact casting. Myo-orthoses provide user friendly and reliable functional electrical stimulation (FES) foot drop correction and may be used as an AFO replacement for some cases of upper motor neuron related DF paralysis or weakness resulting in foot drop.

## Knee Orthoses

Knee orthoses (KOs) are prescribed for support of the tibiofemoral and/or patella-femoral joints. Common designs include neoprene sleeves with buttress pads to control for patellar tracking dysfunction and rigid frame style orthoses with medial and lateral joints for triplanar control. A commonly prescribed KO the compartment unloader style. This KO creates a varus or valgus thrust to open either the lateral or medial compartment of the arthritic knee for pain relief. This type of KO is fabricated as a rigid frame with either 1 or 2 knee joints and an adjustable alignment feature for frontal plane thrust control. Selecting prefabricated vs custom, articulated or nonarticulated including joint type, and the rigidity of the device are primary concerns.

## Knee Ankle Foot Orthoses

Knee ankle foot orthoses (KAFOs) provide support for the lower limb with indications which mirror that of the AFO but, with the direct knee control (Figure 21.20). Mechanical knee joints can either be built as double upright systems (medial and lateral) or as a single upright system with a single knee joint most commonly on the lateral side of the knee. The long mechanical lever arms of the KAFO extending as far as the hip joint proximally and including the foot and ankle distally allow for direct control of the knee joint for frontal plane (varus/valgus), sagittal plane (flexion/hyperextension), or transverse plane (rotation) limits. Foot and ankle control options remain the same as for the AFO (articulated or nonarticulated; free motion, DF assist, or limited motion). Knee joints can be organized as either single axis or polycentric and based on the mechanical resistance to stance phase flexion, that is, knee buckling prevention (Figure 21.21). The majority of knee joints have a 0 or

**Figure 21.20** KAFO.

180 degree stop built into the design to prevent hyperextension. Resistance to flexion is commonly either static lock mechanism, floor reaction effect often with posterior offset axes of rotation, or stance control orthotic knee joints which allow selective lock and unlock during the stance and swing phases, respectively. Construction techniques include traditional all metal and leather systems with shoe attachment, molded plastic, and hybrid combinations of metal and plastic construction. The majority of KAFOs are custom due to the complexity of crossing multiple joints and maintaining accurate orthosis and anatomic joint alignment. Additional designs include axial unloading with ischial weight-bearing proximal brims, femoral fracture orthoses, and contracture management designs with either static progressive or dynamic knee joints.

| Knee Joint | Function |
| --- | --- |
| Free motion | Free motion into flexion; 0 degree knee extension stop. |
| Locked | Locked during weight bearing and released for flexion in sitting. Drop locks, lever locks or pawl /bail locks are common. |
| Posterior Offset | Similar to free motion joint with full flexion and 0 degree knee extension stop. The axis of rotation is offset posteriorly to enhance the knee extension torque when weight bearing. |
| Polycentric | Multiple axes of rotation, Allows for more intimate tracking and alignment of the orthotic and anatomic knee joints. Commonly used in knee orthoses for sports. |
| Stance Control | Selective locking in extension during stance and unlocking to allow flexion during swing. Mechanical and electro–mechanical versions available. |

**Figure 21.21**   Orthotic knee joints.

Ambulatory potential and issues of donning and doffing of the KAFO should be addressed prior to prescription particularly when upper limb function is compromised. As the KAFO is concerned with direct control of the knee, the first decision is the knee joint control mechanism (free flexion, posterior offset stability, locked static or locked dynamic stance control). The ankle joint and knee joint control should be considered as system for a balance of stability and mobility with the goal of providing the least restrictive device possible. Knee joint control, ankle joint control, construction, additional straps, and the appropriate footwear make the basic prescription.

## Hip Knee Ankle Foot or Thoses and Hip or Thoses

Orthoses that cross the hip joint fall into 1 of 2 categories: those that extend to the foot and ankle (hip knee ankle foot orthoses, HKAFOs) and those that do not (Hip Orthoses). A separate category of orthoses are the reciprocating gait orthoses (RGOs) (Figure 21.22). The general design of the HKAFO mirrors that of the KAFO but with the addition of a hip joint, pelvic band, and pelvic belt. This addition allows for direct control of hip instability either in the frontal plane to reduce lateral trunk lean (Trendelenburg's Gait or gluteus medius lurch compensation) or in the sagittal plane to limit posterior lean of the trunk. Transverse plane or rotational control is inherent in the design of the

**Figure 21.22**   RGO.

HKAFO with pelvic connection proximally and foot/ankle leverage distally. Unilateral HKAFOs are prescribed for significant paralysis and instability of the entire lower limb and require a high level of custom fitting and user training. Unilateral hip abduction orthoses may be prescribed to limit hip flexion, adduction, and internal rotation following total hip arthroplasty. The RGO is a bilateral HKAFO with a molded spinal extension and mechanical reciprocating leg assist system mounted posterior and proximal to the hip joints. This reciprocating system can be a cable or rocker bar configuration and creates a linked hip flexion force on one side with hip extension of the other. The user creates the reciprocal pattern by unloading one limb and extending the trunk with the assist of the arms pushing on an assistive device (walker or bilateral crutches). This pattern is an alternative to a swing to or swing through pattern for clients with paraplegia. RGO prescription requires a full evaluation and commitment to ambulation training from the client and rehabilitation team. Full ROM, intact skin, managed spasticity and upright posture need to be assessed in advance and complicating issues of orthostatic hypotension and osteoporosis must be ruled out.

## Upper Limb Orthoses

Upper limb orthoses are provided based on issues including the duration of anticipated orthosis use, materials and fabrication techniques, integration of the orthosis into a therapeutic care plan, referral patterns, preferences, and professional availability. Role delineations and the specific function of the orthotists and therapists (physical, occupational, and hand) within the rehabilitation team vary considerably. In general, orthotists provide devices that are intended for long-term use and those that require more complex construction (eg, high temperature plastics and metals). Orthoses fabricated from low temperature thermoplastics, directly molded to the client's limb and fully integrated into a specific therapy treatment program are primarily the responsibility of the therapist.

### Hand Orthosis

Hand orthoses (HOs) have several functions. They are to maintain the palmar arch, to keep the thumb in opposition, to maintain the web space, and to act as a vehicle for the attachment of other orthotic systems and assistive devices. Features of the HO may include an opponens bar, a thumb adduction stop, metacarpal-phalangeal extension stops, interphalangeal joint extension assists, and molded palmar arch support. HOs are often designed to immobilize a specific joint to assist with healing after trauma or over-use type injury. The orthosis may be prefabricated or custom fabricated and composed of a wide array of materials.

### Wrist Hand Orthosis

WHOs may have many of the features of the HO with an extension across the wrist for more control of the hand and direct control of the wrist. WHOs may be categorized as static or dynamic in basic design. Prefabricated wrist stabilization WHOs of the wrist gauntlet style are commonly prescribed for over-use injuries and soft tissue trauma. Static, palmar wrist cock-up WHOs (Figure 21.23) are a very common orthosis and are provided for the passive positioning of the hand and wrist in the

**Figure 21.23** WHO cock up.

functional position following trauma, neurological insult with paralysis or postsurgical reconstruction. Support of the hand and wrist with a WHO following peripheral nerve injury is common with the design and trimlines specific to the injury and paralysis.

An example of a dynamic orthosis is the Tenodesis style WHO (Figure 21.24) which assists prehension through a wrist driven flexor hinge parallelogram linkage system. Wrist extension provides an MP flexion force. The tenodesis WHO is indicated in cases of C6 or C7 quadriplegia primarily but could be used for C5 level cases with either a shoulder operated cable system or other external power source (eg, FES, compressed air) to create wrist extension. Myo-orthoses provide a user friendly and reliable switch operated FES facilitated tenodesis function primarily indicated for C5 quadriplegia.

**Figure 21.24**   WHO tenodesis.

## Elbow Wrist Hand Orthosis (EWHO) and Elbow Orthoses (EOS)

EWHOs provide several functions including positioning the hand in space, providing elbow flexion, elbow, forearm or wrist contracture management, and postoperative elbow, forearm, wrist, and hand stabilization/immobilization. The orthosis can be prefabricated or custom fabricated; static with a set position for all segments or dynamic with static progressive or dynamic joints or a hybrid of the construction types; and fabricated from many types of materials. EOs are commonly prescribed for protection of unstable elbow joints without forearm or wrist deficits.

## Shoulder Elbow Wrist Hand Orthosis

Shoulder-elbow-wrist-hand orthoses (SEWHOs) are often designed for the short-term static immobilization of the shoulder following postoperative reconstruction. One common static and prefabricated SEWHO, often referred to as an Airplane Splint, (Figure 21.25) immobilizes the shoulder in abduction and neutral rotation and with the elbow at 90 degrees so that the hand is placed out to the side and in front of the body. This position is difficult to maintain for prolonged periods. A dynamic type of SEWHO may be prescribed following brachial plexus injury and is designed to support the flaccid arm and may provide cable operated elbow flexion through a harness and powered by scapular abduction of the contralateral limb. The harness and cable control are similar to the Figure 21.8 harness and the cable system of an upper limb prosthesis.

**Figure 21.25**   SEWHO airplane.

## Mobile Arm Support

Mounted to the back of the chair or wheelchair, the mobile arm support (MAS) or balanced forearm orthosis primarily supports the forearm and hand of the user. The MAS consists of a trough for the forearm often with a hand support (or may be modified for WHO use) and a set of hinged linkages with 2 or 3 segments allowing for gravity balanced arm horizontal abduction and adduction within a limited arc. Standard and elevating designs allow for movement at a predetermined height or variable height controlled with elastic bands. The orthosis is not managed (ie, attachment, adjustment, and maintenance) by the client but by an assistant and may be used only for specific activities such as eating, communication, and so on. The primary prescription criteria are partial upper limb paralysis particularly proximal weakness but with preserved elbow flexion power, for example C5 spinal cord injury. Wheelchair design and details of the back require assessment for mounting of the MAS and for proper sitting posture.

## Spinal and Cranial Orthoses

Spinal orthoses are provided for a wide variety of diagnoses. The goals are to provide abdominal support, pain management, control spine position (reposition flexible deformity, support and accommodate fixed deformity, and prevent the progression of deformity), and control spine motion. These goals are primarily accomplished by the reduction of gross spinal motion, the stabilization of individual motion segments, and the application of forces to control the progression of vertebral column deformities. Spinal orthoses are generally categorized by the spinal segments, the gross spinal motions controlled, the level of customization and the materials used to fabricate the orthosis.

## Sacroiliac Orthoses (SIOs) and Lumbar Sacral Orthoses

SIOs are recommended for sacroiliac joint instability due to trauma, over-use or pregnancy. They provide stability by compression directly on the sacrum as the "keystone" of the pelvis, by circumferential compression of the entire pelvis, and by compression and support of lower abdominal muscles. Canvas or other flexible materials are commonly used and the orthoses are often prefabricated.

Lumbosacral orthoses (LSOs) are recommended to manage pathologies in the L2-S1 region. The anterior trimlines extend from the xiphoid process to the symphysis pubis and posteriorly from the inferior angle of the scapula to the sacrococcygeal junction. LSOs can be categorized as either semirigid or rigid. A corset style LSO (Figure 21.26) is a commonly prescribed semirigid spinal orthosis for the relief of low back pain. The corset may be made of fabric or other flexible materials with adjustable closures to ensure a snug fit and rigid horizontal stays or molded plastic inserts for additional stiffness. The corset increases abdominal compression to provide relief of stress on the posterior spinal musculature and thereby provides pain relief.

Rigid spinal orthoses are defined by the plane of motion that is most restricted by the orthosis. The chairback and the LSO knight (Figure 21.27) both control motion in the sagittal plane and are composed of a rigid posterior frame with a pelvic band, a thoracic band, and a pair of paraspinal uprights. In addition, they both have a corset front which creates abdominal compression to further support the lumbosacral spine. They differ in that the LSO knight also provides restriction of frontal plane motion with the addition of a pair of lateral uprights. The Williams extension and coronal plane control LSO is constructed with a similar rigid posterior frame but, with oblique bars replacing the paraspinal bars, mobile attachments at the thoracic band and lateral bars, and an inelastic pelvic strap. The design allows flexion of the lumbar spine and limits extension. The Williams LSO is prescribed for the treatment of spondylolisthesis. All 3 of these LSOs are traditionally constructed of leather covered metal bands and are custom fabricated. Prefabricated thermoplastic versions are available. Custom molded thermoplastic body jacket style LSOs are available and provide rigid tri-planar motion limitation due to the rigid materials and the intimacy of fit over the pelvis.

**Figure 21.26** LSO corset.

**Figure 21.27** LSO knight.

## Thoracic Lumbar Sacral Orthoses

TLSOs are recommended to manage pathologies in the T3-S1 region. They have anterior trimlines that extend from the sternal notch to the symphysis pubis and posteriorly from the spine of the scapula to the sacrococcygeal junction. TLSOs can be categorized as either semirigid or rigid. A corset style TLSO is a commonly prescribed semirigid spinal orthosis for the relief of lumbar and/or thoracic spine pain. Similar to the LSO corset, the TLSO corset relies on abdominal compression to provide relief of stress on the posterior spinal musculature and thereby provide pain relief. They differ in that the TLSO includes a posterior extension to the spine of scapula with shoulder straps used to create an extension force on the thoracic spine and limit flexion. As in the LSO versions, leather covered metal bands are the traditional materials; however, foam covered thermoplastic versions are now common. A corset front is also used to create abdominal compression to further support the spine. Custom molded thermoplastic body jacket style TLSOs (Figure 21.28) are available and provide the most effective rigid tri-planar motion limitation due to their rigidity and the intimacy of fit over the pelvis and trunk. The body jacket style TLSOs can be fabricated as bivalve or anterior over-lap style for donning. Hyperextension style TLSOs are specifically designed for T10-L2 anterior compression fractures and are designed to prevent flexion and allow extension of the thoracolumbar spine. They are generally a rigid, pre fabricated frame design using a classic 3 point pressure system with body contact via a sternum pad, pubic pad, and a thoracolumbar pad. TLSOs for the management of scoliosis (Figure 21.29) have the primary goal of preventing the progression of the spinal deformity. They achieve this goal through end point control, transverse loading, curve correction, and the combined effect. These techniques are all done in an effort to increase the critical loading capabilities of the spinal column.

## Cervical Thoracic Lumbar Sacral Orthoses

Cervico-thoracic-lumbo-sacral orthoses (CTLSOs) provide control of the entire spine for stabilization following multilevel trauma or post-surgical reconstruction.

## Cervical Orthoses

Cervical orthoses (COs) can be generally categorized as flexible, semirigid, or rigid. They provide control

**Figure 21.28** TLSO body jacket.

**Figure 21.29** TLSO scoliosis.

primarily of sagittal plane motion (flexion more than extension) and to a lesser extent frontal plane motion (lateral flexion) but do not limit transverse plane rotation movements well. The soft foam collar is a simple, prefabricated, flexible CO often prescribed as a general kinesthetic reminder. The Philadelphia collar and similar orthoses (Figure 21.30) are popular semirigid COs for use with stable mid-cervical injuries or used after weaning out of a more rigid orthosis. Poster style rigid COs (2 and 4) (Figure 21.31) are described based on the number of rigid bars or posts used to support the head on the shoulders and upper thorax. They are used primarily for sagittal plane control either with a stable spine following trauma or postoperatively when rigid fixation is required in the C3-C6 region of the cervical spine.

**Figure 21.30** CO Philadelphia.

**Figure 21.31** CO 4 poster.

## Cervical Thoracic Orthoses

Cervicothoracic orthoses (CTOs) are used to extend the region of immobilization to the lower cervical and upper thoracic levels and are indicated for pathologies in the C1-T2 region. CTOs control flexion more effectively than extension due to the longer mechanical anterior lever arms. They are commonly prescribed for stable fractures, flexion injuries in the C3-T1 region, extension injuries in the C3-C5 region, general postoperative stabilization, and after weaning out of HALO use. The Sternal Occipital Mandibular Immobilizer (SOMI) is an example of a CTO and is an alternative to the poster style CO. It is preferred when donning in supine is required as there are no posterior bars. The SOMI specifically limits flexion and is most effective in the C1-C5 region.

The HALO (Figure 21.32) is a rigid CTO used for unstable cervical injuries and particularly for upper cervical spine instability (occiput-C2). The halo ring is fixed into the skull with 4 screws and into 2 or 4 bars which then attach to a rigid vest for shoulder and upper thorax loading.

# ■ WALKING AID

The elderly sick often have difficulty in walking. Rehabilitation aims at allowing them to walk without gadgets, but if they are to walk on their own they may need a walking-aid of some type. Walking aids are helpful for patients who have chronic problems, including hip and knee arthritis, as well as those who have acute injuries, such as ankle sprains and leg fractures. Finding the right type of walking aid will help the patients along the way. Which type is needed is based on several factors. A physical therapist can make a recommendation that suits patients' need. They will assess gait, balance, cognition, cardiovascular fitness, musculoskeletal challenges, and any neurological conditions.

**Figure 21.32** HALO.

Patients may also benefit from an occupational therapy assessment of the living area and work environment. Different walking aids may be needed if there are stairs patients must negotiate, as well as their mode of transport (car, public transportation, etc.) A combination of different types may be recommended for different purposes.

Many people may resist using walking aids because they are not convenient or they feel a stigma attached to needing one. However, they have been shown to reduce fall injuries.

### Single-Point Cane

A single-point cane is helpful for many conditions where a little extra support can alleviate pain and discomfort. A cane is the simplest way to lend some support to the leg, though it is not an appropriate option when weight must be completely removed from the extremity. A single-point cane is a good choice if patient's problem is arthritis. Be sure to know which hand to hold the cane with. The general rule is hold the cane with the hand on patient's strong side and move the cane at the same time as patient's weaker leg. Canes and walking sticks come in a wide variety of designs. However, they do need to be sized correctly and have a grip that patient can use comfortably.

### Quad Cane

A quad cane is a good option for people who need more stability than a standard single-point cane can offer, but who do not need the full support of a walker. They are a good choice if the patient have a neurological impairment, significant weakness, or balance problems.

### Crutches

Crutches allow the patient to completely remove weight from the extremity. Crutches require good stability and upper body strength, so they are often less useful to elderly patients. However, crutches can provide both excellent support and freedom for those with ample strength.

Using crutches takes getting used to, but a few simple steps can help patient get around. If you have been treated for an injury or had surgery, be sure to get instructions or training before you leave the facility. Your crutches need to be fitted for the correct height, and there are several tricks to using them safely.

### Walker

A walker is the most supportive walking aid, though it's also the most cumbersome. It is an excellent option for those with poor balance or less upper body strength. Newer types of walkers have many options and features that can make the device more convenient to use. Factors to consider when looking for a walker include foldability, weight capacity, handle height, heaviness of the walker itself, and width.

The standard walker must be lifted and moved with each step. For those with limited upper body strength, walkers may have wheels or glides on two or all four legs so it can slide between steps rather than needing to be picked up. Walkers with four wheels are called rollators and often have a brake of some type for safety, as well as a seat so that you can take a rest when you are tired.

### Knee Walker

The knee walker is simple to use, and one of the easiest ways to get around safely and quickly without placing weight on your leg. Many people who have a hard time using crutches, and don't want to be slowed down by a walker, will find the knee walker a worthwhile investment.

## ■ SUMMARY

The complete multidisciplinary rehabilitation team includes the prosthetist, orthotist, and Pedorthist. These health care professionals are uniquely trained to provide orthoses, prostheses, and pedorthic services. Three primary issues are to be considered in the fabrication of an orthotic or prosthetic device: (1) the detailed selection of components and materials, (2) the level of customization, and (3) the process of evaluation and provision of the device. Evaluating a patient for and prescribing a prosthesis begins with a functional assessment. Specifically, assessing the potential of the client to use a prosthesis and thereby determine the appropriate prosthesis design necessary to achieve the goal of maximizing pain-free functional independence. The population of upper limb prosthesis users is quite different than lower limb prosthesis users representing a very small minority of the limb loss population. This is primarily due to limited number of upper limb amputations and much higher prosthesis rejection rate. An orthosis is a device, applied to the exterior of the body, for the purpose of supporting, correcting, aligning, or improving the function of moveable parts of the body or reducing pain of the head, spine, or extremities. The prescription and design of a lower limb orthosis begins with a clear diagnosis and physical exam including functional assessment and gait analysis.

## ■ IMPORTANT TERMINOLOGY

prosthetics    修复学
orthotics    矫形学
orthoses    矫形器
amputation    截肢术
rehabilitation    康复
lower limb prostheses    下肢假肢
prosthesis disarticulation knee    膝离断假肢

Syme ankle disarticulation prostheses   赛姆假肢

transtibial prosthesis   小腿假肢

transfemoral prostheses   大腿假肢

hip disarticulation prosthesis   髋离断假肢

transradial prosthesis   前臂假肢

ankle foot orthosis (AFO)   踝足矫形器

knee ankle foot orthoses (KAFOs)   膝踝足矫形器

shoulder-elbow-wrist-hand orthoses (SEWHOs)   肩肘腕手矫形器

# ■ QUESTIONS

1. What is the basic components of lower limb prostheses?

2. What is the primary issues to be considered in the fabrication of an orthotic or prosthetic device?

3. Why the upper limb prosthesis users are quite different from lower limb prosthesis users?

4. What is the purpose of an orthosis?

5. What are the hand orthoses (HOs) functions?

# ■ REFERENCES

1.  Gailey R, Roach K, Applegate E, et al. The amputee mobility predictor: an instrument to assess determinants of lower-limb amputee's ability to ambulate. Arch Phys Med Rehabil. 2002; 83: 615-627.

2.  Kuiken T. Targeted Reinnervation for Improved Prosthetic Function. In: Bussell M, Kraft G, eds. New Advances in Prosthetics and Orthotics. Physical Medicine and Rehabilitation Clinics of North America. Philadelphia, PA: Saunders; 2006: 1-13.

（刘四海）

# Chapter
# 22

# *SPINAL CORD INJURY REHABILITATION*

## ■ SPINAL CORD INJURY EPIDEMIOLOGY

12 000 new spinal cord injuries (SCIs) occur in the United States every year. The vast majority are men under the age of 40. The most common cause of SCI is motor vehicle collisions. Over the age of 45, the most common cause is falls. Violence (primarily gunshot wounds) accounts for 15% of the SCIs in the United States. The most common levels of injury are C5 for complete SCI and T12 for incomplete injuries. Most injuries occur from C4 to C7, T4 to T6 and at the thoracolumbar junction (T10-L1). Non-traumatic causes of SCI are detailed in Table 22.1.

**TABLE 22.1** ▪ Non-traumatic causes of SCI

- Spinal stenosis
- Cancer—most commonly breast, lung, or prostate
- Transverse myelitis
- MS
- Syringomyelia
- Vascular ischemia (thoracoabdominal aneurysms can result in injury to the artery of Adamkiewicz causing T12-L1 ischemic injury)

### Anatomy and Neuro-anatomy

The vertebral column is composed of 7 cervical, 12 thoracic, 5 lumbar, 5 sacral, and 4 coccygeal vertebrae. The spinal cord is protected within the vertebral foramen, and initially occupies the entire length of the vertebral canal. The spinal cord segments, especially in the thoracic and lumbar regions, do not line up with their corresponding vertebral level, and explain why a fracture of T12 for instance results in a L1-2 NLI. At the caudal end, the spinal cord is conical in shape and is known as the conus medullaris. The lumbar and sacral nerve roots descend some distance within the vertebral canal in order to exit from their respective intervertebral foramina. These nerve roots resemble a horse's tail, and are termed the cauda equina (CE). The lumbar cistern extends from the caudal end of the spinal cord (L2 vertebra) to the second sacral vertebra. The subarachnoid space is widest at this site and is therefore most suitable for the withdrawal of cerebrospinal fluid (CSF) by lumbar puncture, usually performed between the L3 and L4 lumbar vertebrae.

Thirty-one pairs of spinal nerves (8 cervical, 12 thoracic, 5 lumbar, 5 sacral, and 1 coccygeal pair) emerge from the spinal cord. At and below the thoracic level, the nerve roots exit just caudal to the corresponding vertebra while in the cervical region the nerve roots exit through the intervertebral foramina just rostral to the corresponding vertebra. This is due to the fact that there are eight cervical nerve roots and only seven cervical vertebrae; the C8 nerve root exits through the intervertebral foramen just rostral to the first thoracic vertebra.

The spinal cord has two enlargements: cervical and lumbar. The cervical enlargement includes the C5-T1 nerve roots to form the brachial plexus which innervates the upper extremities (UEs). The lumbar plexus (roots L1 to L4) and lumbosacral plexus (L4 to S2) emerge from the lumbar enlargement and innervate the lower extremities (LEs). The sacral spinal nerves emerge from the conus medullaris and contain PS and somatic motor fibers innervating the muscles of the bladder wall and external sphincter, respectively.

The spinal cord receives its blood supply from one anterior and two posterior spinal arteries (PSAs) as well as anterior and posterior radicular arteries. The anterior spinal artery (ASA) arises in the upper cervical region and is formed by the union of two branches of the vertebral arteries. The ASA supplies the anterior two thirds of the spinal cord including the gray matter, anterior and anterolateral white matter. The ASA varies in diameter according to its proximity to a major radicular artery. It usually is narrowest in the T4-8 region of the spinal cord. There are two PSAs that originate from the vertebral artery. The PSAs supply the posterior one third of the spinal cord consisting of posterolateral and posterior white matter of the spinal cord.

The blood supply from the anterior and posterior arteries is sufficient for the upper cervical segments. Segmental arteries that arise from the aorta supply the ASA and PSAs in the thoracic and lumbar regions. The radicular arteries arise from the vertebral, cervical, intercostal, lumbar, and sacral arteries and supply the remaining segments of the spinal cord. The major radicular artery that supplies the lumbosacral enlargement of the spinal cord is known as the artery of Adamkiewicz. It usually arises from the left intercostal or lumbar artery at the level of T6-L3 and provides the main blood supply to the lower two thirds of the spinal cord. There are less radicular arteries that supply the midthoracic region of the spinal cord and are smaller in diameter and therefore create a "watershed zone" of the spinal cord at this level. With clinical situations where there is low blood flow to the spinal cord (ie, clamping of the aorta for surgery above the renal artery), this level of the cord is most affected (T4-6 level).

The internal structure of the spinal cord is such that a transverse section of the spinal cord reveals a butterfly-shaped central gray matter surrounded by white matter. The gray matter of the spinal cord contains cell bodies and primarily neurons, dendrites, and myelinated and unmyelinated axons. Autonomic neurons are located laterally and exit by the ventral root and innervate smooth muscle. Lower motor neurons (LMN) are located ventrally, exit by the ventral roots and innervate striated muscle. The white matter consists of ascending and descending bundles of myelinated and unmyelinated axons (tracts or fasciculi). The ascending pathways relay sensory information to the brain while the descending pathways relay motor information from the brain.

Sensory tracts or ascending pathways are composed of axons from peripheral sensory nerves whose cell bodies are located in the dorsal root ganglion (DRG) and ascend toward the brainstem. Receptors for pain and temperature enter the spinal cord and synapse in the dorsal horn of the gray matter. The fibers cross over within one to two vertebral segments, then travel in the lateral spinothalamic tract and ascend to the ventral posterolateral (VPL) nucleus of the thalamus. The fibers then ascend in the internal capsule to reach the postcentral gyrus, which is the primary somatic sensory area of the brain. Pressure and light touch (LT) fibers enter the cord in the same fashion, and pass into the ipsilateral dorsal white column and bifurcate. One branch immediately enters the dorsal horn gray matter, synapses, and crosses over within one to two segments, while the other branch remains ipsilateral, and ascends in the dorsal column for as many as ten spinal segments. The ipsilateral branch ultimately enters the dorsal horn, synapses, and crosses over to join the other branch in the ventral white column, forming the ventral spinothalamic tract. These axons travel in the same pathway as the lateral tract to reach the postcentral gyrus, which interprets these sensations.

The posterior columns transmit three different sensations; proprioception, fine touch, and vibration sense. Their nerve fibers reach the DRG and immediately pass into the ipsilateral dorsal white columns and ascend to the medulla. Axons that enter the cord at the sacral, lumbar, and lower thoracic levels are situated in the medial part of the dorsal column (ie, the lower part of the body) called the fasciculus gracilis. Those axons that enter at the thoracic (above T6) and cervical levels are situated in the lateral part of the column (from the upper part of the body) and are termed the fasciculus cuneatus. Axons of each fasciculus synapse in the medulla and form a bundle termed the medial lemniscus, which ascends to the postcentral gyrus.

The cerebellum is the control center for the coordination of voluntary muscle activity, equilibrium, and muscle tone. The spinocerebellar tract is a set of axonal fibers originating in the spinal cord and terminating in the ipsilateral cerebellum that conveys information to the cerebellum about limb and joint positions (proprioception).

The lateral corticospinal tract is the main tract for voluntary muscle activity. Its origin is the precentral gyrus of the frontal lobe of the brain. Their axons descend through the internal capsule to the medulla oblongata. Approximately 80% to 90% of the axons cross at the pyramidal decussation to the contralateral side of the medulla and descend in the lateral white columns of the spinal cord, in the lateral corticospinal tract. At each level of the spinal cord, the axons from the lateral tract peel off and enter the gray matter of the ventral horn and synapse with secondary neurons. The 10% to 20% of uncrossed axons that continue down on the same side of the cord travel in the ventral corticospinal tract. The axons of the ventral tract then cross over at the corresponding level of muscles that it innervates. Both tracts travel from the precentral gyrus to the ventral horn as a single uninterrupted neuron and are termed upper motor neurons (UMN), while the secondary neurons that they synapse on, are termed lower motor neurons.

## ■ SCI CLASSIFICATION

The American Spinal Injury Association (ASIA) has established examination guidelines that are currently the universal standard for the examination and evaluation of SCI patients. This assessment involves the evaluation of both the sensory and motor system in a uniform fashion. The initial examination should be performed within the first week post injury. For prognostic purposes, the ASIA evaluation should be repeated when the patient is out of spinal shock (reflexes return). Repeat testing is recommended since patient effort and condition at examination can vary and for improving reliability. Multiple evaluations done over several days are considered superior to one single examination.

The ASIA classification and examination has 3 basic components.

### Sensory

The sensory system is evaluated using both pin prick and light touch on the right and left sides. Scoring is described in Table 22.2. A physician should perform pin prick evaluation using a standard unused safety pin. The sharp edge is used to determine a patient's ability to sense the sharp and the dull safety cover of the pin if the patient is able to sense dull sensation. Physicians should perform a light touch evaluation with a wisp of cotton. The control for examination is the face, unless facial injury is noted or suspected.

**TABLE 22.2** ▪ Sensory scoring system

| Score | Description |
| --- | --- |
| NT | Not Testable: used when a level cannot be tested due to secondary factors (cast, cognitive impairment, or other factors) |
| 0 | Inability to register a difference between sharp and dull on pin prick or unable to sense light touch |
| 1 | Ability to register a difference but the sharp is not as precise as that noted on the face. Regarding light touch face is more precise than testing area. |
| 2 | Patient notes sensation is the same on their face and on the dermatomal level being tested. * |

*If hyperesthesia is present the level is given a grade 1 and not 2.

## Motor

The motor system is evaluated based on assessment of specific myotome groups with the patient in a supine position. At levels where motor testing is not feasible (thoracic), the motor is assumed to correspond to the sensory examination. Motor scoring is detailed in Table 22.3.

The most caudal myotome tested with manual muscle test findings equal to or greater than 3/5 with the segment proximal noted to be normal (5/5) is the motor level. For levels where there is no motor testing, the level would correspond to the last normal sensory level.

**TABLE 22.3** ▪ Motor scoring system

| Score | Description |
|---|---|
| NT | Not Testable: used when a level cannot be tested due to secondary factors (cast or other mobilization, spasticity or contracture) |
| 0 | Absent |
| 1 | Palpable or visible contraction |
| 2 | Active movement, full range of motion with gravity eliminated |
| 3 | Active movement, full range of motion against gravity |
| 4 | Active movement full range of motion against gravity and some resistance |
| 5 | Active movement full range of motion against gravity and normal resistance |
| 5* | Muscles by examiners judgment has NL strength but factors preclude full ROM or NL function |

## Anal Sphincter

The sphincter is tested for voluntary anal contraction through digital examination and is graded as present or absent.

## ■ ASIA IMPAIRMENT SCALE

The sensory, motor, and anal sphincter contraction evaluation provides key information used to determine the patients' relative impairment levels and the ASIA Impairment Rating. Table 22.4 describes the multiple levels and scores that are determined through the examination. The ASIA impairment scale ranges from A to E with A indicating the most severe findings and E representing a normal exam. Details for scoring are described in Table 22.5.

**TABLE 22.4** ▪ Various SCI impairment levels

| | |
|---|---|
| Sensory Level | It's the most caudal dermatome level with both pin prick and light touch scoring 2/2 |
| Motor Level | The most caudal myotome tested whose manual muscle test was noted to be equal to or greater than 3/5 with the segment proximal noted to be normal (5/5) on testing |
| Neurologic Level of Injury (NLI) | The most caudal level where motor and sensory are intact |
| Sensory Index Score (112 maximum) | Summary of all the sensory scores for both light touch and pin prick |
| Motor Index Score (100 maximum) | Summary of motor testing 25 points for each limb and 100 for all 4 extremities |
| Zone of Partial Preservation (ZPP) | The segments below the NLI with noted preservation of sensory or motor findings reserved for complete SCI |

**TABLE 22.5** ▪ ASIA impairment scale

| Grade | Description | Injury Type |
|---|---|---|
| ASIA A | Complete injury | Sensory and motor complete |
| ASIA B | Incomplete injury with no motor function preserved below the NLI but some sensory including Sacral 4-5 preservation is present | Sensory incomplete Motor complete |
| ASIA C | Incomplete injury with sensory sacral sparing and motor function preserved below the NLI. This may be >3 levels below the NLI but<50% of the muscles below the NLI have motor score of ⩾3 | Sensory incomplete Motor incomplete |
| ASIA D | Incomplete injury with sensory sacra sparing and motor function preserved >3 levels below the NLI and greater then >50% of the muscles below the NLI must have a motor score of ⩾3 or Voluntary anal contraction is present | Sensory incomplete Motor incomplete |
| ASIA E | Normal: Motor and sensory functions are normal | Normal |

## ■ SPINAL CORD INJURY SYNDROMES (FIGURE 22.1)

### Brown-Sequard Syndrome

Incomplete SCI as a result of damage to the lateral half of the spinal cord (hemisection) resulting in damage to the corticospinal tracts and dorsal column, which cross at the level of the brain stem leading to a loss of proprioception and motor function (paralysis) ipsilateral to the lesion. The spinothalamic tracts cross at the spinal level resulting in loss of pain and temperature sensation on the contralateral side.

### Anterior Cord Syndrome

Damage to the anterior two-thirds of the spinal cord as the result of disruption in blood flow to the anterior spinal artery. This can occur as a result of trauma, embolus, hypotension, or arterial occlusion. On rare occasions, it can occur as a result of aortic clamping during surgery. Patients present with absence of motor and pain sensation below the level of the injury. Blood supply through the posterior spinal artery spares the dorsal columns resulting in normal proprioception below the level of the injury.

### Central Cord Syndrome

The most common of the SCI syndromes occurring primarily in older individuals. This injury is typically the result of a cervical hyperextension injury usually in the presence of spondylosis and is characterized by disproportionately weak upper

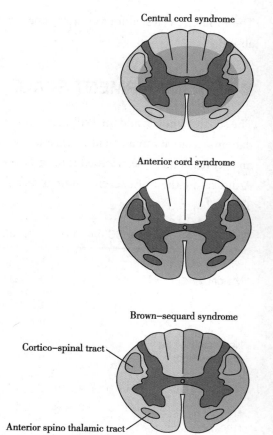

Central cord syndrome

Anterior cord syndrome

Brown–sequard syndrome

Cortico–spinal tract

Anterior spino thalamic tract

**Figure 22.1**   Common incomplete SCI syndromes.

extremities compared to lower extremities. Sensory loss below the level of the injury is variable.

## Conus Medullaris Injury

A syndrome characterized by a mixed upper motor neuron and lower motor neuron presentation. Clinical findings include areflexic bowel and bladder and sensory loss in a saddle distribution with or without lower extremity weakness.

## Cauda Equina Syndrome

This is not a true SCI but involves damage to multiple lumbosacral nerve roots that form the cauda equina and thus upper motor neuron signs are absent. Clinical presentation is similar to conus medullaris injury with bowel and bladder involvement. Asymmetric pain and sensory loss are usually present in the distribution of the nerve roots involved. Reflexes are absent distal to the injury level.

## Prognosis after SCI

For the purpose of determining prognosis, examinations at or within 24 hours of injury are not as accurate as those done at 72 hours. Evaluation of pin prick has better reliability than light touch examination and return of pin prick sensation is the best sign of recovery enabling better predictability.

The review of a patient's reflexes can help determine prognosis. In incomplete SCI, deep tendon reflexes tend to have larger amplitudes compared to complete injuries.

The presence of an abnormal plantar response at 72 hours has a high correlation with complete SCI and portends a poor prognosis. Presence of a crossed adductor response (contralateral adduction and internal rotation to a patellar tap or knee jerk), which is absent in complete injuries, correlates with a greater likelihood of motor recovery in the lower extremities. The absence of the bulbocavernosus reflex within 72 hours after injury suggests a lower motor neuron injury.

Most upper extremity recovery occurs in the first 2 to 6 months post injury with greatest gains occurring in the first 3 months. Motor recovery can continue up to and into the second year post injury; with average functional plateau for complete and incomplete at 12 to 18 months and 9 to 12 months, respectively [1]. Recovery potential based on initial motor scores is summarized in Table 22.6.

**TABLE 22.6 ▪ Review of observational reports on recovery**

| Initial Motor Scores | Motor Recovery Potential |
| --- | --- |
| 1-2/5 | >95% reach 3/5 |
| Key muscles and some immediate adjacent level with 0/5 | 50%-60% will reach 1/5 |
| Adjacent muscles 1 level away from 0/5 | Up to 25% can reach 3/5 |
| Adjacent muscles 2 levels away from injury | <10% recover 1/5 strength |

## Acute SCI

In acute SCI, prehospital management includes standard ACLS protocols with care directed at ensuring proper spinal stabilization at the event scene. All patients should be assumed to have a SCI or bony instability until proven otherwise. The goal of initial stabilization is to minimize acute injury and prevent progression of direct injury and damage to the spinal cord from indirect causes. Direct and indirect causes of SCI are summarized in Table 22.7.

**TABLE 22.7** ▪ Examples of direct and indirect causes of SCI

| Direct | Indirect |
|---|---|
| Foreign Body (bullet, knife) | Hypo-perfusion |
| Bony compression | Metabolic overload |
| Tumor | Thrombus |
| Instability | Local toxic metabolites |
| Fracture | |
| Mass compression | |

**SCI Pearls**

- Complete SCI usually recover one level distal to their initial NLI. Complete SCI above T9 normally do not regain lower extremity motor function.
- Complete SCI below T9, amongst these individuals 33% recover some lower extremity function.
- Nontraumatic SCI patients have shorter length of stay and lower incidence of spasticity, orthostasis, pressure ulcer, dysreflexia, DVT, and pneumonia.
- More likely to continue to work if: young, lower level of injury, less severe injury, educated, driven, and married.
- Consider concomitant brain injury if there is new cognitive impairment, frontal signs, disparity of upper and lower body tone and spasticity, or paradoxical breathing.

## Neurogenic Shock

Acute SCI interrupts the sympathetic nervous system below the level of injury resulting in vasodilatation. If the injury is proximal to the sixth level of the thoracic spine the result is cardiovascular disregulation with a significant loss in systemic vascular resistance. If the injury is proximal to the first thoracic level the patient loses the ability to have compensatory increases in their cardiac rate. These issues result in the classic SCI neurogenic triad; often coexisting with hypovolemia: hypotension, bradycardia, and hypothermia.

## Spinal Shock

Spinal shock is the loss of spinal reflexes with flaccid paralysis, hypotonia, areflexia, with loss of bowel and bladder reflexes and sphincter control. The absence of muscle tone and normal vascular reflexes below the level of injury causes impaired blood-pressure control leading to orthostasis and orthostatic hypotension. Spinal shock is considered resolved when the distal reflexes start to return; delayed plantar reflex followed by the return of the bulbocavernosus reflex. The earlier the return of deep tendon reflexes the better the prognosis. Following resolution of spinal shock, patients can be noted to have the onset of spasticity, hyperreflexia, and clonus.

## Neurogenic And Spinal Shock Management

A patient who is noted to be in shock should be treated with invasive monitoring, volume resuscitation, and vasopressors to maintain blood pressure. Invasive monitoring is important to prevent pulmonary edema and respiratory damage secondary to over-hydration. The uncontrolled sympathetic discharge in acute SCI can cause extravasation of fluid from pulmonary vasculature.

The disruption that occurs between the spinal cord and the sympathetic nervous system leads to bradycardia especially in the first several weeks post injury. In the initial stages of SCI management, monitoring bradycardia and providing supportive care is necessary. In some patients, especially those with injuries at the upper thoracic and cervical area, bradycardia may be serious enough to require transvenous pacing (temporary or permanent). It is important to remember that bradycardia in SCI patients is not a result of atrial dysfunction but a result of uninhibited vagal parasympathetic stimulation on the heart.

Hypotension occurring as a result of spinal and neurogenic shock can result in mean arterial pressure (MAP) around 55 and systolic blood pressure of 90 mmHg or lower. Cardiovascular support with intravenous fluids and pressors can be used to maintain a MAP above 85 and a systolic blood pressure above 110 mmHg. This is important to maintain spinal-cord perfusion.

While there is discussion of the use of hypothermia and even membrane stabilizing agents [2] to slow the metabolism within the spinal cord, decrease progression of further spinal-cord damage and/or help mildly injured cells to recover; there is no definitive evidence available to demonstrate that these techniques result in improved long-term outcomes.

# ■ ACUTE SCI EVALUATION

**X-ray**: Used for initial screening of the spine and evaluation of bony structures.

**CT scan**: Allows for further evaluation of bony structure and central canal when fractures or abnormalities are suspected but not clearly visualized on x-ray. It is the evaluation of choice to determine bony encroachment within the spinal canal. Contrast can be used to evaluate for spinal cord and nerve compression.

**MRI**: Magnetic resonance imaging (MRI) can be used in the acute and subacute stages following SCI to evaluate spinal cord integrity, determine localization, and identify presence of intraspinal and extra spinal hemorrhage and edema. Several findings on MRI are associated with poor prognosis [3,4]:

- Presence of spinal-cord hemorrhage
- Larger length of spinal-cord hemorrhage
- Greater expanse of edema proximal to distal
- Spinal cord compression
- Abnormalities are noted to expand more than one vertebral segment

**MRI STIR**: Imaging can be used to evaluate for edema within the cord in acute injury. Bony fracture can be visualized as a hyper-intense signal with the marrow.

**T2 GRE**: Is the best tool to evaluate for acute cord hematoma.

**MRA**: Used to evaluate for vertebral artery injury.

## Treatment

### Methylprednisolone

Three separate trials of the US National Acute Spinal Cord Injury Study (NASCIS) [5,6] looked at the effects of methylprednisolone after SCI. NASCIS 2 trial results demonstrated significant differences on outcomes when high-dose methylprednisolone was initiated within 8 hours of injury at 30 mg/kg bolus followed by 5.4 mg/kg•hr for 23 hours [7,8]. NASCIS 3 reported improved benefit when methylprednisolone was extended to 48 hours post injury and initiated 3 to 8 hours post injury [6]. Methylprednisolone administration is considered a treatment option in both the Neurosurgical Guidelines and the Spinal Cord Medicine Consortium Clinical Practice Guidelines [9,10]. Emergency medical personnel usually have methylprednisolone available and immediate administration to patients with suspected injury is considered standard protocol [9,11]. Use of methylprednisolone varies due to concerns regarding post infusion side effects. The NACIS' evidence is considered by some to be insufficient (especially for complete SCIs). Others are concerned about the side effects of steroids, specifically, steroid induced myopathy, which has been associated with both the 24-hour and the 48-hour protocols [12]. Steroid utilization has also been shown to cause hyperglycemia, gastritis, and pneumonia in some patients who receive the 48-hour infusion. The 48-hour infusion has also been associated with increased risk of infection. The risk of side effects versus benefit needs to be considered [7].

## Common Medical Complications after SCI

### Pulmonary

The leading cause of mortality in the first year after SCI is pulmonary complications with all levels of injury being at risk [6,12]. Contributing factors to pulmonary complications include atelectasis, hypoventilation, and inability or difficulty managing secretions. SCI injuries with damage at C1-3 will require 24-hour ventilator support post injury with a backup ventilator/portable ventilator and supportive devices. Those with SCI at C5 and below usually do not require long-term ventilation support. The requirements for patients with injuries at the fourth cervical level are variable.

Without the tone of the abdominal wall to provide support and assist in coughing and expiration, SCI patients generally have decreased expiratory capacity and may not be able to generate the peak cough expiratory flow (PCEF) of 5 to 6 liters or more, which is needed to clear secretions properly. Due to the segmental innervations of the intercostal muscles, patients with higher level injuries have more severe impairments of cough and exhalation. Spinal cord patients with high-level injuries eventually lose their expiratory reserve (vital capacity is equal to inspiratory capacity). Without proper PCEF secretions can accumulate and also impair ventilation and subsequent oxygen and carbon dioxide exchange. These factors can lead to infections of the lung and death.

Given the loss of expiratory ability, the need to perform pulmonary toileting and to teach assisted cough maneuvers is important to maintain good pulmonary hygiene, prevent infection, and other pulmonary complications.

### Abdominal Binders

It provides support to the abdominal cavity pushing against the abdominal contents and improving diaphragmatic support and positioning thus assisting in expiratory function and coughing especially while upright.

### Secretion Management

Secretion management is a very important component of SCI management. The basic types of secretion management assistance include: postural drainage, percussion, vibration, and cough assistance techniques or devices. All of these techniques are designed to help mobilize and loosen secretions. Prior to these therapies, bronchodilators administration can be considered to facilitate opening of the airways and improve drainage and/or expectoration of secretions.

There are 10 standardized positions for postural drainage (Figure 22.2). Commonly, patients are placed in a Trendelenburg position (head down) between 10 to 45 degrees to assist in drainage. This can be done independently or in conjunction with other modalities. If performed in the morning, the benefits may continue into the night reducing overall secretion accumulation. Precautions must be employed due to the potential for position associated increases in blood flow return which can lead to cardiovascular complications given the inability to regulate sympathetic and parasympathetic responses. If patients have active infections, extra caution should be used due to risk for increases in flow of secretions from diseased to healthy lobes of lung.

Chest percussion therapy can be performed manually or with machine assistance by trained physical or respiratory therapists. During the expiratory phase, a therapist or mechanical device (at 5 Hz) rhythmically strikes the chest wall in the area where drainage assistances is desired. Manual chest percussion is performed by hand while mechanical percussion involves the use of specially designed machines for time periods that vary dependent upon individual tolerance (1-5 minutes).

**Figure 22.2**  Summary of postural drainage positions.

Vibration therapy is used throughout the respiratory cycle not just the expiratory phase. The machine runs at 10 to 15 Hz for similar time frames as mechanical percussion. These machines can be more costly; but in patients with a high volume of secretions and/or poor clearance prevention of complications justifies its use.

Insufflation-exsufflation devices are highly effective in the removal of secretions. Positive pressure is provided during inspiration resulting in insufflation. This increases the patient's vital capacity which must be a minimum of 1 200 to 1 500 ml to allow for an effective cough (PCEF of at least 5-6 L/sec). The insufflations are provided through masks or directly into endotracheal or tacheostomy tubes. The insufflations are followed by a negative-pressure/controlled suction also called exsufflation. This mechanical technique creates a PCEF of 7 to 11 L/s, which is necessary for proper clearance of secretions. Oral suctioning is used to remove secretions in the oral cavity and posterior oropharynx. Suctioning of airway secretions must be performed using a sterile technique and with caution due to propensity for cardiac abnormalities, pulmonary edema, increased intracranial pressure, tracheal, and/ or mucosal damage.

### Active-Assist Cough

A manually assisted cough is performed with the application of an external force to various sites of the trunk during a cough or the expiratory phase. This requires the assistance of another individual (clinician, nurse, or personal assistant) to facilitate the cough and expiration. Active-assist cough maneuvers include side-lying abdominal thrust assist, costophrenic assist, anterior chest compression assist, or counter-rotation assist. Contraindications include rib fractures, recent abdominal or thoracic surgery, ileus, or the presence of inferior vena cava filters (which can be dislodged by these maneuvers).

### Self-Assist Cough

A self-assisted cough is also possible. To perform this type of cough, the head and trunk are quickly flexed starting from an initial position of relative extension. Contraindications are similar to those for active assist cough.

## Cardiovascular

The interruption in the mechanics of the cardiovascular system in acute and chronic SCI is critical and can lead to several medical problems including secondary injury and/or death. Common cardiovascular sequelae in SCI are summarized in Table 22.8.

**TABLE 22.8** ▪ Cardiovascular issues in spinal cord injury

| Cervical and Thoracic | Lumbar |
|---|---|
| Orthostatic hypotension | Orthostatic hypotension |
| Distal venous blood pooling | Distal venous blood |
| (increased DVT risk) Bradycardia Autonomic dysreflexia | pooling (increased DVT risk) |

Patients who have an injury above the T7 level will have disruption of normal cardiovascular control and of the interactions between the parasympathetic and sympathetic nervous systems. In SCI, the sympathetic nervous system customary inhibitory feedback mechanisms are impaired with function present only at the local level with parasympathetic response maintained. As a result of the parasympathetic and sympathetic nervous system dysregulation, SCI at T6 or above results in autonomic dysreflexia.

Injury at T5 or above results in impaired adrenal function causing dysregulation of adrenaline release.

T1 to T4 are the spinal levels that provide innervation to the myocardium and AV nodes. Injuries at T1 or above result in disconnection between the central nervous system and sympathetic nervous system.

Initially, SCI patients have hypotension and bradycardia; occurring during the first several weeks post injury and stabilizing over time with appropriate management. SCI patients have lower MAP and lower systolic blood pressures. The MAP post injury is usually between 55 to 65 mmHg with systemic pressures at 90 to 100 mmHg due to decreased resting systemic vascular resistance. Bradycardia is also common immediately post injury and may continue for up to 8 weeks post injury, especially in cervical and high-thoracic SCI.

### Treatment for Common Cardiovascular Issues

**Orthostatic Hypotension** is common after SCI. Many patients adapt over time to this sequela (several weeks to months). External vascular support of the arterial and venous system with compression stocking, bilateral lower extremity compression wrapping, and abdominal binders is recommended. The principle is to provide support to the venous system, prevent excessive pooling of blood in the lower extremities, and improve venous return. During physical therapy sessions a tilt table can be used for short periods of time to facilitate adaptation to the SCI and reduce orthostatic episodes. Initial treatment duration is 5 to 10 minutes. Patients should be monitored for tolerance and medical stability with particular focus on changes in alertness, dizziness, shortness of breath, headaches, nausea, hypotension, changes in heart rate, or respiratory rate.

If any of these occur the tilt table session should be discontinued. If a tilt table is not available, physical therapists can work with the patient by progressively elevating the head of the bed, as tolerated, and by having the patient sit on the edge of the bed or in a wheelchair. These techniques can also be implemented by other team members to improve tolerance and foster adaptation.

Oral or intravenous fluids with or without oral salt supplementation can be used to treat orthostatic hypotension. Vasopressors can also be administered in severe cases but are not recommended for night time or bedtime use as there is a risk of hypertension when in a supine position. Patients with severe bradycardia and hypotension should be evaluated by cardiology for cardiac pacemaker candidacy.

**Autonomic Dysreflexia (AD)** occurs when exposure to noxious stimuli results in disinhibited stimulation of the sympathetic nervous system in patients with injuries at T6 or above. The hallmarks of AD are bradycardia and relative hypertension (20-40 mmHg above baseline). Noxious stimulation below the level of the lesion leads to uncontrolled sympathetic discharge. Sympathetic outflow continues, uninhibited, until the noxious stimulus is eliminated. Peripheral vasculature will constrict resulting in increased venous return which in turn elevates blood pressure. Increases in venous return trigger carotid baroreceptors, activate vagal circuitry, and thus, bradycardia ensues.

Treatment of AD requires immediate elimination of the noxious stimulus. Most important is the prevention of cardiac arrhythmias, seizures, ischemic/hemorrhagic stroke, retinal hemorrhages, pulmonary edema, and death.

## Signs of AD

- Flushing and sweating above the level of lesion (parasympathetic signs)
- Piloerection below the level of injury (sympathetic signs)
- Paroxysmal hypertension 20 to 40 mmHg above baseline
- Headache or nasal congestion
- Bradycardia
- Anxiety

## Common Causes

- Obstructed, twisted, or kinked indwelling urinary catheter
- Distended bladder
- Distended or impacted rectal vault or bowel
- Urinary tract infection
- Fracture
- Ingrown toenails
- Other noxious stimuli (heterotopic ossification, pain, pressure ulcer, and acute abdominal pathology, among others)

## Treatment

Immediately
- Loosen clothes.

- Release abdominal binder.
- Remove compression stockings.
Secondary
- If an indwelling urinary catheter is present, inspect the tubing carefully for twists or kinks and flush to determine if obstruction is present.
- Perform bladder scanning to evaluate for distension.
- In the absence of an indwelling urinary catheter, catheterize the bladder while using lidocaine gel to prevent further noxious irritation.
- Perform a rectal exam. If rectal vault is full of stool, perform manual evacuation.
- Check skin and digits for any visible abnormality or possible noxious cause (ie, ingrown nail).
- If no cause is found or systolic blood pressure is above 150 mmHg, consider using a short acting anti-hypertensive agent.
    - Nitropaste 2.5 to 5.0 cm is preferred since it is easy to remove once noxious stimulus is removed.
    - Other choices
        - Nifedipine 10 mg PO, may repeat q 30 to 60 minutes as needed.
        - Clonidine patch 0.1 can also be used in cases of sustained hypertension. Clonidine is a good alternative since the patch can be removed after the AD episode is treated. Patients should be monitored since rebound tachycardia is possible.
    - Severe cases
        - Hydralazine (intravenous or oral) 10 to 20 mg
        - Nitroprusside IV
- Patients can develop temporary hypotension which should be managed as follows:
    - Trendelenburg positioning
    - Intravenous fluids
    - Removal of topical antihypertensives.

## Deep Vein Thrombosis (DVT)

Endocrine changes along with venous pooling increase the potential for systemic venous thrombosis. The use of low molecular weight heparin is preferred over unfractionated heparin in SCI patients. While comparison showed equal rates of DVT, the incidence of pulmonary embolism and bleeding was higher in patients using unfractionated heparin [13]. Treatment is recommended for a total of 6 to 8 weeks post injury. In high-risk patients, those with confirmed DVT, or those who have contraindications to anticoagulation, inferior vena cava (IVC) filter placement should be considered. It is important to remember that IVC filters do not prevent DVT. In addition, manual-assisted cough maneuvers cannot be performed after placement.

## Bladder

SCI patients will typically have an indwelling urinary catheter at the time of admission to a rehabilitation hospital or unit. A bladder program is initiated when the patient is medically stable and no longer requires intravenous fluids or antibiotics and/or monitoring of input and output [9]. The goal of bladder management is to prevent high volumes within the bladder, which increases the risk of urinary reflux to the kidney, resulting in kidney damage and/or infection.

During the spinal shock period, the bladder is flaccid often with some preservation of sphincter tone. As reflexes return, patients with injury above the conus medullaris (upper motor neuron injury) will have continued sphincter tone or heightened tone. Bladder reflexes usually return as spinal shock resolves leading to bladder contractions in association with increasing urine volumes. These contractions, which are the result of parasympathetic input from the S2-4 ganglion via the pelvic nerve, are normally opposed by inhibition of contraction or bladder relaxation a result of sympathetic stimulation (T10-L2) or beta adrenergic stimulation via the hypogastric nerve. Stimulation of bladder contraction and inhibition of bladder contraction occur normally with simultaneous relaxation or contraction of the bladder neck and sphincter, respectively. In some SCI patients, this process does not occur, known as bladder-sphincter dysynergia. Dysynergia creates a high-pressure system, which places the patient at risk for reflux of urine into the ureters and subsequently into the kidneys. Chronic retrograde flow of urine into the kidneys can lead to renal failure. Proper bladder management seeks to maintain low bladder volumes to prevent secondary complications.

An indwelling catheter serves to continually drain the bladder maintaining a low-pressure system. Clean intermittent catheterization (CIC) is the preferred method for bladder management in SCI patients. Level of injury and hand dexterity should be considered when making a decision regarding how to best manage the bladder; indwelling catheter versus CIC. With the use of assistive devices, males with injuries at C6 or below and females with injuries at C7 or below can perform CIC. Urinary volumes should be kept below 500 ml each time catheterization is performed. Consumption of oral fluids should be adjusted to ensure volumes are kept within this range, especially overnight. In the inpatient setting bladder scanning can provide important clinical information to enable the physician to determine the proper frequency of catheterization and whether oral fluid intake needs to be adjusted. It is important to consider that during the acute post injury period large volumes of intravenous fluids are given that may accumulate in the interstitial space (ie, third space accumulation). As SCI patients are mobilized during rehabilitation, fluid will normally shift from the intersitial space into the blood vessels. Thus, SCI patients tend to require more frequent catheterization during the first 2 weeks of their rehabilitation course than they will need later on.

Other considerations for bladder management include sphincterotomies, ventral continent stomas, and suprapubic catheters. These options can provide independence for patients when intermittent catheterization is not possible or for those who have difficulty accessing the perineum for catheterization.

Urinary bacterial colonization is common in SCI patients. Prophylactic antibiotics for prevention of urinary tract infection are not recommended [14]. Treatment should be implemented only after confirmation of a symptomatic infection. Clinical signs of infection include development of autonomic dysreflexia, cloudy or malodorous urine, fever, lethargy, and general malaise. Infections with stone forming organisms (most prominently proteus, but also serratia and klebsiella) should be treated. Additional information on neurogenic bladder management is presented in Chapter 11.

## Gastrointestinal

Impaired or disrupted innervation of the small and large intestine and anal sphincter results in a lower motor neuron syndrome in injuries to the cauda equina or upper motor neuron bowel in SCI at or above the conus medullaris. This results in increased bowel transit time placing patients at increased risk for ileus and peristalsis changes. Monitoring for signs of abdominal distention, decreased or absent bowel sounds, changes in bowel activity, nausea, vomiting, or abdominal pain is necessary, and symptoms should prompt further evaluation. Abdominal X-rays series, ultrasound for identification of gallstones or pancreatic cysts, along with liver and pancreatic blood panels should be considered when symptoms are present.

Prophylactic treatment is highly recommended with $H_2$ blocker or proton pump inhibitors [15]. The typical treatment span should be limited to less than 4 weeks (unless other factors are present) to reduce the risk of clostridium difficile infections [16]. The reader can refer to Chapter 13 for details on neurogenic bowel management.

# ■ OTHER ISSUES

**Heterotopic Ossification (HO)** is the abnormal formation of a new bone around joints and within muscles. Common sites include hips, shoulder, elbow, and knees. It is most likely to occur within the first 6 months after SCI. Evaluation includes X-rays of the affected area(s) and monitoring of serum alkaline phosphatase levels. Triplephase bone scan can be used when there is high level of suspicion and X-rays are negative since it can detect HO within the first 1 to 2 weeks.

**Hypercalcemia:** Immobilization hypercalcemia occurs due to increased osteoclastic activity and bone resorption in the immobilized limbs. Initially bone resorption will result in hypercalciuria. If the kidney is unable to keep up with excretion of serum calcium, hypercalcemia will develop. Patients with SCI, especially males, are at high risk for hypercalcemia secondary to higher bone density and larger bone mass. This commonly occurs between 2 weeks and 6 months after injury with achievement of calcium steady state within 6 months from the time of injury. Bone density scans after 6 months usually reveal decreased bone density below the level of the injury. Evaluation of parathyroid, thyroid, and vitamin D levels should be performed along with initial serum calcium levels. Common signs and symptoms of hypercalcemia include lethargy, fatigue, nausea, anorexia, muscle cramps, polydipsia, and polyuria. Initial treatment should include aggressive intravenous hydration with or without the addition of diuretics such as furosemide. An indwelling catheter is useful during treatment. In severe cases, those with levels lesser than 12.0 mg/dl, therapy with intravenous bisphosphonates should be considered.

**Osteoporosis:** SCI patients will lose close to 25% of their bone mass within 3 months post injury and 33% by 14 months post injury due to increased osteoclastic activity and decreased osteoblastic activity. This leads to initial loss of trabecular bone; loss of cortical bone occurs over time. Bone density should be evaluated periodically using traditional methods. Treatment should include calcium and Vitamin D supplementation and weight-bearing exercises. Bisphosphonates should be considered for confirmed osteoporosis.

**Skin Care/pressure ulcers:** Pressure relief is a critical aspect in management of those with SCI. Knowledge and monitoring of sites prone to skin breakdown is extremely important (heels, hips, occiput, sacrum, shoulders, and spine of scapula). As soon as spine stabilization is verified, a turning schedule (every 2 hours) should be initiated.Use of heel, occipital, and sacral protection is recommended along with careful monitoring of these areas and education in high-risk patients. Pressure areas can also include the ischium, lateral malleoli, and superior calf in wheelchair users. SCI patients should perform weight shifts every 15 minutes or offloading every 15 minutes for 45 seconds to ensure proper blood flow to weight-bearing areas. This can be accomplished manually or by using wheelchairs with tilt-in-space capabilities.

## Thermoregulation

SCI disrupts some of the body's thermoregulation mechanisms including shivering, vasoconstriction, and vasodilation by disrupting connection with the hypothalamus.

Patients with spinal injury are prone to episodes of hypothermia and hyperthermia. It is not uncommon for patients to experience a lower temperature below the level of the lesion. Environmental changes are necessary to maintain adequate temperature control.

# ■ FUNCTIONAL OUTCOMES AFTER SCI

**C4** is a key level for independent respiratory function potentially allowing SCI patients to breathe without mechanical ventilation.

**C5** adds key muscles for shoulder function and elbow flexion along with partial innervation of brachialis and brachioradialis. This allows for mobility independence with the use of power wheelchairs with specialized controls and feeding with adaptive equipment.

**C6** preservation enables patients to perform active wrist extension and subsequently tenodesis grip. The tendons of the thumb, index, and finger flexors will shorten and wrist extension results in opposition of the thumb and index finger. This movement is key for tasks requiring finer control of the hand such as clean intermittent catheterization. Patient with this level of injury can be independent with manual wheelchair mobility and with bladder care.

**C7** preservation of the triceps function allows for elbow extension. Patients can perform weight shifts, transfers, and some meal preparation independently in addition to the functions mentioned above.

**C8** preservation allows dexterous use of the hands. Patients with this level of injury are able to perform self-care activities and mobility using a manual wheelchair independently.

**High thoracic levels.** Patients with high thoracic injuries are able to be independent with all self-care including bladder and bowel management, feeding, transfers, and wheelchair mobility.

**Low thoracic levels:** These patients have complete independence in basic care along with high-level wheelchair activities. It is possible for these patients to have the ability to ambulate household distances with knee-ankle-foot orthoses (KAFOs) and forearm crutches and/or walkers. Lumbar 1-2 levels: Patients with high lumbar injuries have preserved quadriceps and hip flexor function, which enables ambulation for short distances with ankle-foot orthoses AFOs or KAFOs with assistive devices.

**Lumbar 3-4 levels:** Patients can perform knee extension and some ankle dorsiflexion. Patients should be able to ambulate both household and community distances, but will require (AFOs) and assistive devices.

**Lumbar 5 and below:** Patients should be completely independent in all activities although bladder function may be affected.

# ■ SUMMARY

Spinal cord injury refers to the structural and functional damage of the spinal cord, which caused by various reasons such as trauma, myelitis, cancer, resulting in motor, sensory and autonomic nerve dysfunction below the impairment level. The most common levels of injury are C5 for complete SCI and T12 for incomplete injuries. Spinal cord injury includes Brown-Sequard syndrome, Anterior Cord Syndrome Central Cord Syndrome, Conus Medullaris Syndrome and Cauda Equina Syndrome. ASIA assessment involves the evaluation of sensory and motor system, and anal sphincter contraction in a uniform fashion, and ASIA impairment scale ranges from A to E with A indicating sensory and motor complete injury and E representing normal motor and sensory functions. The main factors for early prediction of the prognosis of spinal cord injury include the initial level of nerve injury, muscle strength, and the degree of neurological damage. Acute SCI interrupts the sympathetic nervous system below the level of injury resulting in classic SCI neurogenic triad, including hypotension, bradycardia, and hypothermia. Spinal shock is the loss of spinal reflexes with flaccid paralysis, hypotonia, areflexia. For the management of neurogenic and spinal shock, patients should be treated with invasive monitoring, volume resuscitation, and vasopressors to maintain blood pressure. The common complications after spinal cord injury include pulmonary complications (atelectasis, hypoventilation, and inability or difficulty managing secretions), cardiovascular sequelae (orthostatic hypotension, bradycardia, deep vein thrombosis and autonomic dysreflexia), neurogenic bladder, neurogenic bowel, heterotopic ossification, hypercalcemia, osteoporosis, pressure ulcer, hypothermia and hyperthermia. Effective prevention and management of complications is necessary for rehabilitation of spinal cord injury. The functional outcomes after spinal cord injury are related to neurologic level of injury. Patients with different neurologic level of injury are able to perform self-care activities independently or depend on others or assistive device. The higher levels are accompanied by worse independence.

## ■ IMPORTANT TERMINOLOGY

spinal cord injury 脊髓损伤

Brown-Sequard syndrome 脊髓半切综合征

multiple sclerosis 多发性硬化

neurologic level of injury 神经损伤水平

zone of partial preservation 部分保留区

anterior cord syndrome 前柱综合征

central cord syndrome 中央索综合征

conus medullaris syndrome 圆锥综合征

cauda equina syndrome 马尾综合征

spinal shock stage 脊髓休克期

bulbocavernosus reflex 球海绵体反射

neurogenic shock 神经源性休克

orthostatic hypotension 直立性低血压

autonomic dysreflexia 自主神经反射异常

bradycardia 心动过缓

spasticity 痉挛

deep vein thrombosis 深静脉血栓

clean intermittent catheterization 清洁间歇导尿

neurogenic bladder 神经源性膀胱

heterotopic ossification 异位骨化

pressure ulcer 压疮

## ■ REVIEW QUESTIONS

1. How to assess the patient's plane of nerve injury?
2. What is each grade on the ASIA impairment scale A-E represents?
3. What are the spinal cord injury syndromes? Describe each one.
4. How to determine the prognosis after spinal cord injury?
5. What are the common complications after spinal cord injury and how should they be treated?
6. What are the rehabilitation methods after spinal cord injury?
7. Please describe the functional prognosis for different levels of neurological damage after spinal cord injury.

## ■ REFERENCES

1. Ditunno JF, Flanders A, Kirshblum S, Graziani V, Tessler A, et al. Predicting outcome in traumatic SCI. In: Kirschblum S, Campagnolo DI, DeLisa JA, eds. Spinal Cord Medicine. Philadelphia, PA: Lippincott Williams & Wilkins; 2002: 108-122.
2. Friedman, Somal, Gittler. Dysesthetic pain as a predictor of motor recovery in incomplete SCI [Abstract]. Archives of Physical Medicine and Rehabilitation. 82(9):1291.

3.  Shepard MJ, Bracken MB. Magnetic resonance imaging and neurological recovery in acute spinal cord injury: observations from the National Acute Spinal Cord Injury Study 3. Spinal Cord. 1999;37(12):833-837.

4.  DeVivo M, Stover S. Long-term survival and causes of death. In: Stover S. et al. eds. Spinal Cord Injury Clinical Outcomes from the Model Systems. Gaithersburg, MA: Aspen; 1995:289-316.

5.  Bracken MB, Shepard MJ, Holford TR, et al. Administration of methylprednisolone for 24 or 48 hours or tirilazad mesylate for 48 hours in treatment of acute spinal cord injury. Results of the third national acute spinal cord injury randomized controlled trial. National Acute Spinal Cord Injury Study. JAMA. 1997;277:1597-1604.

6.  Coleman WP, Benzel D, Cahill DW, et al. A critical appraisal of the reporting of the National Acute Spinal Cord Injury Studies (II and III) of methylprednisolone in acute spinal cord injury. J Spinal Disord. 2000;13(3):185-199.

7.  Nesathurai S. Steroids and spinal cord injury: revisiting the NASCIS 2 and NASCIS 3 Trials. J Trauma. 1998;45(6):1088-1093.

8.  Hugenholtz H. Methylprednisolone for acute spinal cord injury: not a standard of care. CMAJ. 2003;168(9):1145-1146.

9.  Consortium for Spinal Cord Medicine. Early Acute Management in Adults with Spinal Cord Injury: A Clinical Practice Guidelines for Health-Care Providers. Washington, DC: Paralyzed Veterans of America; 2007.

10.  Eck JC, Nachtigall D, Humphreys SC, Hodges SD. Questionnaire Survey of spine surgeons on the use of methylprednisolone for acute spinal cord injury. Spine. 2006;31:E250-E253.

11.  Qian T, Guo X, Levi AD, Vanni S, Shebert RT, Sipski ML. High-dose methylprednisolone may cause myopathy in acute spinal cord injury patients. Spinal cord. 2004;43:199-203.

12.  Jackson AB, Gromes TE. Incidence of respiratory complications following spinal cord injury. Arch Phys Med Rehabilitation 1994;75:270-275.

13.  Consortium for Spinal Cord Medicine. Prevention of Thromboembolism in Spinal Cord Injury. 2nd ed. Washington, DC: Paralyzed Veterans of America; 1997.

14.  Morton SC, Shekelle PG, Adams JL, et al. Antimicrobial prophylaxis for urinary tract infection in persons with spinal cord dysfunction. Arch Phys Med Rehabil. 2002;83:129-38.

15.  Simon RK, Hoyt DB, Winchell RJ, Holbrook T, Eastman AB. A risk analysis of stress ulceration after trauma. J trauma 1995;39:289-293.

16.  Dial S, Delaney JA, Barkun AN, Suissa S. Use of gastric acid suppressive agents and the risk of community-acquired Clostridium difficile-associated disease. JAMA. 2005;294:2989-2995.

（许　涛）

# *STROKE REHABILITATION*

## ■ INTRODUCTION

Stroke remains one of the most common rehabilitation problems in the world today. Stroke comprises over half of the neurologic admissions to community hospitals and is a leading cause for long-term disability.

There is strong evidence that intensive post stroke rehabilitation significantly improves functional outcomes. For every 100 patients receiving organized inpatient multidisciplinary rehabilitation, extra 5 returned home independently. Patients receiving specialized stroke services, including rehabilitation services, had a significantly greater probability to survive and live at home up to 10 years after their strokes. Patient satisfaction is significantly better when clinicians comply with stroke rehabilitation guidelines, even after controlling for patient functional outcome[1].

However, effective stroke rehabilitation does not depend exclusively on the types of therapies a stroke survivor receives. Evidence-based treatments have demonstrated that the risk of stroke recurrence can be significantly reduced. There are also a number of pharmacological treatments based on small studies that suggest that functional outcomes from stroke can be improved when combined with intensive rehabilitation. Finally, consensus-based opinions among rehabilitation professionals have guided clinicians in standards of care when evidence from formal trials is absent. This chapter combines all levels of evidence to formulate practical orders that optimize medical and rehabilitation care of the stroke survivor.

## ■ SECONDARY STROKE PROPHYLAXIS

### Antiplatelet and Anticoagulant Agents

Every stroke survivor admitted for rehabilitation must be considered for secondary prophylaxis of stroke. Stroke survivors with non-cardioembolic ischemic stroke or transient ischemic attack (TIA), monotherapy consisting of aspirin 50 to 325 mg by mouth daily or clopidogrel 75 mg by mouth daily, or the combination of aspirin 25 mg and extended-release dipyridamole 200 mg by mouth twice daily are acceptable options for initial therapy to reduce the risk of recurrent stroke and other cardiovascular events [2]. The combination of aspirin and extended-release dipyridamole is recommended over aspirin alone, but should be titrated using one tablet of aspirin/extended-release dipyridamole with aspirin 81 mg for 7 days to reduce the risk of headache. Combination therapy of aspirin and clopidogrel is not routinely recommended for secondary prophylaxis, unless there is a specific indication (ie, coronary stent or acute coronary syndrome) as the addition of aspirin to clopidogrel increases the risk of cerebral hemorrhage.

In most stroke survivors with cardioembolic ischemic stroke (eg, atrial fibrillation, acute myocardial infarction and left ventricular thrombus, dilated cardiomyopathy, valvular heart disease), anticoagulation with adjusted-dose warfarin (target INR, 2.5; range, 2.0-3.0) is recommended. Stroke survivors with an acute myocardial infarction and confirmed left ventricular mural thrombus should be treated with oral anticoagulation for at least 3 months and up to 1 year. A stroke survivor with rheumatic mitral valve disease with or without atrial fibrillation should add aspirin 81 mg by mouth daily to anticoagulation therapy. A stroke survivor with ischemic cardiomyopathy should add aspirin (preferably in the enteric-coated form) in doses up to 162 mg by mouth daily together with oral anti-coagulant therapy. A stroke survivor with a mechanical prosthetic heart valve despite adequate therapy with oral anticoagulants should be treated with adjusted-dose warfarin (target INR, 3.0; range, 2.5-3.5) along with aspirin 75 to 100 mg by mouth daily. If the stroke survivor is unable to take oral anticoagulants, aspirin 325 mg by mouth daily is recommended. A stroke survivor with mitral valve prolapse, mitral valve calcification, or aortic value disease may be treated with antiplatelet therapy only. A stroke survivor without atrial fibrillation who has mitral regurgitation resulting from mitral valve calcification may be treated with either antiplatelet or warfarin therapy. Antiplatelet agents should not be routinely added to warfarin because of the additional risk of bleeding.

When patients taking antithrombotic agents suffer a hemorrhagic stroke, the decision to restart antithrombotic therapy depends upon the risk of recurrent hemorrhage, the risk of arterial or venous thromboembolism, and the overall state of the patient. If the hemorrhagic stroke survivor who requires warfarin has a very high risk of thromboembolism, warfarin therapy may be restarted 7 to 10 days after the onset of the hemorrhage. If the stroke survivor has a lower risk of cerebral infarction (eg, atrial fibrillation without prior ischemic stroke) and a higher risk of amyloid angiopathy (eg, elderly patients with lobar hemorrhage), or if overall neurological function is very poor, an antiplatelet agent may be chosen over warfarin to prevent recurrence of an ischemic stroke.

## Antihypertensive Agents

Hypertension is the most important treatable risk factor in ischemic stroke. In hemorrhagic stroke, treating hypertension is the most important step to reduce the risk of recurrent intracerebral hemorrhage. Because elevation in blood pressure following a stroke is likely a physiological response to brain ischemia [3], aggressive antihypertensive management should begin approximately 7 to 10 days post stroke, unless early treatment is indicated. In hemorrhagic stroke, hypertension should be treated early to prevent vasogenic edema due to the disruption of the blood-brain barrier in the ischemic area around the hemorrhage [4].

Health benefits have been associated with average blood pressure reductions of 10/5 mmHg, and normal BP levels have been defined as less than 120/80 mmHg by JNC-7.(Class Ⅱa, Level of Evidence B). However, absolute target blood pressures should be individualized in stroke survivors since it is unclear below what blood pressure cerebral perfusion may be compromised. At present, available data support the use of a diuretic agent or the combination of a diuretic and an angiotensin-converting enzyme inhibitor (ACEI). The choice of specific drugs and targets should be based on specific patient characteristics (eg, extracranial cerebrovascular occlusive disease, renal disease, cardiac disease, and diabetes mellitus). In addition, lifestyle modifications (eg, sodium restriction and weight loss) should be included as a part of a comprehensive antihypertensive program.

## Antihyperlipidemia Agents (Statins)

Hyperlipidemia is not as well established as a risk factor for recurrent stroke. However, a recent study demonstrated that statin therapy was effective for stroke survivors and without known coronary heart disease to reduce the risk of cardiovascular events and recurrent stroke [5]. In stroke survivors with or without coronary heart disease or symptomatic atherosclerotic disease, statin therapy with a target LDL-C level of 100 mg/dl is recommended. In stroke survivors who are at very high risk or have multiple risk factors, statin therapy with a target LDL-C level of 70 mg/dl is recommended. Stroke survivors with low HDL cholesterol may be considered for treatment with niacin or gemfibrozil.

## Antihyperglycemic Agents

Diabetes is a significant risk factor for stroke. However, data are sparse regarding the secondary stroke prevention of survivors with diabetes. Nevertheless, glucose control is recommended to near-normoglycemic levels among diabetic stroke survivors to reduce microvascular and possibly macrovascular complications. The goal for hemoglobin A1c should be less than 7%.

In addition to glucose control, more rigorous control of blood pressure and lipids should be undertaken in diabetic stroke survivors. While all major classes of antihypertensive agents are suitable for blood pressure control in this population, ACEIs and angiotensin receptor blockers are recommended as first-choice medications because they are more effective in reducing the progression of renal disease. With respect to hyperlipidemia, LDL cholesterol (LDL-C) targets are recommended as low as 70 mg/dl.

## Lifestyle Changes

Secondary stroke prevention also depends upon significant lifestyle changes. Stroke survivors who smoke, have heavy alcohol consumption, or use illicit drugs (eg, cocaine) should be counseled to stop the use of these substances. Stroke survivors should be encouraged to reduce weight through reduced caloric intake, increased physical activity, and behavioral counseling to a body mass index of 18.5 to 24.9 kg/m² and a waist circumference less than 80 cm for women, and 90 cm for men. Clinicians should encourage physical activity of at least 30 minutes of moderate-intensity physical exercise most days to reduce risk factors and comorbid conditions that increase the likelihood of recurrence of stroke. A supervised exercise program may be recommended.

## ■ SECONDARY STROKE COMPLICATIONS

### Contracture Prevention

Because of the development of the flexor synergy pattern in the upper limb and the extensor synergy pattern in the lower limb, one must evaluate range of motion in the affected limbs frequently to prevent contractures. Range of motion exercises without traction should be performed to prevent brachial plexus or other nerve injury. A shoulder splint in 45 degrees of abduction may prevent positioning in adduction and internal rotation at night. A shoulder support during ambulation may prevent traction on the brachial plexus. An armrest in the wheelchair may help to position the arm in a more neutral position. A resting hand splint may help to stretch the wrist and finger muscles if tone begins to develop. A pressure-relief ankle-foot orthosis may prevent foot drop both in bed and in the wheelchair. We can use some drugs like botulinum toxin to reduce the tone if the patient's muscle tension is very high.

### Deep vein thrombosis and Pulmonary Embolism

Deep vein thrombosis (DVT) may occur in up to 20% to 75% of stroke survivors[6]. Clinical signs and symptoms, such as pain, swelling, and warmth of the extremity, are at best marginally diagnostic. Prevention of DVT and pulmonary embolism (PE) is essential in ischemic and hemorrhagic stroke survivors with restricted mobility. Treatment includes heparin 5000 units every 8 to 12 hours, enoxaparin 30 mg subcutaneously every 12 hours, or enoxaparin 40 mg subcutaneously daily. For stroke survivors who have contraindications to anticoagulant therapy, intermittent pneumatic compression (IPC) devices, and elastic stockings are used. Prophylaxis may be discontinued once the patient is ambulating consistently in or out of the parallel bars[7].

Prophylaxis for DVT and PE is not contraindicated for hemorrhagic stroke survivors. Initially, IPC devices should be used. In stable patients, anticoagulant prophylaxis with heparin or enoxaparin may begin as early as the second day after the onset of the hemorrhage but not later than the third or fourth day from onset. Hemorrhagic stroke survivors who develop an acute proximal venous thrombosis, particularly those with clinical or subclinical pulmonary emboli, should be considered for acute placement of a vena cava filter. The decision to add long-term antithrombotic therapy several weeks or more after placement of an inferior vena cava filter must take into consideration the etiology of the hemorrhage, associated conditions with increased arterial thrombotic risk (eg, atrial fibrillation), and the overall health and mobility of the patient.

## Constipation

Strokes may disinhibit the reflex mechanisms for emptying the bowels, and sensation or cognitive impairments may prevent control of defecation. Diets should include adequate fluids and fiber. A bowel program may start with docusate 100 mg by mouth every 12 hours. If a laxative is needed, senna 17.2 mg by mouth at 12 p.m. may be started to target a bowel program for the evening hours. If a suppository or enema is required, it should be given in the evening after dinner to take advantage of the gastrocolic reflex.

## Bladder Dysfunction

A variety of voiding disorders may be observed after stroke [8]. Since many stroke survivors are transferred to the rehabilitation unit with indwelling catheters, a decatheterization protocol should be initiated immediately after admission. Once the catheter is removed, postvoid residuals (PVRs) by bladder scan or catheterization should be obtained at least every 8 hours to assess bladder emptying. If the bladder scan is greater than 400 cm$^3$, intermittent catheterization should be performed to prevent bladder stretching. If the patient voids, but PVR volumes are greater than 100 cm$^3$, pharmacologic therapy should be considered. As long as PVRs are abnormal or changes in medications are made, PVRs should be monitored to ensure that bladder function is normalizing. Associated conditions such as urinary tract infection, fecal impaction, and reduced mobility should be evaluated and treated [9]. Toileting every 2 to 4 hours during the day, and fluid restriction after dinner may prevent incontinence in a majority of patients [10]. External catheters may decrease the incidence of enuresis. Intermittent or indwelling catheterization may be necessary in stroke survivors with areflexic bladders.

## Pressure Ulcers

Pressure ulcers result from both extrinsic (pressure, shear forces, friction, and moisture) and intrinsic [anemia, contractures, spasticity, diabetes, malnutrition (vitamins B, C, K; zinc), edema, and obesity] etiologies [11]. In supine position, common locations of pressure ulcers include the heels, sacrum, and occiput. In sitting, they may occur in the ischial tuberosities. General measures to prevent pressure ulcers include adequate nutrition and hydration, as well as proper incontinence care. In bed, appropriate mattresses may distribute pressure, and pressure-relief ankle-foot orthoses may prevent ankle contractures as well as boots provide pressure relief to the heel and foot. If stroke survivors require assistance in bed mobility, they should be turned at least every 2 hours. In wheelchairs, patients should be issued appropriate cushions to distribute pressure, and if possible, should be taught techniques of pressure relief.

## Dysphagia

Swallowing dysfunction may occur in up to one-third of patients with cortical or brainstem lesions[12]. Complications of poststroke dysphagia include malnutrition and aspiration. Symptoms associated with aspiration include dysphonia and an impaired gag reflex associated with impaired cough [13,14]. If dysphagia is suspected, evaluation by a speech-language pathologist should take place as soon as possible.

## Depression

Depression occurs in 25% to 79% of stroke survivors in the acute medical or rehabilitation setting, but less than 5% receive psychotherapeutic or medical intervention [15]. Depression may be related to mourning the loss of function or to the alteration of function of catecholamine-containing neurons. Diagnosis is usually clinical, and treatment includes psychotherapy and medications. While there are no definitive studies to support nor refute the routine use of pharmacotherapeutic and psychotherapeutic treatments for depression after stroke [16], a neuropsychological evaluation should take place on admission or as soon as depression is suspected. If the diagnosis of major depression is confirmed, pharmacologic therapy with a serotonin-specific reuptake inhibitor should be initiated.

## ■ NEUROSTIMULANT THERAPY

Pharmacological interventions also may have a role in motor recovery. Methylphenidate, a mild central nervous system stimulant whose mode of action is not well understood, may decrease depression and improve function in the early stages after stroke [17]. Side effects with these drugs may include appetite suppression, hypertension, and cardiac arrhythmias. Also, the seizure threshold may be reduced in those who have a history of epilepsy.

Other small studies have demonstrated the potential of some drugs to improve function after stroke. Fluoxetine may help to facilitate motor recovery independent of its effect as an antidepressant [18]. A course of single-dose levodopa over 3 weeks demonstrated significant improvements in motor recovery [19]. The use of amantadine significantly improved walking cadence and length of heel-to-toe movements [20]. At the same time, drugs such as clonidine, prazosin, neuroleptics and other dopamine receptor antagonists, benzodiazepine, phenytoin, and phenobarbital actually may impair motor recovery, although the reasons are not fully understood [21].

## ■ ASSESSMENT OF STROKE REHABILITATION

### Assessment of the Severity of Brain Damage

1. Glasgow Coma Scale.

2. National Institutes of Health Stroke Scale (NIH stroke scale, NIHSS) of the United States: NIHSS is internationally recognized and most frequently used stroke assessment scale, with 11 test items, low scores indicate mild neurological impairment, high scores show that the degree of neurological damage is severe.

### Motor Function Assessment

1. Brunnstrom motor function assessment method: Brunnstrom divided the motor function recovery of stroke hemiplegia into 6 stages, and evaluated the motor function recovery of the patients according to the changes in the muscle tension and movement patterns of the upper limbs, hands and lower limbs. Brunnstrom stage 1 is that the patient has no voluntary movement; Brunnstrom stage 2 is that the patient begins to have voluntary movement, which can elicit joint reactions and joint movements; Brunnstrom stage 3 is that the patient's abnormal muscle tone is significantly increased, and joint movements can occur at will; Brunnstrom stage 4 is the patient's Abnormal muscle tone begins to decline, its common movement pattern is broken, and separate movements begin to appear: Brunnstrom stage 5 means that the patient's muscle tone gradually

recovers, and fine movements appear; Brunnstrom stage 6 means that the patient's motor ability is close to normal, but the movement speed and accuracy worse than the healthy side.

2. Fugl-Meyer assessment method: The Fugl-Meyer assessment method mainly includes limb movement, balance and sensory scores, and joint passive range of motion scores (including total scores of motion and pain).

## Evaluation of Balance Function

1. Three-level balance detection method: The three-level balance detection method is often used clinically. Level Ⅰ balance means that the patient can maintain a sitting or standing balance under static conditions without external force; level Ⅱ balance means that the patient does not move on the support surface (under the condition of sitting or standing), the patient can maintain balance when one or several parts of the body move; Level Ⅲ balance means that the patient can still maintain balance in the sitting or standing position under the condition of external force or external interference.

2. Berg Balance Scale: The Berg Balance Scale is the most commonly used scale in stroke clinical rehabilitation and research. A high score indicates good balance function, and a low score indicates poor balance function.

## Assessment of Activities of Daily Living

Assessment of activities of daily living is a commonly used functional assessment in clinical rehabilitation of stroke, and its methods mainly include Barthel index and functional activity questionnaire (FAQ).

## Quality of Life Assessment

The assessment of quality of life (QOL) is divided into three types: subjective orientation, objective orientation and disease-related QOL. The commonly used scales include life satisfaction scale, WHOQOL-100 scale and SF-36 scale.

## Assessment of Other Dysfunctions

Evaluation of other functional impairments includes sensory function evaluation, cognitive function evaluation, aphasia evaluation, dysarthria evaluation, cardiopulmonary function evaluation, and psychological evaluation.

# ■ REHABILITATION GOAL AND METHODS OF STROKE REHABILITATION

## Acute Phase Rehabilitation

The acute stage of stroke usually refers to 1 to 2 weeks after the onset of stroke, which is equivalent to Brunnstrom stage 1 to 2. In this stage, the patient has no active movement of the affected limb to the recovery of muscle tension, and there are weak flexors and extensors in common. Sports rehabilitation treatment is based on routine neurology or neurosurgery treatment (including treatment of primary disease, treatment of comorbidities, control of blood pressure, blood sugar, blood lipids, etc.), and starts 48 hours after the patient's condition is stable. The rehabilitation treatment in this period is a first-level rehabilitation, and its goal is to promote the recovery of muscle tone and the emergence of active activities in the limbs of the hemiplegic side through passive activities and active participation, as well as the correct placement of the limbs and the conversion of body positions (such as turning over, etc.), Prevent possible complications such as pressure ulcers, joint swelling, deep vein thrombosis of lower extremities, urinary system and respiratory tract infections. Various sensory stimuli, psychological counseling, and other related bedside rehabilitation (such as swallowing function training, vocal organ exercise training, respiratory function training, cardiopulmonary rehabilitation training, etc.) on the hemiplegic side can help improve the impaired function of stroke patients. At the same time, actively control related risk factors (such as high blood pressure, high blood sugar, high blood fat, and atrial fibrillation, etc.), and do a good job in secondary prevention of stroke.

## Resume Early Rehabilitation

The early stage of stroke recovery (subacute stage) refers to 3 to 4 weeks after the onset, which is equivalent to Brunnstrom stage 2 to 3. The patient moves from the weak flexors and extensors of the affected limb to the spasticity, and the patient can actively move Affected limb, but muscle activity is common movement. The rehabilitation treatment in this period is secondary rehabilitation, and its goal is to prevent common complications and secondary prevention of stroke. In combination, pay attention to reducing muscle spasticity in the hemiplegic limb and avoid strengthening abnormal movement patterns (flexor spasticity pattern in upper limbs and extensor muscle spasticity pattern in lower limbs). At the same time, it cooperates with corresponding rehabilitation treatment for other functional impairments of patients.

## Mid-Term Rehabilitation

The middle stage of stroke recovery generally refers to 4 to 12 weeks after the onset of stroke, which is equivalent to Brunnstrom stage 3 to 4. In this stage, patients have obvious muscle spasm in the affected limb and can actively move the affected limb, but the muscle activities range from joint exercise to muscle spasm. Relief, selective muscle activity begins. The rehabilitation treatment in this period is the transition from the second-level rehabilitation to the third-level rehabilitation. Its goal is to strengthen coordination and selective voluntary movement, combined with activities of daily life to strengthen the practical functions of the upper and lower limbs, and at the same time pay attention to inhibiting abnormal muscles tension. The focus of motor function training for stroke patients should be on the restoration of normal motor patterns and motor control. A considerable number of hemiplegia patients have motor impairment related to sensory loss. Therefore, rehabilitation training to improve various sensory functions is very important for motor function recovery.

## Post Recovery Rehabilitation

The late stage of stroke recovery generally refers to 4 to 6 months after the onset of stroke, which is equivalent to Brunnstrom stage 5 to 6. In this stage, most of the muscle activities of patients are selective and can move independently, and they are never affected by joint movements of limbs. Muscle spasms disappeared and dissociative movements were smooth with good coordination but at a slower pace. The rehabilitation treatment in this period is a three-level rehabilitation, and its goal is to suppress spasticity and correct abnormal movement patterns. Improve motor control, promote fine motor, improve motor speed and practical walking ability, master activities of daily living skills, and improve quality of life.

## Rehabilitation in the Sequelae

The post-stroke sequelae period refers to the period in which the functional impairment caused by brain damage will not be significantly improved for a long time after various treatments in 1 to 2 years after onset. The main causes of sequelae of stroke are serious brain damage, failure to carry out early and standardized rehabilitation treatment in time, unreasonable treatment methods or functional training guidance resulting in misuse syndrome, risk factors (hypertension, hyperglycemia, hyperlipidemia) control If it is not ideal, it will cause the aggravation or recurrence of the primary disease. The common sequelae of stroke are mainly manifested as poor motor control of the affected upper limbs and hand dysfunction, aphasia, dysarthria, facial paralysis, dysphagia, difficulty walking (including hemiplegic gait, affected foot drop, etc.), incontinence, vascular dementia etc.

The rehabilitation treatment in this period is three-level rehabilitation, and the recovery of residual and existing functions should be strengthened, that is, compensatory functional training, including the application of orthotics, walking frames and wheelchairs, as well as environmental modification and necessary vocational skills training, so as to Adapt to the needs of daily life. At the same time, pay attention to prevent further aggravation of abnormal muscle tone and contracture. Avoid the occurrence of disuse syndrome, osteoporosis and other complications, help patients get out of bed and carry out appropriate outdoor activities, pay attention to more communication with patients and necessary psychological counseling, stimulate their awareness of active participation, and play the role of family and society role.

## Method

1. Activities on the bed and beside the bed: a. upper limb lifting movement b. bedside sitting and bedside standing c. alternate flexion and extension of both lower limbs, d. bridge movement.

2. Sitting activities: a. sitting balance training b. weight bearing on the affected upper limbs c. functional activities of the upper limbs d. functional activities of the lower limbs.

3. Standing activities: a. standing balance training, b. weight bearing on the lower limb of the hemiplegic side (single leg weight bearing) c. up and down steps.

4. Weight-loss walking training can be carried out on the premise that the lower limbs of the hemiplegic side cannot adapt to single-leg support. The training can reduce the weight of the lower limbs by supporting part of the body weight, and make the lower limbs of the affected side bear weight as soon as possible, providing symmetrical weight transfer for both lower limbs. Repeat for a full walking cycle with added safety to your training.

5. Robot-assisted walking training needs to be carried out under the premise that the patient can adapt to the standing position. The weight-bearing degree of the patient on the power platform can be adjusted with the help of the robot weight reduction system, and the patient is driven to walk through the driving device connected to the leg or foot. It can improve walking ability and at the same time ensure the symmetry of gait in training.

6. Parallel bar walking can be performed on the premise that the lower limbs on the hemiplegic side of the patient can adapt to single-leg support. In order to avoid insufficient hip extension, knee hyperextension or knee weakness on the hemiplegic side, the therapist should give help and guidance on the hemiplegic side. If the dorsiflexion of the affected ankle is insufficient, an ankle-foot orthosis may be worn to prevent possible hemiplegic gait.

7. For indoor walking and outdoor activities, if the patient can perform alternate lower limb movements relatively smoothly, indoor walking training can be performed first, and a cane can be added if necessary to increase the stability of walking. The principle of stair climbing training is that the healthy leg goes up first when going up the stairs, and the hemiplegic leg goes down first when going down the stairs. The therapist can give appropriate help and guidance on the hemiplegic side. When the patient's physical strength and the movement control ability of the lower limbs on the affected side are good, outdoor activities are feasible, but it must be noted that it should be accompanied by a therapist at the beginning.

8. Compulsory exercise therapy (constraint - induced movement therapy, CIMT) is mainly used for the recovery of upper limb function in stroke patients. The classic compulsory exercise therapy consists of three parts: repetitive task training, adaptive task training for the purpose of improving daily life ability, and continuous restriction of the unaffected limb. During the treatment, the patients are required to limit the activities of the upper limbs of the non-affected side for 90% of the waking time, and at the same time carry out training for 6 hours a day for 2 to 3 weeks.

9. The focus of physical factor therapy is to target the extensor muscles of the hemiplegic upper limb (such as triceps and forearm extensors) to improve the functions of elbow extension, wrist extension, and finger

extension; Muscle and peroneus longus and brevis, to improve knee flexion and ankle dorsiflexion, commonly used methods include functional electrical stimulation, myoelectric biofeedback, and low-intermediate frequency electrical stimulation.

10. Occupational therapy selects occupational activities that are suitable for the individual according to the patient's functional status, and improves the patient's ability to perform activities of daily living and adapt to social life. Occupational activities generally include: Activities of daily living: the level of daily living ability is an important indicator reflecting the effect of rehabilitation and whether patients can return to society. Basic activities of daily living (such as active movement, eating, personal hygiene, changing clothes, bathing, walking and toileting, etc.) and applied activities of daily living (such as housework, use of transportation, cognition and communication, etc.) should be included. Motor functional activities: increase the patient's muscle strength, endurance, balance and coordination, and joint range of motion through corresponding functional activities. Training on the use of auxiliary devices: In order to make full use of and exert existing functions, auxiliary devices can be configured to help improve the patient's functional mobility.

11. The application of walking frames and wheelchairs for elderly people with relatively poor walking ability, in order to ensure safety, walking frames can be used to increase the support surface and improve the stability of walking. If the degree of paralysis of the lower limbs is severe, those who cannot walk independently can use a wheelchair instead of walking to expand the range of activities of the patient.

12. Speech therapy for stroke patients with dysarthria or aphasia, speech function training should be performed early to improve the patient's communication ability and contribute to the improvement of their overall functional level.

# ■ SUMMARY

Stroke is one of the most common rehabilitation problems in the world. Stroke treatment is a multidisciplinary treatment involving neurology, psychiatry, rehabilitation therapy and rehabilitation engineering, as well as home nursing. In this chapter, we will learn the medication principle of anti-platelet and anticoagulant agents, how to decrease plasma lipids, what is better selection for patients with hypertension, how to control the blood glucose, how to prevent the complications of stroke such as dysphagia, contracture, deep vein thrombosis, pulmonary embolism, constipation, bladder dysfunction and depression. Finally, we present a process involving medical, diet, nursing, evaluation, rehabilitation training, orthoses and walkers. All of these reflect everything we do in stroke patient treatment.

# ■ REVIEW QUESTIONS

1. What are the risk factors of stroke?
2. How to prevent the shoulder pain after stroke?
3. Please describe the functional assessments after stroke.
4. What is the therapy goal and principles after stroke?
5. Which kind of medicals should be used to prevent recurrent stroke?

# ■ IMPORTANT TERMINOLOGY

stroke 脑卒中
rehabilitation 康复

antiplatelet agents   抗血小板药

assessment   评估

contracture prevention   预防挛缩

bladder incontinence   尿失禁

prophylaxis   预防

# ■ REFERENCES

1. Reker DM, Duncan PW, Horner RD, et al. Postacute stroke guideline compliance is associated with greater patient satisfaction. Arch Phys Med Rehabil. 2002;83(6):750-756.

2. Adams RJ, Albers G, Alberts MJ, et al. Patients with stroke and transient ischemic attack. Update to the AHA/ASA recommendations for the prevention of stroke. Stroke. 2008;39;1647-1652.

3. Wallace JD, Levy LL. Blood pressure after stroke. JAMA. 1981;246(19):2177-2180.

4. Lavin P. Management of hypertension in patients with acute stroke. Arch Int Med. 1986;146(1):66-68.

5. Amarenco P, Bogousslavsky J, Callahan A Ⅲ, et al; Stroke Prevention by Aggressive Reduction in Cholesterol Levels (SPARCL) Investigators. High dose atorvastatin after stroke or transient ischemic attack. N Engl J Med. 2006;355:549-559.

6. Turpie AG. Prophylaxis of venous thromboembolism in stroke patients. Sem Thrombosis Hemostasis. 1997;23(2):155-157.

7. Bromfi eld EB, Reding MB. Relative risk of Deep venous thrombosis or pulmonary embolism post-stroke based upon ambulatory status. J Neuro Rehab. 1988;2(2):51-56.

8. Borrie MJ, Campbell AJ, Caradoc-Davies TH, Speers GFS. Urinary incontinence after stroke: a prospective study. Age Ageing. 1986;15:177-81.

9. Linsenmeyer TA, Zorowitz RD. Urodynamic findings of patients with urinary incontinence following cerebrovascular accident. NeuroRehabil. 1992;2(2):23-26.

10. Sogbein SK, Awad SA. Behavioural treatment of urinary incontinence in geriatric patients. CMA J. 1982;127:863-864.

11. Nurse BA, Collins MC. Skin care and decubitus ulcer management in the elderly stroke patient. PM&R State of the Art Rev. 1989;3(3):549-562.

12. Veis SL, Logemann JA. Swallowing disorders in persons with cerebrovascular accident. Arch Phys Med Rehabil. 1985;66(6):372-375.

13. Linden P, Siebens AA. Dysphagia: predicting laryngeal penetration. Arch Phys Med Rehabil. 1983;64:281-284.

14. Horner J, Massey EW. Silent aspiration following stroke. Neurology. 1988;38:317-319.

15. Gordon WA, Hibbard MR. Poststroke depression: an examination of the literature. Arch Phys Med Rehabil. 1997;78(6):658-663.

16. Hackett ML, Anderson CS, House AO. Interventions for treating depression after stroke. In: The Cochrane Library, Issue 1. Chichester, West Sussex: John Wiley & Sons, Ltd; 2005.

17. Grade C, Redford B, Chrostowski J, Toussaint L, Blackwell B. Methylphenidate in early poststroke recovery: a double-blind, placebo-controlled study. Arch Phys Med Rehabil. 1998;79(9):1047-1050.

18. Dam M, Tonin P, De Boni A, et al. Effects of fluoxetine and maprotiline on functional recovery in poststroke hemiplegic patients undergoing rehabilitation therapy. Stroke. 1996; 27(7):1211-1214.

19. Scheidtmann K, Fries W, Muller F, Koenig E. Effect of levodopa in combination with physiotherapy on functional motor recovery after stroke: a prospective, randomised, double-blind study. Lancet. 2001;358(9284):787-790.

20. Baezner H, Oster M, Henning O, Cohen S, Hennerici MG. Amantadine increases gait steadiness in frontal gait disorder due to subcortical vascular encephalopathy: a double-blind randomized placebo-controlled trial based on quantitative gait analysis. Cerebrovasc Dis. 2001;11(3):235-244.

21. Goldstein LB. Common drugs may influence motor recovery after stroke. The Sygen in Acute Stroke Study Investigators. Neurology. 1995;45(5): 865-871.

（吴　毅）

# TRAUMATIC BRAIN INJURY REHABILITATION

## ■ INTRODUCTION

The term traumatic brain injury (TBI) refers to injury to the brain caused by an external force. Open TBI involves disruption of the dura mater, whereas the dura mater remains intact during a closed TBI. Primary causes of injury include diffuse axonal injury (DAI), petechial hemorrhages, contusions, and cranial nerve injuries. Secondary causes of injury following TBI may include intracerebral hemorrhage, intracerebral edema, hypoxia, excitotoxicity, and oxidant injury. During a TBI, the rapid acceleration and deceleration of the brain within the skull results in DAI within the brain. DAI may or may not be visible on neuroimaging studies. DAI may result in generalized deficits including loss of consciousness, coma, confusion and incoordination [1].

It is estimated that 1.5 million people per year experience TBI in the United States. Three percent of these injuries are fatal. Ninety percent of these injuries are classified as mild. Falls are the leading cause of TBI, followed by motor vehicle collisions, and blunt trauma (including assaults and sports related injuries). Alcohol is involved in more than 50% of TBI cases [2].

The best Glasgow Coma Scale (GCS) score within the first 24 hours following injury is used to classify TBI as mild (GCS 13-15), moderate (GCS 9-12), or severe (GCS 3-8) [1].

Older age, longer length of coma, and prolonged duration of posttraumatic amnesia have consistently been shown to be predictors of poor outcome following TBI. Following severe TBI (ie, Initial GCS <8), severe disability is unlikely (<10% chance) when coma lasts less than 2 weeks or when posttraumatic amnesia lasts less than 2 months. Good recovery is unlikely (<10% chance) when coma lasts longer than 4 weeks, posttraumatic amnesia lasts longer than 3 months, or patient is older than 65 years of age [2].

The Rancho Los Amigos Cognitive Scale is used to describe the stages of cognitive recovery following TBI [1]. Severe TBI may result in coma. The term coma refers to a cognitive state in which there is a lack of wakefulness. The patient's eyes remain closed, and there is no electroencephalogram evidence of a sleep-wake cycle. A patient in a minimally conscious state demonstrates evidence of a sleep-wake cycle and awareness of environmental stimuli (eg, sustained visual fixation and pursuit, purposeful movements, emotional responses to salient stimuli, command following, and verbalization). Coma emergence programs are designed to encourage cognitive recovery by providing patients with a wide variety of environmental stimuli. Progression from coma to minimally conscious state is identified through multiple examinations at different times, by a variety of clinicians, with a variety of stimuli [3].

The majority of individuals who survive mild brain injuries (ie, concussions) recover well without residual cognitive deficits. Unfortunately, a significant minority develop post concussive syndrome. Postconcussive syndrome is associated with physical, cognitive, and emotional problems including headaches, dizziness, fatigue, visual disturbances, light and noise sensitivity, cognitive impairments, depression, anxiety, and irritability. Symptom-based treatment may include analgesics, antidepressants, education, reassurance, and cognitive remediation [3].

# THEORIES OF NEUROLOGIC RECOVERY

The leading theories of neurologic recovery following TBI involve central nervous system reorganization (neuroplasticity) through unmasking and sprouting. Unmasking theorizes that several potential synaptic pathways exist for the execution of a single neurologic function. During optimal brain activity, the most efficient (primary) synaptic pathway executes the neurologic function, and parallel pathways are masked. Following a TBI, a lesion may develop affecting the primary pathway, resulting in the unmasking of a less efficient parallel pathway, which then takes over execution of the neurologic function. Sprouting theorizes that when a lesion occurs, unaffected neurons in the surrounding area create new synapses that take over for the affected neuron [1].

Research data demonstrates that intensive therapy emphasizing cognition enhances cognitive recovery following TBI. Although research data is not definitive, widely used medications with theoretical potential to enhance cognitive recovery following TBI include dopamine agonists (ie, amantadine and bromocriptine) and acetylcholine agonists [1].

# BEHAVIOR MANAGEMENT

Agitation, decreased arousal, and depressed effect are among the most common undesirable behaviors that interfere with functional recovery following TBI. Sources of agitation, decreased arousal, and depressed effect include the brain lesion itself, premorbid personality, withdrawal, hypoxemia, pain, overstimulation by staff and environment, sleep-wake cycle disturbance, medical issues (cardiac, pulmonary, infection), medications, and physical restraints. It is important to measure the frequency of the target behavior to determine the efficacy of treatment interventions [4,5].

Agitation may be reduced by limiting environmental stimuli and by creating a structured daily routine. Medications such as inderal, trazodone, seroquel, depakote, and tegretol are used to decrease agitation. Haldol and benzodiazepines have the potential to slow cognitive recovery, and should be avoided if at all possible. A stimulating and optimistic atmosphere may assist individuals with decreased arousal and depressed effect. Amantadine and bromocriptine are used to improve arousal and attention. Serotonin reuptake inhibitors have been shown to be safe and effective in the treatment of depression following TBI [4,5].

When managing undesirable behaviors, an organized approach to medication intervention is recommended. Start low and go slow. Provide an adequate therapeutic trial. Perform continuous reassessment (identify and measure the target behavior). Monitor drug-drug interactions. Change strategy if symptoms intensify [4,5].

# MEDICAL COMPLICATIONS

Medical complications, including hydrocephalus, dysautonomia, hyponatremia, heterotopic ossification (HO), venous thromboembolism (VTE), aspiration pneumonia, and spasticity, may result in unexpected functional decline and instability following TBI [1].

Hydrocephalus is commonly caused by cerebral atrophy associated with ventricular dilation and results in progressive cognitive decline. Neuroimaging findings consistent with hydrocephalus include the absence of sulci, enlarged ventricles, and periventricular lucency [1].

Dysautonomia involves paroxysmal increases in heart rate, temperature, and blood pressure caused by surges of epinephrine and norepinephrine following TBI. Decerebrate and decorticate positioning can also occur. Centrally acting beta-blockers (eg, inderal) are indicated for management of heart rate, temperature, and blood pressure. In addition, evidence supports the use of bromocriptine in managing long-standing dysautonomia. Nitroprusside derivatives should be avoided, because they cause intracerebral vascular dilation, which may result in increased intracranial pressure. Hypotension has been associated with worse outcomes and should be avoided following TBI [1].

Hypotonic hyponatremia is common following TBI. It may be due to the syndrome of inappropriate antidiuretic hormone (SIADH) or cerebral salt wasting (CSW). In SIADH, hyponatremia is dilutional. It is due to excessive water retention by the kidneys without an inciting disturbance in sodium balance. It is characterized by higher than normal urine osmolality and low plasma osmolality. Antidiuretic hormone (ADH) is not appropriately suppressed in response to low plasma osmolality; thus, further water retention ensues. Treatment includes fluid restriction to approximately 1 L/d, sodium supplementation, and diuresis. Demeclocycline is reserved for chronic SIADH. In CSW, there is excessive sodium excretion, possibly secondary to impaired renal reabsorption. CSW is characterized by low urine and plasma osmolalities. CSW is treated with fluid repletion with hypertonic saline. Less commonly occurring is diabetes insipidus, where there is a lack of ADH secretion, which results in polydipsia and polyuria. Treatment is with desmopressin [1].

HO, formation of lamellar bone in soft tissue, commonly involves the shoulder, elbow, and hip regions in TBI survivors. Risk factors include prolonged coma, spasticity, and bone fractures. Signs and symptoms include increased warmth and edema, decreased range of motion, and worsening contractures. Early detection of HO is with triple phase bone scan. Serum alkaline phosphatase is elevated in HO, but is a nonspecific finding. Creatine phosphokinase may be more valuable in the management of HO, because levels are elevated acutely, and decline when treatment for HO is successful. HO is treated with etidronate disphosphonate at 20 mg/kg · d for 2 weeks, followed by 10 mg/kg · d for 10 weeks and concurrent non-steroidal anti-inflammatories (ie, indomethacin). Surgical excision of HO is usually delayed until full maturation of the ectopic bone, which usually requires 12 to 18 months. Recurrence of HO is common [1].

TBI survivors are at increased risk for VTE. Deep vein thrombosis (DVT) is among the most commonly occurring forms of VTE. Signs and symptoms include pain in the extremity, warmth, and swelling. If a DVT is suspected, bilateral venous ultrasounds of the lower extremities should be obtained. VTE prophylaxis includes low molecular weight heparin at 40 mg once daily, unfractionated heparin 5000 units 3 times daily, or oral warfarin. When anticoagulation is contraindicated, pneumatic compression devices, compression stockings, and inferior vena cava filters may be used for individuals who develop a DVT [1].

Cranial nerve dysfunction and lack of coordination may result in dysphagia and aspiration pneumonia following TBI. Silent aspiration is common; therefore, modified barium swallow studies are more valuable than bedside swallow evaluations. One of the best treatments for swallowing dysfunction is to modify the consistency of food and drink. Using strategies such as a simple chin tuck, or elevating the head of bed during mealtime can also reduce aspiration risk [1]. Formal evaluation by a speech-language pathologist is recommended if aspiration is suspected.

Spasticity is a velocity-dependent increase in muscle tone. Spasticity commonly develops in days to weeks following TBI. If spasticity develops, aggressive joint range of motion is indicated. Medications including dantrium and baclofen may be indicated if spasticity causes pain or interferes with functional activities. Centrally acting antispasmodics (eg, valium and flexeril) should be avoided due to cognitive side effects [1].

# ■ PAIN MANAGEMENT

Headaches and neuropathic pain syndromes are common following TBI. An appropriate diagnostic work up is necessary to identify potential sources of pain (eg, extension of intracranial hemorrhage, bone fracture, HO, thromboembolism, abscess, peripheral neuropathy, radiculopathy, etc). Due to cognitive side effects, it is best to avoid narcotics when managing post TBI pain. Less sedating analgesics such as acetaminophen, nonsteroidal anti-inflammatories, and neurogenic agents are better options for pain management following TBI.

## ■ SEIZURE MANAGEMENT

Posttraumatic seizures are classified as immediate, early, or late. Following TBI, immediate seizures occur within 24 hours, early seizures occur after 24 hours but within 7 days, and late seizures occur more than 7 days following TBI. The risk of late seizures increases with biparietal contusions, dural penetration with metal fragments, multiple intracranial surgeries, subdural hematoma with evacuation, midline shift greater than 5 mm, and multiple or bilateral cortical contusions. Seizure prophylaxis is recommended for all TBI survivors with a GCS less than 12. Seizure prophylaxis should be discontinued 7 days following closed TBI, if the survivor has only immediate seizures or if the survivor remains seizure free. TBI survivors who experience early or late seizures should be treated with antiepileptic medications for at least 12 months. Although phenytoin is commonly used for seizure prophylaxis in the acute phase, it may slow cognitive recovery. Consider other antiepileptic agents when extended seizure prophylaxis is indicated [6-8].

## ■ BOWEL AND BLADDER MANAGEMENT

Incontinence is common following TBI. It has been associated with prolonged length of stay in acute rehabilitation and poor functional outcome. Bowel incontinence may be due to an uninhibited neurogenic bowel, lack of awareness of the need to defecate, or the inability to communicate the need to defecate secondary to impaired cognition or aphasia. In order to minimize fecal incontinence, it is important to develop a daily bowel program that provides consistent timing of fecal evacuation. If dysphagia occurs and gastrostomy or jejunostomy feeding is required, high fiber supplementation or fiber-rich enteral feeds may be used to bulk the stool and prevent diarrhea. Stool softeners (eg, colace) may be used to prevent constipation. Laxatives (eg, senna) may be used to promote peristalsis and move fecal material through the colon. Suppositories (eg, dulcolax or glycerin) may be scheduled daily for effective bowel evacuation. Following TBI, urinary incontinence is most commonly related to neurogenic bladder dysfunction. In a healthy brain, the corticopontine mesencephalic nuclei allow bladder storage; the pontine mesencephalic pathway coordinates bladder contraction and sphincter relaxation; and the pelvic and pudendal nuclei mediate the parasympathetic micturation reflex. Disruption of any of these pathways may result in incontinence due to a hyper-reflexic bladder wall with an uninhibited micturation reflex [9]. Initial treatment for urinary incontinence may include an indwelling catheter, which should be discontinued as soon as possible to prevent urinary tract infection and urethral erosion. Following catheter removal, post void residuals should be monitored every 6 hours to assess bladder emptying. Intermittent catheterization should be employed for postvoid residuals greater than 250 cm³. Alpha adrenergic antagonists (eg, flomax) can be used to aid in relaxation of the bladder neck. If bladder storage capacity is limited by hyperreflexia, anticholinergic medications (eg, ditropan) may be indicated [9].

## ■ DISPOSITION

Recovery following TBI may continue for 3 to 24 months. Although resources to support physical recovery are commonly available, resources to support cognitive recovery may be extremely limited. Most insurers provide financial support for physical rehabilitation, but cognitive rehabilitation is excluded from many insurance policies. Because of cognitive deficits and safety concerns, TBI survivors may require 24-hour supervision for a prolonged period of time. Social workers and case managers are valuable advocates and can help identify the resources available to TBI survivors for community reentry.

# ■ ASSESSMENT OF TBI REHABILITATION

## Assessment of the severity of craniocerebral injury

The degree of brain injury is mainly reflected by the degree of consciousness disorders, and the depth and duration of coma are indicators to determine the severity of TBI. The Glasgow Coma Scale (CGS) is widely used internationally to assess the consciousness status during acute injury. This method checks the three indicators of eye-opening response, speech response, and motor response in patients with traumatic brain injury, determines the scores of these three reactions, and then accumulates the scores as the basis for judging the severity of the injury. GCS can provide a simple, objective, and quantitative assessment of coma and its depth, and also has prognostic significance.

## Cognitive impairment

Cognitive function mainly involves memory, attention, understanding, thinking, reasoning, intelligence, and psychological activities, belonging to the category of advanced activities in the cerebral cortex. Cognitive impairment includes changes in consciousness, memory impairment, hearing comprehension abnormalities, spatial discrimination disorders, apraxia, agnosia, neglect, body image disorders, cortical blindness, and intellectual impairment.

## Behavioral disorders

Mainly judged based on symptoms, such as aggression, impulsiveness, loss of self-control, lack of motivation and severe obsessive compulsion, malaria, etc.

## Speech disorders

Please refer to Chapter 3, Section 3 for methods for assessing speech impairment. The characteristics of speech disorders in patients with traumatic brain injury are: ①Speech disorder: In the disorientation stage, it is mainly disoriented speech, manifested as disorientation, unable to recognize characters, time, location, etc., answering incorrectly, but without obvious vocabulary and grammar errors, not cooperating with the examination, and not realizing whether the questions answered by oneself are correct. ②Articulation disorders are common. ③Naming disorders are also common and persist for a long time aphasia: Unless directly affecting the speech center, true aphasia is relatively rare, with approximately 50% of aphasia being named aphasia. Additionally, poor understanding of complex data is also common.

## Movement disorders

There are various types of motor disorders that can be caused by craniocerebral injury. Decreased muscle strength and limited joint activity can affect motor function, while abnormal muscle tone can affect motor control. It can also include balance and coordination disorders, ataxia, tremors, and delayed motor response. Please refer to Chapter 3 for relevant evaluation methods.

## Ability to engage in daily activities

Due to the fact that many patients with brain injury have cognitive impairments, it is advisable to use assessments that include cognitive items when assessing activities of daily living, such as the assessment of independent living ability. Please refer to Chapter 3.

## Outcome of craniocerebral injury

The Glasgow Outcome Scale (GOS) was used to predict the outcome of brain injury.

# ■ REHABILITATION GOAL AND METHODS OF TBI REHABILITATION

## Early rehabilitation treatment

After craniocerebral injury, appropriate non-surgical treatment is indispensable, regardless of surgery or not. So non-surgical treatment plays a very important role in treatment, and comprehensive treatment measures should be taken. Early rehabilitation management can help prevent complications such as twinning, pressure ulcers, ectopic ossification, and neurogenic intestinal and bladder problems. If these complications are not actively prevented, they will cause great difficulties in the recovery of motor function, and even become irreversible, seriously hindering the recovery of surviving patients in the future.

1. Rehabilitation goals: stabilize the condition, improve the patient's awakening ability, promote amnesia recovery, prevent complications, and promote functional recovery.

2. Rehabilitation treatment

(1) Medication and surgical treatment: The purpose is to reduce cerebral edema, treat hydrocephalus, clear hematoma, and monitor cerebral pressure and perfusion. Generally speaking, once the patient's condition (including underlying diseases, primary diseases, comorbidities, complications, etc.) stabilizes for 48-72 hours, even if the patient is still in a state of consciousness that has not yet recovered, rehabilitation treatment should be considered.

(2) Supportive therapy: Provide a high protein and calorie diet to avoid hypoproteinemia, enhance the body's immune system, promote wound recovery, and repair and functional reconstruction of nerve tissue.

(3) Maintain a good posture: Keep the patient in a comfortable, spasmodic, and contracture resistant position.

(4) Awakening promotion therapy: upright posture training, limb massage, passive movement, and rapid brushing, tapping, squeezing, and ice stimulation of the skin on the hemiplegic limb, which has a certain stimulating effect on the brain and helps to maintain and restore the range of joint activity. Some constantly changing colorful lights can also be used to stimulate the retina, cerebral cortex, etc.

(5) Evacuate and drain phlegm to keep the respiratory tract unobstructed: use an empty palm to pat the patient's back from the bottom of the lungs upwards to the tip of the lungs each time they turn over, to help the patient expel phlegm; guide patients to perform posture sputum drainage.

(6) Maintain the elasticity of muscles and other soft tissues to prevent contractures or joint deformities: Practice passive joint range of motion, stretch muscle groups and other soft tissues that are prone to shortening, twice a day to maintain the flexibility of joints and soft tissues.

(7) Early activity: Once the vital signs are stable and conscious, patients should be assisted in deep breathing, active limb movements, bed mobility, and sitting and standing exercises as soon as possible and gradually.

(8) Physical factor therapy: For patients with flaccid paralysis, low-frequency pulse electrical stimulation

therapy can be used to enhance muscle tone, stimulate motor or sensory nerves that control muscles, and enhance limb motor function.

(9) Application of orthopedic braces: If exercise and training cannot make the muscles actively elongate, orthopedic braces should be used to fix the joints in a functional position; Provide assistance to those with weaker muscle strength to maintain normal exercise.

(10) Hyperbaric oxygen therapy: Timely improvement of cerebral circulation after traumatic brain injury, maintenance of relatively stable cerebral blood flow, prevention of insufficient or excessive perfusion, will be beneficial for reducing secondary damage and promoting brain function recovery. The role of hyperbaric oxygen in this regard cannot be underestimated.

## Rehabilitation treatment during recovery period

The brain is an advanced central nervous system and an important organ for learning. After varying degrees of brain injury, cognitive impairment occurs to varying degrees, resulting in learning difficulties. With the repair of injuries and training, new things can still be learned. Rehabilitation therapy is also a learning process.

1. The rehabilitation goal is to reduce patients' directional disorders and speech disorders, improve memory, attention, thinking, organization, and learning abilities: to maximize the recovery of sensory, motor, cognitive, language function, and self-care abilities, and improve quality of life.

2. Rehabilitation therapy for TBI is a diffuse, multi-site injury that impairs physical movement, cognition, behavior, and personality.

There are many differences in the way, scope, and severity of damage. The interaction between cognition and behavior further increases its complexity.

In the rehabilitation of traumatic brain injury, treatment such as exercise, language, and psychology can be found in Chapter 5, Rehabilitation of Stroke.

(1) Treatment of cognitive impairment: Patients in the recovery phase generally have a certain degree of motor and cognitive impairment.

In addition to motor dysfunction, it is often accompanied by cognitive disorders such as memory difficulties, lack of concentration, difficulty in thinking comprehension, and decreased judgment

Functional training is the training to improve intelligence and should run through the entire process of treatment. At present, the cognitive rehabilitation methods for TB1 mainly include occupational therapy, computer-aided and virtual cognitive rehabilitation, electromagnetic stimulation, etc. There is no unified and fixed model for the training and treatment of cognitive impairment.

Formulas and methods, as patients' cognitive impairment manifestations are complex and diverse, must be flexible and varied according to the specific situation of the patient.

The method is to utilize as many beneficial environmental factors as possible to provide patients with benign stimuli, in order to promote the improvement of their cognitive function.

1) Memory training: Memory is the imprint left in the brain by things that have been perceived, experienced, and done in the past. It is the reflection of past experiences in the human brain and the process of the brain receiving, storing, and extracting information. Short-term memory refers to the ability to keep information for 1 minute to 1 hour; long-term memory refers to the ability to keep information for 1 hour or more. Improving memory function can be assisted by using 30 mg of nimodipine (nimotop) three times a day; or huperzine A (haboyin) 100 μg 3 times a day. When conducting memory training, pay attention to slow progress. The training ranges from simple to complex, breaking down memory tasks into zero parts, and then gradually concatenating them. The duration of each training session should be short, requiring patients to remember less information and present it for a longer time. Gradually increase the amount of information

in the future. When patients succeed, timely reinforcement, encouragement, and confidence should be given. This repeated stimulation and training improves memory ability.

2) Attention training: Attention is the direction and concentration of psychological activities towards certain things. TBI patients often cannot pay attention or concentrate enough time to handle an activity task, and are easily distracted by external environmental factors.

3) Thinking training: Thinking is the most complex form of psychological activity, the highest stage of cognitive process, and the brain's summary and indirect reflection of objective things. Thinking includes various processes such as reasoning, analysis, synthesis, comparison, abstraction, and generalization, which are often manifested in human problem-solving. Provide targeted training based on the patient's cognitive impairment.

(2) Treatment of perceptual disorders: There are three methods for treating perceptual disorders, namely functional training, conversion training, and sensory motor training, with the former being the most commonly used.

1) Functional training method: In functional training, treatment is a learning process that considers the abilities and limitations of each patient. The focus of treatment should be on correcting the patient's functional problems, rather than focusing on the causes of these problems. The method used is compensation and adaptation. To compensate for existing problems, it is the first necessary to let patients understand their own shortcomings and their meanings, and then teach them the skills to use the existing perceptual function. Adaptation refers to the improvement of the environment. During training, attention should be paid to using simple and easy to understand instructions, establishing routine methods, doing each activity in the same order and manner, and constantly repeating the practice.

2) Transfer training method: It is an activity practice that requires certain perceptual participation, which has an improvement effect on other activity abilities with the same perceptual requirements. The use of specific perceptual activities such as sample copying, 2D and 3D building blocks, and puzzles can promote the improvement of ADL.

3) Sensory motor method: By delivering targeted sensory stimuli and guiding subsequent movements, we can influence the brain's sensory input modes, particularly in cases of unilateral neglect, which predominantly affects the left side. To address this, engage patients in activities that stimulate the neglected side, alter their environment, and encourage attention to the hemiplegic side. For instance, place essential items such as food, lights, telephones, and televisions on the hemiplegic side of the patient. Position yourself on the hemiplegic side when conversing with them. Encourage physical and visual activities that cross the body's midline, making the patient aware of the neglected side.

For visual spatial recognition, simplify the patient's environment by placing only a few frequently used items in drawers and bedside tables. Highlight these items with bright colors. Utilize verbal cues and tactile guidance to practice identifying specific items among many, and repeat these exercises to reinforce learning. Challenge patients to differentiate between objects with similar shapes and demonstrate their uses.

To improve the identification of spatial relationships, start with simple, graded activities. Begin by practicing the selection of one appropriate item from a painting with two items, then progress to selecting one item from a painting with three items, and finally, practice choosing one item from an entire painting. Gradually increase the complexity of the stimuli to approximate a more typical level.

For spatial location training, practice tasks such as placing a pen into a cup, arranging items according to specific instructions, and describing the relative positions of two items. Through this targeted training, patients' perceptual functions are expected to show significant improvement.

(3) The treatment of behavioral disorders: TBI patients have a variety of behavioral disorders. The purpose of treating behavioral abnormalities is to eliminate their abnormal and socially unacceptable behaviors and

promote their prosocial behavior. The treatment methods are as follows:

1) Creating an environment suitable for behavioral therapy: Environmental arrangements should ensure an increase in the probability of appropriate behavior occurring and minimize the probability of inappropriate behavior occurring. A stable and restricted residence and structured environment are key to changing bad behavior.

2) Medications: Some medications have certain effects on patients' motor control, motor speed, cognitive ability, and emotions. Multiple applications of drugs that are effective in improving behavior and suppressing post traumatic seizures with minimal side effects, such as carbamazepine and acetazolamide.

3) Behavioral therapy: Behavioral disorders can be divided into positive and negative behavioral disorders. Positive behavior disorder often manifests as attacking others, while negative behavior disorder often manifests as feeling low, indifferent, and unwilling to do something that can be accomplished. The treatment principles are: ①Encourage all appropriate behaviors; ②Refuse to reward inappropriate behavior that is still ongoing; ③Eliminate all rewarding stimuli within a short period of time after each inappropriate behavior occurs; ④Apply predeclared penalties after inappropriate behavior occurs; ⑤Provide the patient with aversive stimulation after extremely serious or stubborn adverse behavior occurs.

### Rehabilitation treatment for sequelae

After clinical treatment and formal early and recovery rehabilitation treatment, TBI patients have achieved varying degrees of improvement in various functions, but some patients still have varying degrees of functional impairment. Therefore, the rehabilitation in the sequelae period mainly includes community rehabilitation, family rehabilitation, occupational rehabilitation, and social rehabilitation, etc.

Rehabilitation goals enable patients to learn to cope with situations of functional impairment, learn new methods to compensate for functional impairment, enhance their independence and adaptability in various environments, and return to society, to ultimately improve ADL ability, social participation ability, vocational skills, and quality of life.

## ■ SUMMARY

TBI is common rehabilitation problems in the world. TBI treatment is a multidisciplinary treatment involving neurology, psychiatry, rehabilitation therapy and rehabilitation engineering, and home nursing. In this chapter, we will introduce the theories of neurologic recovery, how to control the emotion of the patients, how to prevent the following complications and sketch the pain management, seizure management, Bowel and bladder management. Finally, we give a process involving medical, diet, nursing, evaluation, rehabilitation training, orthoses and walkers. All these present everything we do in TBI patient treatment.

## ■ IMPORTANT TERMINOLOGY

traumatic brain injury (TBI)　创伤性颅脑损伤
diffuse axonal injury (DAI)　弥漫性轴索损伤
neuroplasticity　神经可塑性
hydrocephalus　脑积水
dysautonomia　自主神经功能紊乱
heterotopic ossification (HO)　异位骨化
venous thromboembolism (VTE)　静脉栓塞

bowel and bladder management 膀胱与肠道管理
Behavior management 行为治疗

# ■ REVIEW QUESTIONS

1. Please state the seizure management after TBI.
2. How to assess the prognosis of a TBI patient?
3. Please describe the functional assessments after TBI.
4. What is the therapy goal and principles after TBI?
5. Which states the medical complications after TBI?

# ■ REFERENCES

1. Cifu DX, Kreutzer JS, Slater DN, Taylor L. Rehabilitation after traumatic brain injury. In: Braddom RL, ed. Physical Medicine and Rehabilitation. 3rd ed. Philadelphia, PA: Saunders Elsevier; 2007:1133-1174.

2. Brown AW, Elovic EP, Kothari S, Flanagan SR, Kwasnica C. Congenital and acquired brain injury. 1. Epidemiology, pathophysiology, prognostication, innovative treatments, and prevention. Arch Phys Med Rehabil.2008;89:S3-S8.

3. Kwasnica C, Brown A, Elovic E, Kothari S, Flanagan S. Congenital and acquired brain injury. 3. Spectrum of the acquired brain injury population. Arch Phys Med Rehabil.2008;89:S15-S20.

4. Flanagan SR, Kwasnica C, Brown AW, Elovic EP, Kothari S. Congenital and acquired brain injury. 2. Medical rehabilitation in acute and subacute settings. Arch Phys Med Rehabil. 2008;89:S9-S14.

5. Elovic E, Kothari S, Flanagan SR, Kwasnica C, Brown AW. Congenital and acquired brain injury. 4. Outpatient and community reintegration. Arch Phys Med Rehabil. 2008;89:S21-S26.

6. Anonymous. Antiseizure prophylaxis for penetrating brain injury. J Trauma. 2001;51:S41-S43.

7. Chang BS, Lowenstein DH. Practice parameter: antiepileptic drug prophylaxis in severe traumatic brain injury: report of the Quality Standards Subcommittee of the American Academy of Neurology. Neurology. 2003;60(1):10-16.

8. Teasell R, Bayona N, Lippert C, Villamere J, Hellings C. Post-traumatic seizure disorder following acquired brain injury. Brain Inj. 2007;21(2):201-214.

9. Chua K, Chuo A, Kong KH. Urinary incontinence after traumatic brain injury: incidence, outcomes and correlates. Brain Inj. 2003;17(6):469-478.

（吴　毅）

# WHEELCHAIR PRESCRIPTIONS

## ■ INTRODUCTION

Prescription of assistive devices is a major component of rehabilitation. Of these devices, wheelchairs are one of the most essential; designed to fit and cater to the individual's specific needs. As "durable" medical equipment (DME), wheelchairs are intended to last for years, making the thoroughness of the evaluation process even more important. Wheelchairs function as the primary means of short or long-term locomotion for patients who are non-ambulatory or who have very poor endurance. Mobility may be an independent (active) or dependent (passive) process. Often, this is the only way for these individuals to partake in activities, which are necessary and meaningful. For the average manual wheelchair user, time spent in the wheelchair is estimated at 9.2 h/d [1].

Therefore, wheelchair prescription is an essential component of patient care for this population and works best when performed conjunctively by select healthcare professionals (physiatrist, specialized occupational and/or physical therapist, wheelchair vendors, and patient/ family). This process must incorporate a comprehensive evaluation and consideration of the wheelchair user(s) activity demands to preserve and ultimately promote functional independence and health.

## ■ WHEELCHAIR EVALUATION

Determining an appropriate wheelchair prescription requires an understanding of the fundamentals of wheelchair design including those factors that impact mobility and those that influence posture within the seating system. To ensure favorable results, a thorough evaluation process must be conducted to determine the client's needs and goals, both short and long-term.

Other factors to consider include body habitus, environments, impairments, comorbid medical conditions, endurance (both endurance for mobility and postural endurance), behavior, posture, balance, transfer status, muscle tone, range of motion, and financial resources among others. It is often necessary to prioritize a patient's needs during an evaluation. No piece of equipment solves all client concerns, and compromise is often necessary.

Patient involvement and education should be performed from the onset of the evaluation process and continue on through the time of delivery and shortly after to maximize patient satisfaction and understanding. To ensure the accuracy of measurements and identify postural impairments, the wheelchair evaluation process should be conducted on the mat, both in the supine and seated positions [2]. The mat assessment allows the examiner to determine general joint mobility, alignment/positioning including asymmetries, muscle length, and physical function [2,3]. It serves as a useful way to assess for deformities, both permanent (managed by adaptation) or malleable (managed through correction when possible) of the spine or pelvis. Careful measurement of patient body dimensions and appropriate prescription of a wheelchair to meet body measurements is of primary importance during seating evaluation.

## Wheelchair Dimensions

**1. Seat depth** is measured from the back of the buttocks to the popliteal region. Ideally, there should be approximately 2.5 to 5.0 cm between the popliteal space and the anterior aspect of the seating surface[4]. When obtained correctly; forces are dispersed evenly through the pelvis and the femurs. If too shallow, the user is at risk for skin breakdown and maladaptive posturing (excessive hip abduction or flexion). In contrast, if too deep, there is a tendency for skin breakdown (popliteal fossa and calves) and posterior pelvic tilt positioning.

**2. Seat width** is measured as the distance from the most lateral aspect of one buttock to the other (at the widest point) and must guarantee appropriate support for the greater trochanters. It is generally recommended for the seat width to be around 2.5 cm greater than the pelvic width[4]. If too wide, wheelchair propulsion is more challenging usually requiring greater than normal amounts of shoulder abduction. Conversely, a seat that is too narrow provides ineffective support/pressure relief and may lead to integumentary compromise in addition to compensatory, unwanted postural changes (pelvic rotation to remove pressure from the lateral hips). In addition to body dimensions, other factors impact clinical reasoning when determining an appropriate seat width for a patient. Of course, doorway clearance must be considered; particularly for the negotiation of home and other environments.

**3. Lower leg length** is measured from the most posterior aspect of the heel to the popliteal region. It is critical that there is at least 2.5 cm between the ground and the foot rests for clearance[4]. However, caution must be taken to avoid elevation of the distal femur. The rear portion of the footrest must be designed to promote front wheel (caster) mobility. Elevating or angled foot rests and seat height are adjusted for accessibility.

**4. Back height** is determined by measuring from the buttock to the inferior angle of the scapula. When the back is too high, scapulohumeral motion is restricted because the back of the chair extends beyond the inferior angle of the scapula interfering with wheelchair propulsion. At times, a higher back may be preferred; as in cases of poor trunk control or in power or manual tilt and recline chairs, which require frequent seat-to-back angle changes.

In wheelchair dimensions assessment, for some specific patients these dimensions may be helpful[2]:

(1) Hip-to-occiput measurement: Used for headrest positioning.

(2) Chest depth: Measurement taken for lateral thoracic supports or anterior thoracic support components.

(3) Arm rests: Placement and design can be variable based on client needs and can assist with postural alignment. Positioning is determined by measuring from the sitting surface to the elbow.

(4) Trunk width at the inferior border of the ribs, at the nipple line, and at the acromion process: these measurements are particularly important when selecting appropriate back rests and lateral thoracic supports, and more so when fabricating custom seating components to accommodate for a severe postural deformity.

(5) Knee width: In patients with significant hip abduction contractures, this measurement may differ significantly from hip width and be an important consideration in seating and positioning.

It is extremely important to consider how the wheelchair will be used to avoid the prescription of a chair that is incompatible with a client's daily roles and environment. Additional considerations for wheelchair use include time spent in the chair, mobility needs, mode of transportation (automobile vs public transportation), the ability of the chair to allow for growth (pediatric population), patient age, and need for additional devices (ventilator, oxygen, and tank). It is also tremendously helpful to survey the family and/or caregivers.

For those spending long periods of time in a wheelchair, it's important to plan for the chair to support either independent or dependent pressure relief.

It is critical to educate the client about the convenience and portability aspects of the intended wheelchair. Portability needs are variable depending on the client. Many clients prefer wheelchairs which can be folded for travel. In contrast, chairs with rigid frames can be placed in an automobile, albeit not without compromising vehicle seating capacity. However, folding frame chairs tend to be less stable than rigid frame chairs, and lose mechanical efficiency during manual propulsion due to the greater number of moving parts.

For pediatric patients, it is important that the wheelchair frame enables growth. Otherwise, replacement is required more frequently due to the child outgrowing his/her chair.

Environmental considerations are also fundamental to the success of the wheelchair prescription. The environment includes not only the home, but also other settings such as one's school, community venues.

The wheelchair vendor-prescriber relationship is fundamental. Vendors serve as the primary point of contact after equipment has been fitted and delivered. As the patient's needs change and/or the wheelchair requires maintenance and/or repair, the vendor can assist in directing these services.

Medical factors also play a major role in the overall evaluation and prescription process. Of these, the most commonly addressed include muscle tone, range of motion, edema, strength/movement patterns, skin integrity/wound history and future risk for integumentary problems, cognitive status, weight, neurologic impairments (seizures, ataxia, and dystonia), behavior (self-injurious behavior, elopement risk), postural considerations (fixed vs flexible deformity, asymmetry, pelvic tilt, scoliosis, and contracture), pain, postural endurance/tolerance, sitting balance, transfers, and complexity of positioning relative to caregiver's ability to assist.

# ■ MOBILITY

Manual wheelchairs are routinely assigned to both independent and dependent users. In contrast, power wheelchairs are usually chosen for those with more severe impairments, albeit those who do have the ability to be independent with alternate methods for propulsion.

## The standard wheelchair

The standard wheelchair found most commonly in hospitals or institutions is ideal for temporary purposes but not typically custom-fitted and should not be considered for prolonged client use. These chairs are too heavy to support extensive self-mobility. Refer to Figure 25.1 for the major components of a standard wheelchair.

## Manual Mobility

Standard manual mobility is well-established and ordinarily quite successful (Figure 25.2A). However, some wheelchair users' mobility options are limited by pain, impaired cardiac/pulmonary status, and poor arm strength and trunk control [5,6].

A number of options exist for alternate manual mobility such as power-assist systems that augment the wheelchair users' physical effort (though adding to the overall weight of the chair), or locomotion generated by the wheelchair user through levers, rims, or by foot propulsion [7]. Another factor to consider is whether a client who is at an independent level for long-distance propulsion should use power-assist technology—a system that may afford better protection against overuse upper extremity injuries [4,5]. Power assist systems augment the user's physical efforts with motor-driven force and greatly reduce the physical demand of prolonged self-mobility [5]. However, they add weight to the wheels of the chair and require more upkeep than a standard wheelchair wheel.

**Figure 25.1**   Standard hospital wheelchair with components highlighted.

A. Push handles; B. Arm rest; C. Skirt Guard; D. Leg rest; E. Foot rest; F. Castors; G. Brake and brake handle; H. Tire with push rim.

**Figure 25.2**   Various manual and power wheelchairs available.

A. Light weight wheelchair with anti-tippers; B. Reclining standard wheelchair; C. Power wheelchair; D. Power scooter; E. Tilt-in-space power wheelchair.

## Powered Mobility

Since the advent of powered mobility approximately 59 years ago, options and means of transportation have improved considerably [8]. There are several types of powered wheelchairs: standard, programmable, lightweight/portable, and customized/motorized. The power mobility evaluation process begins with selection of the most appropriate power base; rear-wheel, front-wheel, or mid-wheel drive. In rear-wheel drive wheelchairs, the rear wheels are larger increasing speed, navigation, and maneuverability; but due to the small front wheels negotiation of uneven terrain may be limited. They also have a larger turning radius creating mobility challenges in small areas. Front-wheel drive mechanisms afford greater control on irregular terrain since the small wheels are located posteriorly, but many users find front-wheel drive chairs awkward, particularly when turning, and at faster velocities the chair can "fish tail" [2].

In mid-wheel drive systems, the rear wheels are situated closer to the mid-point of the chair, increasing driving capacity in indoor as well as outdoor settings where obstacles are present and often, unpredictable (Figure 25.2C). Users must be cautious on rugged terrain so as not to catch the smaller front and rear wheels.

Once the base is selected, powered positioning components such as tilt, recline, lower extremity elevation, total seat elevation, and other more specialized features like standing and stair climbing can be considered. Specialized controls are another consideration at this stage, and may include standard wheelchair electronics (joystick), eye gaze systems, sip and puff systems, voice controls, head controls or specialized hand controls. If the patient intends to drive an automobile while in a wheelchair, seating, positioning, and input accessories must accommodate for leg clearance, steering, adaptive driving controls, and assistive technology/switch access.

Functional mobility and independence can also be augmented, particularly in older adults, by the use of a scooter. Scooters are widely prescribed and offer the user-powered locomotion which is less expensive, uncomplicated and travel compatible. Typically, scooters have either three or four wheels and are powered by a motor that is located posteriorly. Upper extremity strength, mobility, and coordination are necessary for transferring, steering, and breaking. Disadvantages include limited stability due to top-heaviness, larger turning radius, decreased accessibility (counters, sinks, and tables), and inability to accommodate positioning challenges [2].

A scooter is rarely a viable option for in-home mobility unless the home environment is specifically designed for that purpose (Figure 25.2D). Another consideration when using mobility options is the fact that additional training is generally required in order to ensure success, particularly in older adults [2,3].

Given the intricate and often novel control mechanisms, short-term equipment trials are recommended prior to submitting the final order to make certain that the proposed equipment functions as intended and meets the patient's goals. In this stage, relationships with vendors are critical.

## ■ FRAME DESIGN

Options for frame design include fixed back (frame set at approximately 90 degrees to seat), rear wheel posterior off-set, tilt, and recline mechanisms [9].

Tilt and recline systems will be covered in more detail when seating is reviewed. Figures 25.2B and 25.2E show images of recline and tilt systems, respectively. Fixed back chairs are more compact and lightweight. A posterior off-set rear wheel design (3.2 cm) is typically selected for bilateral above-knee amputee patients [9].

In this position, the center of gravity is optimized to account for the lighter load of the residual limbs and to prevent posterior tilting when traversing upward slopes and curbs. Given the wheel position relative to the user, anti-tipping devices are usually recommended and training is essential. Alternatively, the frame can be designed with a seat dump (frame height is higher in the anterior portion than the posterior) to prevent forward motion [7].

## ■ AXLE POSITION

The position of the axle is critical to the overall wheelchair and propulsion mechanics. An axle which is placed in a forward position enables backward tipping to negotiate curbs, but is less desirable for propulsion (seat more posterior in relation to push rim). A high or low positioned axle inversely alters the seat height and typically requires commensurate caster modification.

# ■ TIRES

Tires are extremely important for locomotion and tracking and can be pneumatic with supplemental air needs or firm necessitating less upkeep. Wheels can be either plastic or metal with spokes and vary in size; many options exist for locking using handles of various configurations, lengths, and engagement maneuvers (push vs pull), as needed.

# ■ PUSH RIMS

Push rims also play a major role in maneuverability and propulsion. Available materials include titanium, plastic, and foam with or without extension pieces. Similar to most wheelchair components, hand rim styles and configurations can be chosen according to client specifications. Ratcheting hand rims may be preferred in select cases of impaired manual dexterity.

As opposed to traditional push rim(s) use, lever drive systems can be implemented unilaterally or bilaterally to facilitate transmission of forces via shoulder and elbow muscles from the lever(s) to the wheels. This mechanism is thought to decrease the energy expenditure, fatigue, and wear and tear on distal hand/wrist joints and muscles [7,10].

Whereas, 1-arm drive chairs are beneficial for those who have 1-sided deficits and who are only able to generate a propulsive force with the unimpaired side.

# ■ SEATING AND POSITIONING

Choices for wheelchair seating systems are among the most important considerations when choosing mobility equipment. In this step, a client's needs may be addressed in several ways to promote safety, augment function, alleviate discomfort, and prevent unnecessary medical complications, prescription errors, and client dissatisfaction.

The key to proper positioning is implementation; targeting specific body parts in a logical, sequential fashion. The alignment of the pelvis is most essential given the interdependence of the legs, trunk, head, and shoulder girdle/arms; efforts should proceed accordingly. Neutral positioning is recommended for the pelvis, shoulders, and head, which should also be erect [11]. For the elbows and lower extremities, optimal positioning is pure flexion (90 degrees at hips, knees, and ankles) [4,11].

However, while the above is ideal for a patient whose trunk and limbs do not fit this pattern, it may be counterproductive to force body parts into a configuration that counteracts preexisting body alignment. It may even contribute to worsening of postural deformities and/or skin breakdown.

Reclining chairs allow the wheelchair back to be adjusted to various degrees in a posterior direction with regard to the seat to provide pressure relief and can be either full or semi reclining; however, recline mechanisms add considerable weight to the overall chair. Also, there is an increased risk for shearing forces when maneuvering between the standard and reclining positions increasing the risk of skin breakdown; an important consideration for those with sensory deficits and poor postural control. Additionally, reclined positions tend to exacerbate posterior pelvic tilt and "sacral sitting" which can also lead to skin breakdown. Figure 25.2B shows an image of a reclining wheelchair.

A tilt system adjusts the wheelchair user's orientation in space while maintaining a fixed position[3].

At the same time, it automatically redistributes pressure from one area (the buttocks and posterior thighs) to another area (posterior trunk and head). Tilt can occur in either a forward or backward direction for positioning purposes [12], which is often a more desirable alternative for those with severe spinal curvatures, sensory impairment, inability to perform pressure relief and/or remain upright independently [2]. Figure 25.2E shows the image of a tilting system.

## Components of a Seating System

There are several positioning options including but not limited to cushions, backs, lateral thoracic supports, medial and lateral thigh supports/guides, abductor and adductor pads, as well as lap belts and thoracic supports. Material choices are extensive and should be selected wisely to accommodate seating and positioning specifications.

## Cushions

Cushions function to support body position, distribute pressure, and maintain alignment. When seated, the ischial tuberosities bear a large percentage of a patient's body weight, followed by the greater trochanters, sacrum, and finally the coccyx [13].

There are specialized techniques and a variety of options available for cushion selection and vendor collaboration is essential to this step. Wheelchair cushions may be air or gel filled or composed of foam, plastics, or composite materials. Figure 25.3 shows various types of cushions. Alternatively, cushions can contain combinations of some or all of these materials with options for customization based on individual client needs. Geometric patterns such as planar, angled, or contoured designs are often used to cradle the pelvis and femurs.

The following information is meant to provide a basic introduction to wheelchair cushion selection: Foam cushions (Figures 25.3A and B) are utilized for uncomplicated positioning and pressure relief concerns. Poured or custom-molded foam is often considered for patients with significant orthopedic deformities not suited for prefabricated equipment. Foam tends to be moderately heavy. Other characteristics include poor aeration and a short lifespan of approximately 1 to 2 years.

Air-filled cushions (Figure 25.3E) maximize pressure relief when fragile skin is a consideration and/or if lifestyle necessitates long periods of chair time. They offer dynamic support; a benefit for wheelchair users that adjust their positions frequently. The downfall is the need for extensive maintenance and risk for skin breakdown if over or under filled. Air-filled cushions can also be even more dynamic; consisting of several specifically placed air-filled chambers which serve to intermittently off-load the most pressure sensitive areas by allowing air to flow in and out accordingly.

Cushions with gel inserts (Figure 25.3C) afford excellent pressure relief, but provide poor ventilation and tend to trap heat and moisture, which tends to be quite bothersome in those with intact buttock sensation.

Plastic or composite "honeycomb" cushions (Figure 25.3D) are a good option for patients with incontinence, as they are generally washable and allow good air exchange. However, positioning capacity is rather limited precluding use in those requiring intensive correction.

Anti-thrust cushions often composed of foam or composite materials are generally used to control extensor tone. These cushions have trim lines, which are higher, anteriorly creating an inherent extension, which serves to restrict sliding.

Options also exist for custom fabrication, creating custom molds to accommodate more severe postural deformities that are not well-managed by off-the-shelf cushions.

**Figure 25.3**   Seat cushions.

A. Standard foam; B.High density foam; C. Gel cushion; D. Honeycomb cushion; E. Air cushion with pump.

## Wheelchair Back Supports

Wheelchair backs may be soft or rigid, curved or planar and exist in many heights. Cutouts, integrated lateral thoracic, or lumbar supports, or even multiple-angular adjustments are possible to accommodate significant, fixed deformities. These items may be purchased in standard sizes or custom molded for exact fit.

The following are important considerations when selecting a wheelchair back.

1. Back height: the wheelchair back, as previously described, is usually placed with the top edge 2.5 to 5.0 cm below the inferior angle of the scapula for those independent with mobility, to prevent the back of the chair from impeding scapular movement. Higher backs are generally chosen for those dependent for mobility, such as in tilt or recline chairs and for those who have poor functional trunk control and/or significant orthopedic deformities.

2. Contour backs: are available in many different shapes or styles (planar or curved). Planar backs or mildly curved backs allow closer placement of lateral thoracic supports and limit thoracic kyphosis and scapular protraction. Curved backs also improve comfort in those with existing deformities and/or dependent alignment needs.

3. Fabric versus solid backs: fabric backs are lighter than solid backs and often have adjustable tension, affording mild to moderate trunk support. Fabric backs are appropriate for light-duty wheelchairs and those with limited support needs.

## Additional Positioning Components

Often, supplementary positioning components are required to optimize patient comfort and alignment[4].

1. Lateral thoracic supports

2. Headrests

3. Pelvic guides

4. Removable or permanent lateral (placed on the outside of the thighs to limit adduction)

5. Medial thigh pads (placed between knees to restrict abduction)

6. Medial and lateral thigh supports/guides which restrict hip joint motion (abduction/external rotation and abduction/internal rotation, respectively)

7. Lap belts

8. Anterior thoracic supports

9. Axillary straps

10. Footrests
11. Calf pads/panels

## ■ OTHER CONSIDERATIONS

It is possible to accessorize the wheelchair in different ways depending on a particular client's needs and lifestyle. Baskets, brakes/locks of variable shapes, lengths, and sizes, lap trays, baggage rests/transport devices, receptacles for drinks/assistive devices, attachments for knapsacks/bags, fasteners (tie-downs), and harnesses/straps (upper body, waist) including vests and jackets are items that are available for this purpose.

## ■ SPECIAL TECHNIQUES

There are various pressure-monitoring devices on the market (eg, sphygmomanometer mediated) which aid in cushion selection. An increasingly popular technique is pressure mapping, which can be used to optimize wheelchair seating both as an instructional and diagnostic tool [3].

Several techniques exist for mapping based on feedback from sensors which monitor the amount of pressure displaced by a given cushion which is placed under the buttocks. A digital reading of pressure information is generated and displayed on a computer screen. Pressure mapping is an excellent complement to the standard mat evaluation and increases the likelihood that skin integrity will be protected by a given cushion. Pressure mapping is illustrated in Figure 25.4.

**Figure 25.4**   Pressure mapping showing areas of increased pressure to assist in cushion molding.

A. Normal pressure mapping without areas of increased pressure; B. Increased pressure along the ischial tuberosities.

# ■ EQUIPMENT PROCUREMENT

Standards for reimbursement and medical necessity determination differ depending on the payor source and location. Successful procurement of DME, in this case wheelchairs and seating, often necessitates documentation in a letter format. Letters of medical necessity should discuss the medical diagnosis, comorbidities, and background circumstances including functional status, reason intended equipment is needed as opposed to something less expensive and consequences of not rendering.

# ■ SUMMARY

Wheelchairs are one of the most essential assistive devices and serve as the primary means of mobility for many users whether for short- or long-term purposes. A proper wheelchair prescription necessitates a careful, organized, comprehensive, and interdisciplinary approach involving not only the appropriate healthcare professionals, but also the client, family, and/or caregivers.No piece of wheelchair solves all patients' concerns, so patient involvement and education should be performed from the onset of the evaluation process and continue on through the time of delivery and shortly after to maximize patient satisfaction and understanding. To ensure the accuracy of measurements and identify postural impairments, the wheelchair evaluation process should be conducted on the mat, both in the supine and seated positions.There are various manual and power wheelchairs, and given the intricate and often novel control mechanisms, short-term equipment trials are recommended prior to submitting the final order to make certain that the proposed equipment functions as intended and meets the patient's goals.The design of a wheelchair may involve frame design, axle position, tires, push rims, seating systems, back supports, lateral thoracic supports, headrests, pelvic guides, removable or permanent lateral, medial thigh pads, etc.To perform wheelchair prescription well, special attention must be given to the evaluation, seating, and mobility process in the context of the client's personal goals, demands, and medical condition(s). Otherwise, mobility, functional status, quality of life, and health may be compromised.

# ■ MPORTANT TERMINOLOGY

manual wheelchair　手动轮椅

power wheelchair　电动轮椅

rim　轮圈

axle　轮轴

anti-tippers　防翻轮

front-wheel drive　前轮驱动

mid-wheel drive　中轮驱动

rear-wheel drive　后轮驱动

power scooter　动力踏板车

frame design　框架设计

tire　轮胎

seating systems　座位系统

cushion　坐垫

air-filled cushion　充气式坐垫

wheelchair back supports　轮椅靠背

# ■ REVIEW QUESTIONS

1. Who will be the wheelchairs' clients?
2. What are the differences among front-wheel drive, mid-wheel drive and rear-wheel drive wheelchairs?
3. What factors should be considered when prescribed wheelchairs to old adults and pediatric patients?
4. What are the differences on pressure relief mechanisms between reclining and tilt?
5. What are the assessment points involved on the wheelchair prescription?
6. What are the measurement points involved on the wheelchair prescription?

# ■ REFERENCES

1. Yang YS, Chang GL, Hsu MJ, Chang JJ. Remote monitoring of sitting behaviors for community-dwelling manual wheelchair users with spinal cord injury. Spinal Cord. 2009;47(1):67-71.
2. Sabol TP, Haley ES. Wheelchair evaluation for the older adult. Clin Geriatr Med. 2006;22(2):355-75, ix.
3. Hastings JD. Seating assessment and planning. Phys Med Rehabil Clin N Am. 2000;11(1):183-207, x.
4. Koontz, A. et al. Prescription of Wheelchairs and Seating Systems. In: Physical Medicine and Rehabilitation. Braddom RL. ed.3rd ed. Edinburgh, UK: Elsevier Saunders; 2007.
5. Cooper RA, Fitzgerald SG, Boninger ML, et al. Evaluation of a pushrimactivated, power-assisted wheelchair. Arch Phys Med Rehabil. 2001;82(5): 702-708.
6. Veeger HE, van der Woude LH, Rozendal RH. Effect of hand rim velocity on mechanical efficiency in wheelchair propulsion. Med Sci Sports Exerc. 1992;24(1):100-107.
7. Cooper, R.A. et al. Seating, Assistive Technology, and Equipment. In: Stroke Recovery and Rehabilitation. Stein, J. et al. eds. New York: Demos; 2009.
8. Woods B, Watson N. A short history of powered wheelchairs. Assist Technol. 2003;15(2):164-180.
9. Spiegler JH, Goldberg MJ. The wheelchair as a permanent mode of mobility a detailed guide to prescription. I. frame, armrests and brakes. Am J Phys Med. 1968;47(6):315-316.
10. van der Woude LH, Dallmeijer AJ, Janssen TW, Veeger D. Alternative modes of manual wheelchair ambulation: an overview. Am J Phys Med Rehabil. 2001;80(10):765-777.
11. Trefler E, Taylor SJ. Prescription and positioning: Evaluating the physically disabled individual for wheelchair seating. Prosthet Orthot Int. 1991;15(3):217-224.
12. Michael SM, Porter D, Pountney TE. Tilted seat position for non-ambulant individuals with neurological and neuromuscular impairment: a systematic review. Clin Rehabil. 2007;21(12):1063-1074.
13. Ferguson-Pell MW. Seat cushion selection. J Rehabil Res Dev Clin Suppl. 1990;2(2):49-73.

（许　涛）

# *WOUND CARE*

## ■ WOUND HEALING

The management of chronic wounds is gaining increased attention due to growing awareness of the high cost and morbidity of poorly healing wounds and a better understanding of the pathophysiology of wound healing. As health care providers dedicate themselves to practicing the science of wound care, outcomes will improve. In addition to a greater understanding of the fundamentals of wound healing, there are many emerging technologies that can be helpful to the practitioner treating refractory wounds.

Despite the heavy investment in advanced treatment modalities, good wound care starts with the basics.

## ■ WHAT IS A CHRONIC WOUND?

Chronic wounds are wounds that fail to heal along the normal healing pathway. In order to treat chronic wounds, it is important to recall the normal healing cascade that takes place in a healthy host with an acute injury.

Normal wound healing is a very complex and dynamic process. A simplified description generally divides this process into three overlapping phases: inflammatory, proliferative, and remodeling.

1. **Inflammatory phase**   Some authors subdivide the inflammatory phase into a hemostatic and inflammatory phase. Immediately following an injury, blood and platelets enter the wound to stop the bleeding. Platelets secrete (among many things) histamine, platelet derived growth factor, and transforming growth factor. This causes vasodilation and an influx of neutrophils and macrophages. From days 2 to 4, the macrophages continue to secrete growth factors to promote fibroblast influx into the wound which signals the ending of the inflammatory phase and beginning of the proliferative phase.

2. **Proliferative phase**   The proliferative phase is dominated by the fibroblast and begins about 3 to 5 days after injury and continues for approximately 3 weeks. This is the period when angiogenesis and collagen deposition occurs. Granulation tissue appears in the wound and epithelialization can be observed.

3. **Remodeling phase**   The remodeling phase begins around 3 weeks and can continue for a year after injury. During this time, type III collagen is replaced by type I collagen which crosslinks, and increases the tensile strength of the wound. Chronic wounds are considered healed once epithelialized; however, the tissues will continue to evolve until the remodeling phase is complete.

Once a chronic wound has been identified, the process of returning the patient to the normal healing pathway can begin. As in most areas of medicine, proper treatment requires an initial accurate diagnosis. In almost all cases, a careful history and physical exam should result in a solid diagnosis. One can classify most wounds appropriately by their anatomic location and the patient's past medical history. The diagnosis should go beyond the simple identification of a pressure ulcer and should include an understanding of the underlying anatomic structure that is contributing to the wound as well as any contributing pathophysiology.

The diagnosis should be accompanied by an assessment of the wound bed. The presence of necrosis, exudate, purulence, or granulation tissue should be noted. The viable tissue at the base of the wound should be characterized. Does the wound extend into dermis, subcutaneous fat, paratenon, muscle, tendon, periosteum, or bone? The periwound tissue should also be assessed for signs of cellulitis, maceration, callus, or epiboly (rolled skin edges).

If the wound is on the lower extremity, the arterial and venous systems should be assessed. The clinician will need to determine whether history and physical exam alone is sufficient. Often noninvasive arterial Doppler studies will be necessary to adequately evaluate the lower extremity circulation. Studies have shown that the presence of a palpable pulse does not exclude the possibility of early peripheral arterial disease (PAD) [1].

Offloading is a critical early step in managing chronic wounds. This may require sitting restrictions, frequent repositioning, or nonweight bearing status. Pressure may play a role in less obvious ways from splints, wheelchair leg supports, and poor fitting shoes. It can be helpful to examine the footwear of patients with pedal wounds. Failure to identify the underlying pressure contributing to the wound will result in treatment failure and probably worsening of the wound.

Once a diagnosis has been made and adequate perfusion has been established, wound bed preparation can begin. Debridement can be performed surgically with scalpels, currettes, or hydrosurgery. Alternative forms of debridement include mechanical with dressing changes, chemical with enzymatic agents, or biological with maggots. If feasible, surgical debridement is often preferred. Sharp debridement allows for rapid wound bed preparation and assessment of the depth of injury. Frequent sharp debridements are associated with a faster rate of healing [2]. There may be cases where surgical debridement is not practical or tolerated. These are the preferred times to use enzymatic debridement. Mechanical debridement with wet-dry saline dressings have largely fallen out of favor because it is painful and requires the dressing to dry which violates the principle of maintaining a moist wound bed. Maggot therapy is still used in select cases. It is recognized as a way to relatively painlessly and efficiently remove devitalized tissue from a wound. Although maggots are a legitimate form of wound bed management, the logistics and need for proper disposal of the maggots makes maggot therapy impractical for most medical settings in the United States.

In addition to identifying the cause of injury and preparing the wound bed, the physician managing a complex wound will need to identify any intrinsic or extrinsic barriers to healing (Table 26.1).

**TABLE 26.1** ▪ Barriers to wound healing

| Intrinsic | Extrinsic |
|---|---|
| Edema | Pressure |
| Malnutrition | Infection |
| Ischemia | Poor wound care |
| Radiation injury | |
| Fibrosis | |

# ■ INTRINSIC FACTORS

## Edema

Lower extremity edema will predispose the patient to developing wounds and inhibit the diffusion of oxygen to the skin. Thus it must be controlled in order to assist healing. Edema management involves excluding or managing venous disease and deep venous thromboses (DVTs) and initiating leg elevation, diuretics, and compression therapy when appropriate. Prior to instituting compression therapy adequate arterial inflow should be assured. Layered compression should start at the toes and extend up to the knee, to avoid creating swelling distal to the wraps. Typically layered compression wraps are used while the patient is healing a wound. After healing, the patient is transitioned into compression stockings at a pressure of 25 to 35 mmHg. Lower pressure stockings are less ideal but may have a role when the patient does not tolerate higher levels of compression or only has very mild disease.

## Nutrition

The nutritional status of the patient should be assessed. Patients with significant wounds and under stress should receive 30 to 35 kcal/kg•d. This should include 1.25 to 1.5 g/kg of protein. A well-balanced diet should be encouraged with oral supplements provided as needed. Vitamin and mineral supplements should be given if vitamin deficiency is suspected or dietary intake is poor. Zinc and vitamins A, B complex, and C are particularly important.

Ischemic and radiated tissues may require advanced treatments including revascularization procedures or hyperbaric oxygen (HBO) therapy. The management of wounds associated with PAD is discussed later in the chapter.

## ■ EXTRINSIC FACTORS

Ensuring that the wound care is conducive to healing and addressing issues like infection and pressure are critical to success. Once the wound etiology has been determined, and the wound bed prepared, the dressings can be selected. The goal of the dressing should be to keep the wound bed moist and the periwound tissue dry. In the outpatient setting, the frequency of dressing changes should be determined by the needs of the wound and the patient's resources. Clean, improving wounds can be dressed anywhere from daily to weekly, depending on the drainage and the patients' needs. Patients requiring compression therapy over wounds tend to have their dressings changed every 3 to 7 days. However, early on in therapy, daily wraps may be required. Dressing selection is a dynamic process and the clinician will need to adjust the treatment plan as the wound evolves. Most dressing changes are performed in a clean but not sterile environment. The wound needs to be cleaned of loose exudate and slough. There is little evidence to recommend a particular type of wound cleanser. Saline, sterile water, or tap water can all reasonably be used at the discretion of the health care provider depending on the circumstances[3]. Some patients may report more comfort with one technique over the other.

Once the wound is clean, the dressing can be applied. One of the most frequently prescribed wound dressings is hydrogel and gauze daily. This combination keeps the wound moist, is generally well tolerated and is easy to apply. This is adequate for most wounds with mild drainage. When a more absorbent dressing is needed, hydrofibers or alginates can be selected. If tendon, bone or vital structures are exposed in the wound, special attention should be paid to ensure that they do not desiccate between dressing changes. When bacterial colonization is a concern, a silver impregnated dressing may be considered. Silver dressings tend to be more expensive and so rational use of the products is urged. Like systemic antibiotics, it is appropriate to select a stop date so that patients are not left on silver dressings for unnecessary lengths of time. Cytotoxic agents like iodine, peroxide, and Dakin's solution at standard concentrations should be avoided. Their use may be appropriate in rare, isolated short-term applications when managing gross wound contamination is prioritized over promoting wound healing.

Wound bed infection can be difficult to determine on clinical exam alone. Wounds that are not responding to local care should be reassessed for possible infection. Not all patients with clinically significant bacterial contamination will present with typical signs of infection (ie, fever, erythema, warmth, and leukocytosis). Wound bed infections have been defined by a colonization of greater than 100 000 organisms per gram. Ideally, quantitative cultures should be obtained; however, these tests are not available to all clinicians. As an alternative, semi-quantitative wound swabs have shown some clinical utility. Judicious use of antibiotics is appropriate in patients with a significant clinical suspicion of wound bed infection. As with treating most other infections, antibiotics use should be focused and time limited. The clinician will need to determine whether a wound bed infection should be treated with topical or systemic antimicrobials.

## ■ SPECIFIC WOUNDS

### Pressure Ulcers

Pressure ulcers occur in the sensory- and mobility-impaired patient. Tissue injury typically occurs over bony prominences. Tissue injury is caused by increased pressure on the overlying skin and fat. Areas of high pressure (eg, the ischium in a sitting patient) can be injured in as little as 2 hours, whereas lower pressure sites can tolerate longer periods of weight bearing. Thus offloading must be individualized to the wound. Once identified, these ulcers should be classified by their anatomic location.

In addition to staging the wound, the patient's sitting and weight-bearing history should be obtained. Offloading should be done with the specific anatomic location of the wound in mind. It may be useful to refer patients for pressure mapping. Tetraplegics should be prescribed tilting wheelchairs to allow them to relieve pressure while sitting. For large or worsening wounds, complete offloading may be necessary initially; however, once the wound is stabilized short periods of weight bearing can often be tolerated if adequately padded and time-limited. Moisture and friction will also contribute to wound formation and should be minimized.

Bone infection can be assessed by several methods. If after clinical exam, sedimentation rate, white blood cell count, and plain film X-ray, osteomyelitis is not evident but still suspected MRI's, bone scans or bone biopsies may be needed. When practical, bone biopsies not only assist in the diagnosis, but also aid in the treatment as bone cultures can be obtained at the same time. MRI is surpassing the bone scan as the preferred modality when advanced imaging is needed. The management of wound associated osteomyelitis is variable. Patients who are acutely ill with leukocytosis, fever, and elevated sedimentation rates tend to require long-term, culture-specific antibiotics. However, it is not clear that chronically exposed bone in the absence of acute illness should be treated with systemic antibiotics in all instances. Surgical removal of devitalized or friable bone should be performed; however, it may not be practical to remove all of the involved bone. If the goal is to eradicate bone infection then consideration should be made to providing permanent soft-tissue coverage over the bone so that at the completion of antibiotics the wound is covered with durable soft tissue.

Flap repair for pressure ulcers should be considered for patients whose wounds are unlikely to heal in a timely fashion with good durable tissue. Appropriate surgical candidates respond to local care, comply with the offloading regimen and are motivated to participate in a postoperative program to protect the flap and prevent recurrences. These patients should be assessed for underlying osteomyelitis which can be treated prior to or in conjunction with the definitive surgical repair. Patients should be aware that there are a limited number of local flaps available at each wound site and therefore should only pursue treatment when they are absolutely committed to the treatment course which typically involves surgery followed by 3 to 6 weeks of strict offloading.

Wounds that fail to respond on a weekly basis should be reassessed for adequate offloading, proper dressing selection and infection. Many times patients will report that they are being compliant with their offloading, not realizing that a certain position or activity is contributing to their wound. Large stage 4 wounds may stall after a long period of steady improvement. After ensuring adequate wound bed preparation, offloading and infection control, the patient should be referred to a plastic surgeon for evaluation for flap reconstruction.

## Diabetic Foot Ulcers

The cause of DFUs (diabetic foot ulcers) is often multifactorial. These patients tend to have vascular disease, neuropathy, and impaired granulocytic and chemotaxic activity [4]. Initial attention should be paid to assessing the peripheral pulses. Noninvasive arterial studies can be helpful in determining the presence of PAD. Ankle-Brachial indices (ABIs) can be falsely elevated due to calcified vessels. Toe pressures often provide better information. Acute infection should also be addressed and systemic antibiotics used when necessary (Figure 26.1). The depth of the wound and presence of pus should be determined. Wounds that probe to bone may have concomitant osteomyelitis and further work-up is indicated. Once the tissues involved have been determined, then the wound should be graded according to Wagner's Grading [5].

**Figure 26.1**  DFU with eschar and associated cellulitis.

Much like pressure ulcers, an underlying bony prominence can often be identified (ie, metatarsal head). Identifying pressure points will help in selecting the appropriate offloading device. A consultation with a certified pedorthotist can be very helpful in this regard. The patient's diabetes must be under good control. A hemoglobin A1C can provide insight into the patients' blood sugar control over time. A goal of less than 6.5% to 7% is suggested by leading organizations. Poorly controlled diabetics are at risk of poor wound healing, infection, and major amputation.

## Venous Stasis Ulcers

These wounds generally occur between the mid-calf to just below the malleoli. Venous stasis ulcers (VSUs) typically result from chronic dysfunction of the venous system due to factors related to valvular dysfunction, heart failure, chronic deep venous thromboses, and/or poor calf muscle pump function. Over time, chronic venous insufficiency leads to fibrosis of the subcutaneous tissues.

Venous ulcers tend to have irregular borders and granulating wound beds (Figure 26.2).

These patients may benefit from venous ultrasound work-up to evaluate for valvular incompetence or prominent venous perforators which may be amenable to saphenous

**Figure 26.2**  VSU with granulating bed.

stripping or perforator ligation which can improve healing and decrease the risk of recurrence [6].

Edema management in these patients is critical. Once adequate arterial inflow is determined, layered compression wraps should be used to decrease lower extremity swelling [7]. Leg elevation and lifestyle modification is often necessary. Fluid management for patients with a component of heart failure may also be necessary. Patients with a history of VSUs often require chronic compression to prevent recurrences.

## Arterial Ulcers

PAD ulcers tend to be sharply demarcated and poorly granulating. They are often painful. The vascular work-up is critical for these patients. Often these patients will report a history of intermittent claudication or rest pain. If the patient has significant arterial disease, a vascular surgery consult should be obtained. Revascularization, in general, should precede major debridement. The perfusion of the limb continues to improve for about 3 to 4 weeks after revascularization [8]. If the wound is acutely infected it may not be possible to postpone debridement until after revascularization. ABIs are an appropriate initial diagnostic test for patients suspected of PAD. ABIs of 0.9 to 1.1 are considered normal. Diabetics and patients with heavily calcified vessels may have falsely elevated ABIs. An ABI of 0.5 or less suggests a foot ulcer is unlikely to heal without vascular intervention. Ratios greater than 1.3 should be considered as potentially falsely elevated. ToeBrachial Indices can be useful when ABIs are falsely elevated as digital pressures tend to be less affected by medial calcification [9].

Once the perfusion status has been assessed and addressed, wound care can proceed using the same principles outlined previously.

## ADVANCED TREATMENT MODALITIES

For wounds that do not respond to conventional treatments, these advanced modalities may be useful. These tend to either be cost- or time-intensive treatments and should be used selectively to improve their cost-effectiveness. The following is a brief overview of a few commonly used therapies.

**Sub-Atmospheric Dressings** or negative pressure wound therapy (NPWT). These dressings have been shown to promote granulation tissue formation, control wound drainage and edema, stimulate wound perfusion, and promote wound healing [10]. They should be considered for large wounds, deep wounds or those not responding to conventional treatment. Necrosis and infection should be resolved prior to their use and caution should be taken in anticoagulated patients in those patients with potentially exposed vascular structures. Typically a NPWT dressing will be changed every 48 to 72 hours. Disadvantages of NPWT are that it requires a patient to be attached to a pump (however mobile), the machine or dressing can fail requiring an unscheduled dressing change, and a small percentage of patients will find NPWT to be too painful.

**HBO** has been found to be clinically helpful in advanced Wagner's grade DFUs, radiated tissues, refractory osteomyelitis, and failing flaps and grafts. Its use can be considered in cases where local reversible hypoxia is contributing to the wound and where ischemia is not surgically correctable. Transcutaneous oxygen measurements can be obtained to determine whether the local tissues are ischemic and whether they might respond to HBO. These treatments can be very time consuming (for the patient) and expensive. A typical outpatient hyperbaric center will treat patients for 2 hours a day, 5 days a week for 4 to 8 weeks depending on their diagnosis. The most common complications include barotrauma to the ears and seizures due to oxygen toxicity.

**Cellular therapy**. This is a broad category and includes growth factors, cryopreserved human skin allografts, and cellular synthetic skin substitutes like Apligraft (comprised of human fibroblasts and keratinocytes) and Dermagraft (a biodegradable mesh seeded with human fibroblasts). These therapies tend to be expensive but can be cost-effective when used on appropriately selected patients. These tend to be patients who have failed to improve despite standard wound care and are cleared of infection.

Acellular therapy can consist of decellularized allogeneic or xenogeneic tissue or other biomaterials. These can be appropriate for replacing areas of deficient collagen or promoting cellular ingrowth by providing a collagen scaffold. They may also be used to cover and protect underlying structures and may decrease wound pain.

## ■ CONCLUSION

Wound healing is a highly complex process that involves an orderly sequence of cellular events. Chronic wounds fail to follow this orderly sequence for a variety of reasons. The care of chronic wound patients requires a proper diagnosis and intervention. Initially it may be necessary to evaluate wounds on a weekly basis to ensure that they are responding to treatment. Once steady improvement is observed and the wound is objectively improving, less frequent exams are appropriate. Wounds can be documented by simply measuring length, width, and depth. Although this is often adequate, these measurements may miss small improvements in an irregularly shaped wound. Newer photographic systems provide greater detail by measuring the complete surface area. It is important to have an objective way of measuring and documenting progress. When wounds fail to respond (ie, show no consistant signs of improvement), the treatment plan should be adjusted. A chronic wound can be successfully healed by following a systematic evaluation and management strategy.

## ■ SUMMARY

Wound healing is a highly complex process. Chronic wounds fail to follow this orderly sequence for a variety of reasons. The care of chronic wound patients requires a proper diagnosis and intervention. Adequate treatment requires an initial accurate diagnosis. In almost all cases, a careful history and physical exam should result in a solid diagnosis. Most wounds can be appropriately classified by their anatomic location and the patient's past medical history. The diagnosis should include an understanding of the underlying anatomic structure that is contributing to the wound, as well as be accompanied by an assessment of the wound bed. Once a diagnosis has been made and adequate perfusion has been established, wound bed preparation can begin. Debridement can be performed by various procedures, such as surgery, dressing changes, chemical with enzymatic agents, or biological with maggots. In addition to the diagnosis and wound bed preparation, the physician managing a complex wound will need to identify any intrinsic or extrinsic barriers to healing. Wound bed infection can be difficult to determine, but should be treated properly as its critical influence to the healing. The specific wound need the clinician's more attention in the practice.

## ■ IMPORTANT TERMINOLOGY

wound healing   伤口愈合
chronic wound   慢性伤口
wound bed   伤口创面
debridement   清创术
pressure ulcer   压疮
offloading   减除压迫
flap   皮瓣
diabetic foot ulcers (DFUs)   糖尿病足部溃疡
Wagner's Grading   Wagner 分级

venous stasis ulcers (VSUs)　静脉淤滞性溃疡
peripheral arterial disease (PAD)　周围动脉疾病
intermittent claudication　间歇性跛行
revascularization　再血管化
sub-atmospheric dressings　低压敷料
negative pressure wound therapy　负压伤口治疗
hyperbaric oxygen (HBO)　高压氧
cellular therapy　细胞治疗
acellular therapy　非细胞治疗

## ■ REVIEW QUESTIONS

1.  What are the potential complications of surgical wounds that can be prevented by proper post-operative wound care?

2.  How should chronic wounds be managed with respect to offloading, pressure, and footwear?

3.  What are the common issues in post-operative wound care, and what are the effective methods to promote surgical wound healing?

4.  What are the advanced treatment modalities for surgical wounds, such as negative pressure wound therapy and cell therapy?

## ■ REFERENCES

1.  Collins T, Suarez-Almazor M, Peterson NJ. An absent pulse is not sensitive for the early detection of peripheral arterial disease. Fam Med. 2006; 38:38-42.

2.  Steed DL, Donohoe D, Webster MW, Lindsley L. Effect of extensive debridement and treatment on the healing of diabetic foot ulcers. Diabetic Ulcer Study Group. J Am Coll Surg. 1996;183(1):61-64.

3.  Fernandez R, Griffiths R, Ussia C. Water for wound cleansing. Int J Evid Based Healthc. 2007;5:305-323.

4.  Singer AJ, Clark RAF.Cutaneous wound healing. N Engl J Med.1999;341(10):738-746.

5.  Wagner FW Jr. The dysvascular foot: a system for diagnosis and treatment. Foot Ankle. 1981;2(2):64-122.

6.  O'Donnell T Jr. The present status of surgery of the superficial venous system in the management of venous ulcer and the evidence for the role of perforator interruption. J Vasc Surg. 2008;48(4):1044-1052.

7.  Laura Bolton. Compression in Venous Ulcer Management. J Wound Ostomy Continence Nurs. 2008;35(1):40-49. Copyright 2008, by the Wound, Ostomy and Continence Nurses Society. ISSN publication 1071-5754.

8.  Caselli A, Latini V, Lapenna A, et al. Transcutaneous oxygen tension monitoring after successful revascularization in diabetic patients with ischaemic foot ulcers. Diabet Med. 2005;22(4):460-465. Published Online: January, 2005.

9.  DeAnna Holtman NP, Vivian Gahtan MD. Peripheral arterial perfusion: is it adequate for wound healing? Wounds. 2008;20(8):230-235.

10. Niezgoda JA, Mendez-Eastman S. The effective management of pressure ulcers. Adv Skin Wound Care. 2006;19(suppl 1):3-15.

（曾　岩）